Translation of Evidence Into Nursing and Health Care Practice

Kathleen M. White, PhD, RN, NEA-BC, FAAN, is an associate professor and director for the doctor of nursing practice (DNP) program at the Johns Hopkins University School of Nursing (JHUSON). Dr. White has considerable knowledge base in the research translation field, having been an invited speaker on various aspects of the topic internationally, nationally, and at the state and local levels since 2004 and having coordinated the DNP level Translation of Research to Practice course for the past two semesters at JHUSON. In addition, Dr. White brings a wealth of professional experience from her wide range of funded and grant-supported research, initiatives, and teaching that have spanned nearly 30 years. She has published more than 45 papers, delivered more than 50 scholarly presentations (45 national and 7 internationally), and has been an active member of many policy-setting boards, including the American Nurses Association (ANA) Standards and Guidelines Committee and the Maryland State Patient Safety Committee (appointed). Dr. White serves on two editorial boards, including the journals of *American Nurse Today* and *Nursing Management*, and serves as an associate editor of the *Journal of Policy, Politics, and Nursing Practice*. Since 1999, Dr. White has been credentialed as a certified nurse administrator, advanced, and in 2008, she was inducted as fellow into the American Academy of Nursing.

Sharon Dudley-Brown, PhD, RN, FNP-BC, is an assistant professor of medicine and nursing and codirector of the gastroenterology and hepatology NP fellowship program at JHUSON where, among other courses, she has taught the Translation of Research to Practice DNP course for the past two semesters as well as the Nursing Inquiry for Evidence-Based Practice course. Dr. Dudley-Brown is an expert nurse practitioner, having worked as a family NP since 1992. She has strong clinical roots, having completed her PhD research on a GI clinical topic. She has been an invited speaker on clinical topics both nationally and internationally and has published 10 research articles, five abstracts, and five journal articles on topics related to nursing education. She has received funding for research proposals from the National Institute of Nursing Research (NINR), the Society of Gastroenterology Nurses and Associates (SGNA), the Sigma Theta Tau International (STT), and the Chinese University of Hong Kong, where she taught for 3 years. In addition, Dr. Dudley-Brown has taught at several major university schools of nursing including Thomas Jefferson University, University of Delaware, University of Maryland, and Catholic University of America before joining the JHUSON faculty in 2007. She serves on three editorial boards, including the International Editorial Board of the Journal of Advanced Nursing, Clinical Nursing Research, and the Gastrointestinal Nursing Journal. She is a member of the American Academy of Nurse Practitioners (AANP), STT, National Organization of Nurse Practitioner Faculties (NONPF), and SGNA professional nursing societies.

Translation of Evidence Into Nursing and Health Care Practice

Kathleen M. White, PhD, RN, NEA-BC, FAAN

Sharon Dudley-Brown, PhD, RN, FNP-BC

SPRINGER PUBLISHING COMPANY
NEW YORK

Springer Publishing Company, LLC
11 West 42nd Street
New York, NY 10036
www.springerpub.com

Acquisitions Editor: Margaret Zuccarini
Production Editor: Dana Bigelow
Composition: Absolute Service, Inc.

ISBN: 9780826106155
E-book ISBN: 9780826106162

12 13 14 / 5 4 3

The author and the publisher of this Work have made every effort to use sources believed to be reliable to provide information that is accurate and compatible with the standards generally accepted at the time of publication. Because medical science is continually advancing, our knowledge base continues to expand. Therefore, as new information becomes available, changes in procedures become necessary. We recommend that the reader always consult current research and specific institutional policies before performing any clinical procedure. The author and publisher shall not be liable for any special, consequential, or exemplary damages resulting, in whole or in part, from the readers' use of, or reliance on, the information contained in this book. The publisher has no responsibility for the persistence or accuracy of URLs for external or third-party Internet websites referred to in this publication and does not guarantee that any content on such websites is, or will remain, accurate or appropriate.

Library of Congress Cataloging-in-Publication Data

CIP data is available from the Library of Congress.

Printed in the United States of America by Bradford & Bigelow.

Dr. White and Dr. Dudley-Brown would like to dedicate this book to the doctoral students with whom they have worked—past, present, and future— whose ideas and questions provided inspiration for this book.

Contents

Contributors

Anne E. Belcher, PhD, RN, AOCN, CNE, ANEF, FAAN   Associate Professor, Johns Hopkins School of Medicine, Nursing and Public Health, Baltimore, MD

Barbara B. Frink, PhD, RN, FAAN   Vice President for Clinical Excellence and Informatics, Main Line Health System, Bryn Mawr, PA

Christine A. Goeschel, ScD, MPA, MPS RN   Director, Patient Safety and Quality Initiatives, Johns Hopkins School of Medicine, Nursing and Public Health, Baltimore, MD

Cynda Hylton Rushton, PhD, RN, FAAN   Department of Acute and Chronic Care, Johns Hopkins School of Nursing, Baltimore, MD

Julie Stanik-Hutt, PhD, ACNP, CNS, FAAN   Associate Professor, Johns Hopkins University School of Nursing, Baltimore, MD

Mary Terhaar, DNSc   Assistant Professor, Acting Director, DNP Program, Johns Hopkins School of Medicine, Nursing and Public Health, Baltimore, MD

Joyce Williams, DNP, RN, AFN   Armed Forces Medical Examiner System, Baltimore, MD

Foreword

The need to practice in an evidence-based environment is paramount, particularly given the explosion of new knowledge from basic and clinical research. All health professionals have a moral obligation to ensure that patients receive appropriate and evidence-based care. To accomplish this, we need clinicians who can critically appraise and summarize the evidence, simplify and prioritize it, and design strategies to ensure patients actually receive the therapies. This book guides clinicians to accomplish this last important part of the process, translating the research into practice. As many of us have learned from the research, patients, on average, receive half the recommended therapies. As a result, tens of thousands of patients die needlessly and suffer unnecessary harm, and health care costs skyrocket. Strategies to summarize the evidence and establish best practices to ensure that all patients receive that evidence are needed.

Far too often nurses have been on the sidelines of evidence-based practices, when they, in fact, have a vital role in this process. This role is to ensure that patients get the best care and evidence-based therapies. They also play a vital role in questioning practice and highlighting gaps in new knowledge to provide better care; gaps that should be the focus of research priorities. When we asked nurses in the ICU at Johns Hopkins Hospital about evidence-based practices for ventilator-assisted patients, the nurses initially knew little about the therapies. When asked why they used therapies, the nurses responded, "because the doctor ordered them" rather than, because the evidence says they should get it. This has changed, and now nurses do participate in summarizing the evidence and implementing new evidence at the bedside. However, nurses need to be more engaged in planning for the practice change. This includes the decision making about whether to implement the new evidence and the design of the strategies to translate that evidence into their local practices. This book discusses the current knowledge on translation models and strategies and can serve as an important resource for nurses to engage in these other key steps in the process of translating evidence. Indeed nursing should address evidence-based practice to the same degree that they tackle giving compassionate and holistic care to patients. Our patients deserve nothing less.

Peter J. Pronovost, MD, PhD
Director of the Armstrong Institute for Patient
Safety and Quality
Johns Hopkins Medicine Senior Vice President
for Patient Safety and Quality

Preface

It is widely known that there is a wide gap in time between the generation of research to the implementation of those findings into practice, or the translation or research into practice. This book aims to provide clinicians and administrators in health care with knowledge and strategies to address this problem, and begin to shorten this timeframe and close this "translation gap."

As faculty members designing a translation course for the new Doctor of Nursing Practice (DNP) program at The Johns Hopkins University School of Nursing, we found lots of great resources on evidence-based practice and current journal articles on the emerging science of implementation and translation. However, we were looking for that one great resource on translation and didn't find it. Of course, we were particular in what we were looking for and we wanted it to follow the sequence of the translation course. The resource needed to first include the theoretical perspective on translation to give the students the foundation for their developing expert practices. This theoretical perspective needed to include not only the models and frameworks for translation but also a discussion of the change process. Second, the resource had to include current topics or foci of translation, such as clinical practice guidelines, information technology or health policy to name a few. And finally, we wanted the resource to discuss the practical perspective on the translation of evidence into practice, including content on organizational culture, barriers and facilitators to implementation and a discussion of the how-to's. After developing the content and teaching the DNP translation course once, we found ourselves contemplating the possibility of creating this needed resource for the course. It turned out to be this book!

We hope that you will agree that this book meets an important need as a textbook for DNP students as well as a practical resource for other health professionals leading translation of evidence into practice projects. The two major threads throughout the book are 1) the integration and application of knowledge into practice and 2) the leadership strategies necessary for translation of evidence for both direct and indirect care. Each chapter includes an extensive list of references, current web links, and other applicable resources to enhance learning.

Part I of the book (Chapters 1–3) describes theories and frameworks important to the translation of research into practice. Chapter 1 describes and reviews the key tenets of evidence-based practice frameworks and models being used in nursing today. Chapter 2 defines translation of research to practice and discusses current translation frameworks and the important elements for consideration in any translation effort.

Chapter 3 discusses models of change as they relate to translation of research to practice.

Part II of the book (Chapters 4–9) provides detail on existing evidence for translation in specific areas of nursing and health care practice and describes methods of translation for these specific situations. Chapter 4 discusses the importance of translation of evidence to improve clinical practice, specifically, clinical outcomes, and outlines how the Appraisal of Guidelines for Research and Evaluation (AGREE) collaborative process can be used by clinicians. Chapter 5 describes the current quality and safety environment and the need for translation of evidence to improve quality of care and increase patient safety. Chapter 6 explains the importance of translation of evidence for effective leadership in health care today. Chapter 7 illustrates many innovative strategies used to translate evidence in nursing education. Chapter 8 discusses the difficulties in translation of evidence to health policy and offers strategies to decrease the divide between researchers and policy makers. Finally, Chapter 9 defines the role of information technology (IT) in translation and how IT is a strategy for translation.

The last section of the book, Part III (Chapters 10–15), provides specific strategies and interventions to conduct the translation of evidence into practice. The first chapter in Part III (Chapter 10), Creating a Culture that Promotes Translation, delineates how organizational culture influences the translation of evidence, and steps to address this. Chapter 11, Challenges and Barriers in Translation, offers strategies in the identification, prioritization, and interventions to addresses common challenges in translation, guided by the use of a cascade framework. Chapter 12, Legal and Ethical Issues in Translation, adresses issues of legal risk and fairness in the translation of evidence. Chapter 13, The Project Plan and the Work of Translation, provides detail in the development, planning, and execution of a complex project such as that in translation. Chapter 14, Evaluation of Translation, provides a theory-driven approach to evaluation of translation and translation projects. The final chapter, Dissemination of Translation (Chapter 15), delineates necessary avenues for dissemination, and provides detail of dissemination at multiple levels.

As a companion and follow up to texts on searching for, analyzing and grading the evidence, this text provides details about the next step, which is the translation of the evidence. The translation of evidence has not previously been described in sufficient detail to be practical, which was the driving force behind the development of this book. We trust that you will discover how well this book provides these important details along with the leadership qualities useful in closing the translation gap.

Kathleen M. White and Sharon Dudley-Brown

Acknowledgments

Dr. White would like to thank her family for their continuing support and encouragement over the years for her work.

Dr. Dudley-Brown would like to acknowledge her husband and friends who provided unwavering support and encouragement during this journey.

PART ONE

Translation of Evidence

CHAPTER ONE

Evidence-Based Practice

Kathleen M. White

Evidence-based practice (EBP) is not new. In fact, most contemporary literature credits Dr. Archie Cochrane, a British epidemiologist in the 1970s, with the impetus for moving medicine toward EBP. Cochrane criticized the medical profession and their use of findings from medical research: "It is surely a great criticism of our profession that we have not organized a critical summary, by specialty or subspecialty, updated periodically, of all randomized controlled trials" (Cochrane, 1972).

The implementation of EBP in health care has moved us from a "do something . . . anything" framework of patient care to "Why do we do these things when we don't really know what works?" The Evidence-Based Medicine Working Group (1992), in promoting a new paradigm for medical practice, is often quoted as saying:

> Evidence-based medicine de-emphasizes intuition, unsystematic clinical experi-
> ence, and pathophysiologic rationale as sufficient grounds for clinical decision
> making and stresses the examination of evidence from clinical research. Evidence-
> based medicine requires new skills of the physician, including efficient literature
> searching and the application of formal rules of evidence [in] evaluating the clini-
> cal literature. (p. 2420)

However, the nursing profession also lays claim to the origins of EBP, from Florence Nightingale's collection of epidemiological data that were used to change practice (Titler et al., 2001). Nightingale emphatically taught her nurses that the foundation of clinical practice was to use evidence to guide clinical decision making. Stetler and Marram (1976), in their earliest work on research utilization for nursing, noted that even though tools are available to critique research design, there are no criteria to help the nurse—from critique to application—to decide if and how to use the findings in the nurse's specific work environment. For nursing, the framework for decision making has long been the nursing process: a systematic problem-solving methodology that has served us well. However, this process does not include the step of questioning one's own practice and being able to say "I don't know if what I am doing is really improving the patient's outcome." The evaluation step of the nursing process only takes the nurse halfway to maximizing quality and effectiveness of care.

This chapter discusses the importance of EBP for nursing and presents a summary of key EBP nursing models in use today.

■ WHY EVIDENCE-BASED PRACTICE AND WHY NOW?

Nurses can no longer rely solely on their clinical experience to provide quality care. Nurses routinely need to question their practice and look for alternative methods to improve the processes of care. As the nurse evaluates patient care processes and the outcomes of that care as part of everyday care, he or she must ask whether the best and the most current practices are being used and whether those interventions are producing the best outcomes for the patient. This critical thinking is the foundation for EBP and should be guided by a systematic approach to the evaluation of current practice. EBP in health care today uses a formal process with specific criteria to appraise emerging evidence and methods for incorporating that evidence to inform and change practice.

Why has the emphasis for use of evidence in practice gained so much momentum? The increasing complexity of health care delivery systems has seen five important factors that challenge clinicians to seek and use evidence to guide their practice. The first factor is the high visibility of the *quality and safety movement* in health care. In the midst of ever-increasing health care choices, clinicians want to know what works to increase the quality of care delivered, including the best practices to improve and optimize patient outcomes, the satisfaction with care to optimize the patient experience throughout the continuum of care, and implementing safer systems of care to protect patients from medical error. Recently, it has been recommended that consumers should be included in discussions and implementation of safety and quality initiatives at local levels, and this challenges clinicians to consider the role of patients in these initiatives. For example, proper hand washing before and after patient contact has been consistently shown to decrease the spread of infections. Empowering patients to ask their physician or nurse when they enter their hospital room or clinic suite, "have you washed your hands," directly involves the patient in implementing evidence at the point of care.

The second factor is the *tremendous growth of new knowledge* available to today's health care clinician. As of November 2010, there are 5,511 journals that are indexed in MEDLINE, including journals that are cited as *Index Medicus*, as well as other non-*Index Medicus* journals. There are 4,893 journals indexed in the *Index Medicus* and 618 non-*Index Medicus* journals, such as dentistry, nursing, health care administration, health care technology, history of medicine, consumer health, and HIV/AIDS (https://www.nlm.nih.gov/bsd/num_titles.html). The Cumulative Index to Nursing and Allied Health Literature (CINAHL; n.d.) now includes more than 3,000 journals in its index for nursing and allied health professionals (http://www.ebscohost.com/academic/the-cinahl-database). In 1995, when there were fewer journals than are available to clinicians today, it was estimated that clinicians would need to read 19 articles a day, 365 days a year to stay abreast of the explosion of new information (Davidoff, Haynes, Sackett, & Smith, 1995). The challenge to be updated with new knowledge in health care is even greater today.

The third factor is the research in health care that has shown that there is a *considerable delay in incorporating new evidence into clinical practice* (Balas & Boren, 2000). There are many examples of these delays in implementing knowledge into practice, too numerous to cite here; however, the most famous is that in 1973, there was good evidence for the effectiveness of thrombolytic therapy in reducing mortality in acute myocardial infarction (MI), which is still not uniformly given in a timely fashion to patients who would benefit.

The fourth factor is a result of the growth of new knowledge and the delays in implementing that new knowledge, a resultant *decline in best care knowledge for patient care.* There is so much information available to the clinician and the limited time to read and evaluate it for use in practice. It is widely recognized that the knowledge of best care has a negative correlation with the year of graduation (i.e., the longer the time since graduation, the poorer a person's knowledge of best care practices. EBP techniques, such as systematic reviews of evidence, available to the clinician at websites—such as the Cochrane Collaboration, the Agency for Healthcare Research and Quality (AHRQ), National Guidelines Clearinghouse, and the Joanna Briggs Institute)—synthesize new knowledge and make it available to clinicians to improve best care knowledge.

Finally, *the tremendous consumer pressure* created by an increasingly savvy consumer with online health care information at their fingertips has increased consumer expectations to take part in treatment decisions. Patients with chronic health problems who often access the Internet have considerable expertise in the self-management of their health care. Nurses at the point of care are in important positions to provide up-to-date information to patients, incorporating the best available evidence when patients question the type and quality of care being provided.

These factors mentioned previously demand that the nurse in today's health care system be knowledgeable about their practice and use explicit criteria and methods to evaluate their practice to incorporate appropriate new evidence. However, the research over the last 15 years has been inconsistent on nurses' use of evidence to inform and improve practice.

In one of the earliest studies, Mitchell, Janzen, Pask, and Southwell (1995) studied the use of research in practice in Canadian hospitals and found that only 15% had a research utilization/ EBP program for their nurses and only 38% based changes in practice on research, but that 97% wanted assistance in teaching their nurses about the research process. They also found that only 35% of small hospitals of less than 250 beds had nursing research journals in their library.

In 2000, Parahoo studied nurses' perceptions of research and found that many reported a lack of skill in evaluating research and felt isolated from colleagues who might be available to discuss research findings. The study found that nurses lacked the confidence to implement change and felt that they did not have the autonomy to implement changes. Parahoo also found that organizational characteristics are the most significant barriers to research use among nurses, including lack of organizational support for EBP, noting a lack of interest, a lack of motivation, a lack of leadership, and a lack of vision, strategy, and direction among managers.

In a Cochrane Review, Foxcroft and Cole (2006) reviewed studies that had identified organizational infrastructures that promote EBP to determine the extent of effectiveness of the organizational infrastructure in promoting the implementation of research evidence to improve the effectiveness of nursing interventions. They found only seven case study designs to review. They concluded that there were no studies rigorous enough to be included in the review and recommended that conceptual models on organizational processes to promote EBP need to be researched and evaluated properly.

Pravikoff, Tanner, and Pierce (2005) studied the EBP readiness of registered nurses (RNs) in a geographically stratified random sample of 3,000 RNs ($n = 1,097$) obtained from a nationwide publishing company. The purpose of the study was to examine the nurses' perceptions of their skills in obtaining evidence and their access to tools to obtain that evidence.

Seven-hundred sixty of the RNs were currently in clinical practice. Among that group, the study team found that 61% of the respondents said they needed to seek information at least once per week; however, 67% of those nurses always or frequently seek information from a colleague instead of a reference text, and only 46% were familiar with the term EBP. Additionally, 58% reported not using research reports at all to support their practice, 82% reported never using a hospital library, and 83% reported rarely or never seeking a librarian's assistance. These are large gaps in nurses' skills and knowledge that are necessary for EBP.

In a study to identify the presence or absence of provider and organizational variables associated with the use of EBP among nurses, Leasure, Stirlen, and Thompson (2008) surveyed nurse executives to identify barriers and facilitators to the use of EBP. They found that facilitators to EBP are reading journals that publish original research, joining journal clubs, nursing research committees, facility research committees, and facility access to the Internet. However, the barriers included lack of staff involvement in projects, no communication of projects that were completed, and no knowledge on outcomes of projects.

It is clear from this sampling of studies that EBP is continuing to evolve but not to the extent that is necessary. Nurses must understand the importance of EBP, and health care organizations must invest in resources necessary for nurses to have access to evidence at the point of care. However, a systematic approach to using that evidence is necessary: A formal process that uses specific criteria to appraise evidence to enhance efficiency and effectiveness of practice, and uses methods for incorporating that evidence into practice. There are many good EBP models that have been developed to organize and assist nurses to ask clinical questions, evaluate new evidence, and to make changes in the clinical setting. Each of these models has advantages and disadvantages and they vary in usefulness by setting and context. Gawlinski and Rutledge (2008) suggested that a deliberate process should be followed by an organization to select a model for EBP. They first suggested that a group should be developed to champion the EBP process and that this group should review models by using specific criteria, and summarize the strengths and weaknesses of the models by asking specific questions such as:

What elements of EBP models are important to your organization?
Is the model useful for all clinical situations and populations?
Has the model been tested and disseminated?
Is the model easy to use and who will be the users of the model?

They also suggested that once a model is chosen, the EBP champion group should educate the staff. Dearholt, White, Newhouse, Pugh, and Poe (2008) have gone further suggesting that once the organization decides that an evidence-based foundation for nursing is needed, a model should be chosen that is easy for the staff nurse to use; the administration should also create a strategic initiative around the implementation of EBP for the nursing department, supporting the initiative with resources in terms of time, money, and people.

■ EVIDENCE-BASED PRACTICE CONCEPTUAL FRAMEWORKS AND MODELS

A conceptual framework or model is a guide to an empirical inquiry that is built from a set of concepts, deemed critical to the inquiry, that are related and function to outline the inquiry or set of actions. Frameworks have been used in nursing to guide research and to define the foundation for nursing practice and educational programs. Likewise, models for implementing EBP have also been developed to guide the process. These models vary in detail and in explicit criteria and methods for carrying out an EBP inquiry. However, the following steps or phases are common to most models:

1. Identification of a clinical problem or question of practice.
2. Search for best evidence.
3. Critical appraisal of strength, quality, quantity, and consistency of evidence.
4. Recommendation for action (no change, change, further study) based on the appraisal of evidence.
5. Implementation of recommendation.
6. Evaluation of that recommendation in relationship to desired outcomes.

The chapter continues with a presentation of the key nursing EBP models in use today.

Stetler's Model of Research Utilization

Cheryl Stetler's model of research utilization (Figure 1.1) was one of the original models developed as an EBP for nursing that began to receive attention. She originally developed the model in 1994 and revised it in 2001. The purpose of the model is to formulate a series of critical-thinking and decision-making steps that are designed to facilitate effective use of research findings (Stetler, 2001). The model is an individual practitioner-oriented model rather than an organizational-focused model. The revised model promotes the use of both internal data (such as quality improvement, operational, evaluation, and practitioner experience data) and external evidence (such as primary research and consensus of national experts). The model describes five phases of research utilization. In Phase I, *Preparation*, the nurse searches for and selects research to be evaluated for practice implementation. This step is driven by critical thinking about potential internal and external influencing factors. During Phase II, *Validation*, the nurse appraises the findings of the study using specific methodology and utilization considerations. In Phase III, the *Comparative Evaluation or Decision Making* phase, a decision about whether a practice change can be made is made using four applicability criteria: (a) the substantiating evidence, (b) the fit for implementing the research findings in the setting, (c) the feasibility of implementation, and (d) the evaluation of current practice. Phase IV is when the *translation or application* of the research findings are implemented and the "how to's" of implementation are considered. Phase V, *Evaluation*, requires that processes include different types and levels of evaluation.

Dobbins's Framework for Dissemination and Utilization of Research

In 2001, Dobbins, Cockerill, and Barnsley studied the factors affecting the utilization of systematic reviews. The purpose of their study was to determine the extent to which public health decision makers in Ontario used five systematic reviews to make policy decisions and to determine the characteristics that predict their use. The findings of the study were used to assist health services researchers in disseminating research. Informed by their own research and using Everett Rodgers's diffusion of innovation model, the Dobbins's framework for dissemination and utilization of research (Figure 1.2) was developed for policy and practice. The model illustrates that the process of adoption of research evidence is influenced by characteristics related to the individual, organization, environment, and innovation. The model includes

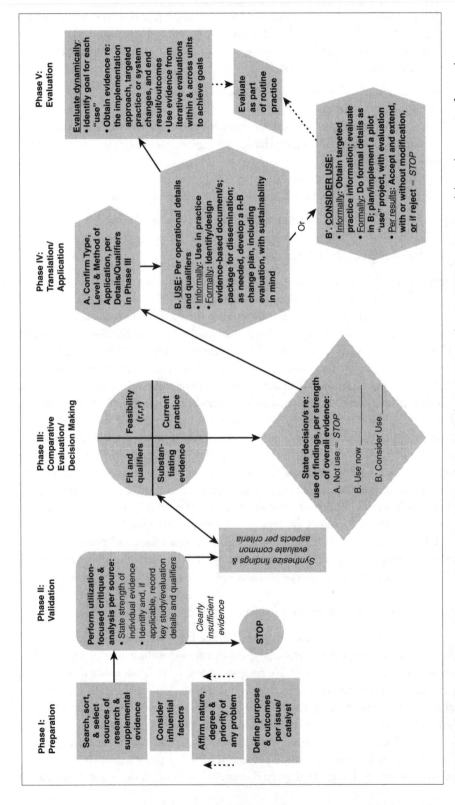

FIGURE 1.1 The Stetler model. From Ciliska, D., DiCenso, A., Melnyk, B. M., & Stetler, C. (2005). Using models and strategies for evidence-based practice. In B. M. Melnyk & E. Fineout-Overholt (Eds.), Evidence-based practice in nursing and healthcare: A guide for translating research evidence into best practice. (2nd ed., in press). Philadelphia, PA: Lippincott Williams & Wilkins. Adapted with permission.

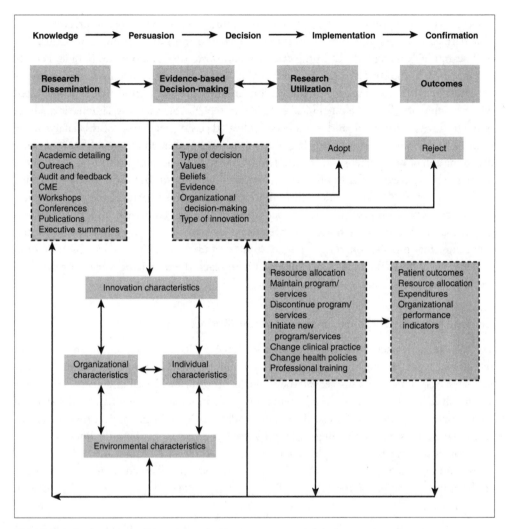

FIGURE 1.2   Framework for research dissemination and utilization. From Dobbins, M., Ciliska, D., Cockerill, R., & Barnsley, J. (2001). Factors affecting the utilization of systematic reviews: A study of public health decision makers. *International Journal of Technology Assessment in Health Care, 17*(2), 203–214. Copyright by Cambridge University Press. Adapted with permission.

five stages of innovation: knowledge, persuasion, decision, implementation, and confirmation. Identified under each of the five stages are the considerations for transferring research to practice in health care (Dobbins, Ciliska, Cockerill, Barnsley, & DiCenso, 2002).

Funk's Model for Improving the Dissemination of Nursing Research

In 1987, the research team of Funk, Champagne, Tornquist, and Wiese, after concluding that there was a huge gap between the conduct of nursing research and the use of research findings to improve practice, developed the BARRIERS scale to assess clinicians', administrators', and academicians' perceptions of barriers to the utilization of research findings in practice. Items were derived from the literature, from research data, and from the Conduct and Utilization of Research in Nursing (CURN) project's research utilization questionnaire (Crane, Pelz, & Horsley, 1977). The BARRIERS scale consisted of 28 items in four categories: characteristics of the adopter, the organization, the innovation, and the communication. The tool was tested with a sample of 1,948 RNs in clinical practice ($n = 924$). Standard psychometric analyses of the tool were performed, and it has been replicated. Using the results of this analysis, the team developed a model for improving research utilization. The Funk model for improving dissemination of nursing research (Figure 1.3) includes three components: the qualities of the research, characteristics of communication, and facilitation of utilization (Funk, Tournquist, & Champagne, 1989). The model delineates three mechanisms to achieve the dissemination of research: (a) hold topic-focused, practice-oriented research conferences; (b) write monographs that are based on the research conference presentations; and (c) develop an information center that provides ongoing dialogue, support, and consultation for the dissemination (Funk et al., 1989). The goal of the approach is to reach the practicing nurse with research results and to provide support and consultation to those doing the research.

Clinical Practice Guideline Implementation Model

The Registered Nurses Association of Ontario (RNAO; 2002) took the lead in Canada in the development of best practice guidelines for nurses. The Nursing Best Practice Guidelines (NBPG) project was funded by the Ontario Ministry of Health and Long-Term Care and involved the development, implementation, evaluation, and dissemination of a series of clinical practice guidelines (CPGs). It became evident early on in the project that the health care organizations were struggling to identify ways to implement the guidelines, and little attention was being paid to implementation strategies. The RNAO established a panel of nurses and researchers, chaired by Alba DiCenso, to develop a planned, systematic approach to the implementation of the CPGs (DiCenso et al, 2004). The likelihood of success in implementing CPGs increases when:

- A systematic process is used to identify a well-developed, evidence-based CPG.
- Appropriate stakeholders are identified and engaged.
- An assessment of environmental readiness for CPG implementation is conducted.
- Evidence-based implementation strategies that address the issues raised through the environmental readiness assessment are used.
- An evaluation of the implementation is planned and conducted.
- Consideration of resource implications to carry out these activities is adequately addressed (DiCenso et al., 2002).

The panel developed an implementation model (Figure 1.4) with an accompanying toolkit for implementing CPGs (http://www.rnao.ca/Storage/12/668_BPG_Toolkit.pdf).

The Johns Hopkins Nursing Evidence-Based Practice Model and Guidelines

The Johns Hopkins Nursing EBP (JHNEBP) model (Figure 1.5) was developed by a collaborative team of nurse leaders from the Johns Hopkins Hospital (JHH) and the Johns Hopkins University School of Nursing (JHUSON) to develop a practical model

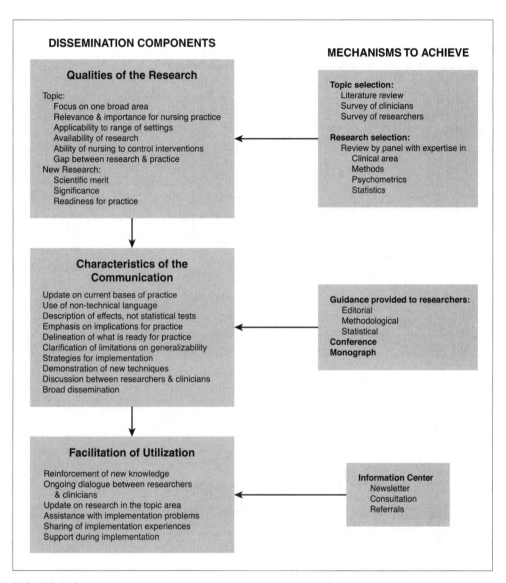

FIGURE 1.3   The Funk research dissemination model. From Funk, S. G., Tournquist, E. M., & Champagne, M. T. (1989). A model for improving the dissemination of nursing research. *Western Journal of Nursing Research, 11*(3), 361–367. Copyright by Sage Publications, Inc. Republished with permission.

to ensure that staff nurses would be able to evaluate current evidence and translate research findings into patient care. The goals of EBP at both the JHH and JHUSON are to:

- Assure the highest quality of care.
- Use evidence to promote optimal outcomes or provide equivalent care at lower cost/time.

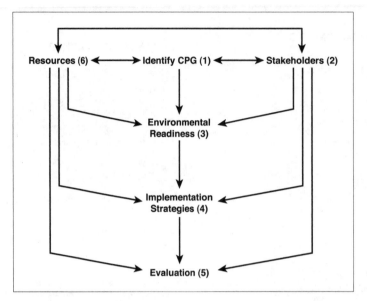

FIGURE 1.4   Clinical practice guideline implementation model. From the Registered Nurses Association of Ontario. (2002). *Toolkit: Implementation of clinical practice guidelines.* Toronto, Canada: Author.

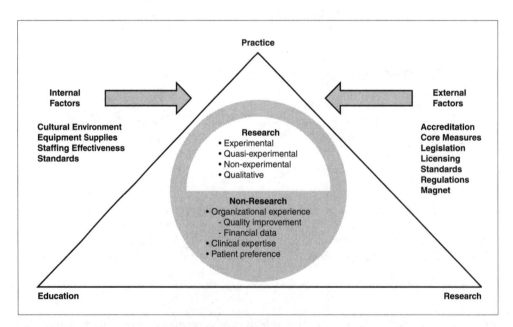

FIGURE 1.5   Johns Hopkins Nursing evidence-based practice conceptual model. From Newhouse, R. P., Dearholt, S. L., Poe, S. S., Pugh, L. C., & White, K. (2007). *Johns Hopkins Nursing evidenced-based practice model and guidelines.* Sigma Theta Tau International.

- Support rational decisions (including structural changes) that reduce inappropriate variation.
- Make it easier to do our job (optimal processes).
- Promote patient satisfaction and health-related quality of life (HRQOL).
- Create a culture of critical thinking and ongoing learning.
- Grow an environment where evidence supports clinical and administrative decisions.

The JHNEBP model is defined as a problem-solving approach to clinical decision making within a health care organization that integrates the best available scientific evidence with the best available experiential (patient and practitioner) evidence, considers internal and external influences on practice, and encourages critical thinking in the judicious application of such evidence to the care of the individual patient, patient population, or system (Newhouse, Dearholt, Poe, Pugh, & White, 2005). The model also includes the three domains of professional nursing: nursing practice, education, and research.

The guidelines that accompany the model describe the three phases in getting to an EBP (Figure 1.6). These three phases are described as the "PET" process, an acronym that stands for the *practice question*, *evidence*, and *translation*.

The first phase or "P" in PET is the practice question and involves five steps:

1. Identify a practice question through the use of the *PICO* format that will help to identify key search terms for the evidence search (Richardson, Wilson, Nishikawa, & Hayward, 1995):

   P – Patient, population, or problem (age, sex, patient setting, or symptoms)
   I – Intervention (treatment, medications, education, and diagnostic tests)
   C – Comparison with other treatments (may not be applicable or may not be apparent until additional reading is done)
   O – Outcome (anticipated outcome)

2. Recruit an interprofessional team.
3. Define the scope of problem including agreement with the team on the patient population, staff involved, and key stakeholders.
4. Assign a team leader.
5. Schedule team meetings.

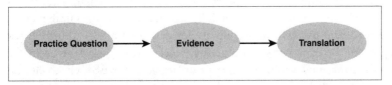

FIGURE 1.6 Evidence-based practice process. From Newhouse, R. P., Dearholt, S. L., Poe, S. S., Pugh, L. C., & White, K. M. (2005). Evidence-based practice: A practical approach to implementation. *The Journal of Nursing Administration, 35*(1), 35–40. Copyright by the Johns Hopkins Hospital/The Johns Hopkins University. Reprinted with permission.

The second phase or "E" in PET is evidence and involves another five steps:

1. Think about key search terms for the evidence search and brainstorm what databases and other places to search for the evidence.
2. Conduct search for evidence.
3. Critique each piece of evidence by rating the strength and the quality of each piece of evidence.
4. Summarize the evidence.
5. Determine the overall strength of the evidence.

The third phase or "T" in PET is translation that includes the following eight steps:

1. Determine the appropriateness and feasibility of translating recommendations into the specific practice setting.
2. Create an action plan.
3. Implement the changes.
4. Evaluate the outcomes.
5. Report the results of the preliminary evaluation to the decision makers.
6. Secure support from decision makers to implement the recommended changes internally.
7. Identify the next steps.
8. Communicate the findings.

This model includes a set of tools for use at each of the phases discussed previously and a project management tool that includes the 18 steps in the PET process. The tools are:

1. Developing a Practice Question.
2. Evidence Appraisal Guideline.
3. Review Tool for Scientific Evidence.
4. Review Tool for Non-Scientific Evidence.
5. Evidence Review Table.
6. Summary of Evidence Review and Recommendations.
7. Project Management Tool

These tools are an added dimension to the model and make its use very practical for the staff nurse.

The Iowa Model of Research-Based Practice to Promote Quality Care

The Iowa model of research-based practice was developed as a decision-making algorithm to guide nurses in using research findings to improve the quality of care (Figure 1.7). It was originally published in 1994 and a revised model in 2001 was based on changes in the health care system and feedback from users, including the use of new terminology and feedback loops, and encouraged the use of nonresearch types of evidence (case studies, etc.) in the absence of research. The Iowa model uses the concept of "triggers" for EBP, either clinical problem-focused or new knowledge-focused triggers often coming from outside the organization. These triggers set an EBP inquiry into motion and at each point in the algorithm, the nurse must answer the algorithm question, consider the organizational context, and the strength and quantity of evidence, while answering several questions:

Are the evidences to change practice sufficient?
Are findings across studies consistent?

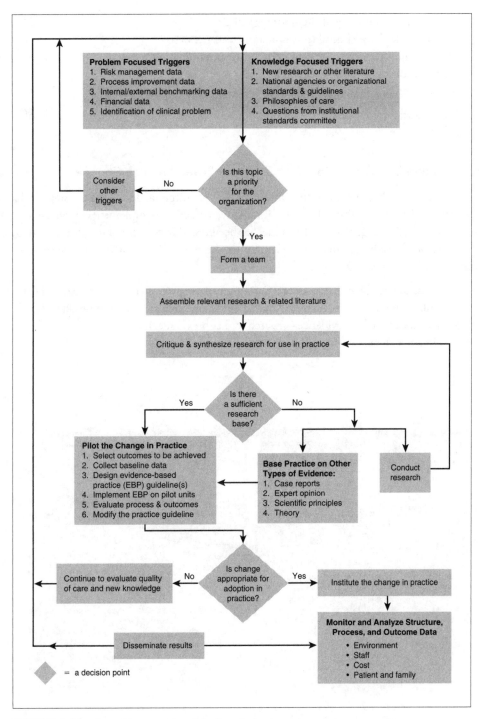

FIGURE 1.7   The 1998 Iowa model of evidence-based practice to promote quality care. Adapted from Titler, M. G., Kleiber, C., Steelman, V. J., Rakel, B. A., Budreau, G., Everett, L. Q., . . . Goode, C. J. (2001). The Iowa model of evidence-based practice to promote quality care. *Critical Care Nursing Clinics of North America, 13*(4), 497–509.

Are the type and quality of the findings sufficient?

Do the studies have clinical (not just statistical) relevance?

Can the studies reviewed be generalized to your population?

Are the findings of the study feasible?

How appropriate is the risk/benefit ratio?

This model emphasizes the use of pilot testing versus the implementation of a practice change.

Rosswurm and Larrabee's Model for Evidence-Based Practice Change

Rosswurm and Larrabee (1999), at the University of West Virginia, developed a 6-step model to facilitate a shift from traditional and intuition-driven practice to implement evidence-based changes into practice (Figure 1.8). The model has been tested in the acute care clinical setting, but the authors think it is adaptable to primary care settings. The following are the six steps in the model (Larrabee, 2009):

1. Assess the need for change in practice by comparing internal data with external data
2. Link the problem with interventions and outcomes (standard interventions, if possible)
3. Synthesize the best evidence (research and contextual evidence)
4. Design a change in practice

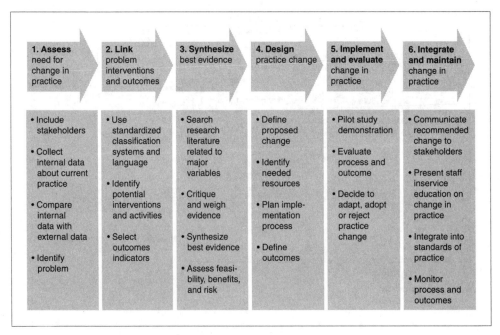

FIGURE 1.8   A model for change to evidence-based practice.
From Rosswurm, M. A., & Larrabee, J. H. (1999). A model for change to evidence-based practice. *Image—The Journal of Nursing Scholarship, 31*(4), 317–322. doi:10.1111/J.1547-5069.1999.TB00510.x. Copyright by Blackwell Publishing. Reprinted with permission.

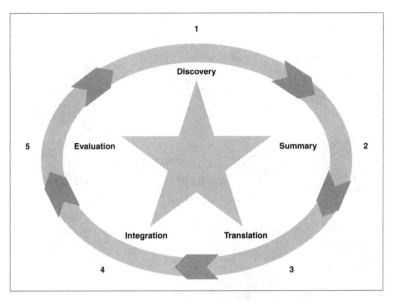

FIGURE 1.9   The ACE Star model of knowledge transformation. Adapted from Academic Center for Evidence-Based Practice, University of Texas Health Science Center at San Antonio. (n.d.). The ACE Star model. Retrieved from http://www.acestar.uthscsa.edu/acestar-model.asp.

5. Implement and evaluate the change in practice, including processes and outcomes
6. Integrate and maintain the change in practice using diffusion strategies

The Ace Star Model of Knowledge Transformation

The Academic Center for Evidence-Based Practice (ACE; n.d.) Star model of knowledge transformation (Figure 1.9) was developed by Kathleen Stevens and staff at the University of Texas Health Science Center in San Antonio to provide a framework for understanding the cycles, nature, and characteristics of knowledge that are used in EBP processes into operation (http://www.acestar.uthscsa.edu/acestar-model.asp). The goal of the process is knowledge transformation that is defined as "the conversion of research findings from primary research results, through a series of stages and forms, to impact on health outcomes by way of [evidence-based] care" (Stevens, 2004). The model promotes EBP by stressing the identification of knowledge types (from research to integrative reviews to translation). This model does not discuss the use of nonresearch evidence. The ACE Star model is depicted by a 5-point star for the five stages of knowledge transformation:

Point 1: Knowledge discovery (knowledge generation)
Point 2: Evidence summary (single statement from systematic review)
Point 3: Translation into practice (repackaging summarized research—clinical recommendations)
Point 4: Integration into practice (individual and organizational actions)
Point 5: Evaluation (effect on targeted outcomes)

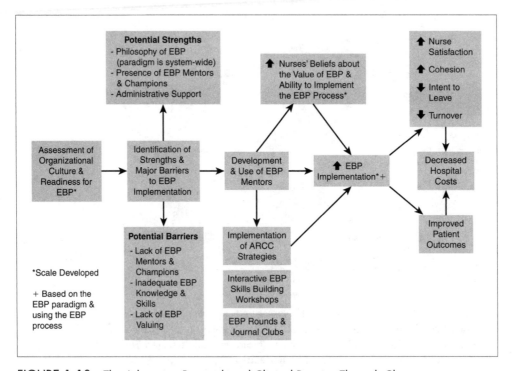

FIGURE 1.10   The Advancing Research and Clinical Practice Through Close Collaboration (ARCC) model. Figure adapted from Melnyk, B. M., Fineout-Overholt, E., Giggleman, M., & Cruz, R. (2010). Correlates among cognitive beliefs, EBP implementation, organizational culture, cohesion and job satisfaction in evidence-based practice mentors from a community hospital system. *Nursing Outlook, 58*(6), 301–308.

Advancing Research Through Close Clinical Collaboration

The Advancing Research and Clinical Practice Through Close Collaboration (ARCC) model (Figure 1.10) was originally developed by Fineout-Overholt, Melnyk, and Schultz (2005) at the University of Rochester Medical Center.

The goals of the ARCC model are as follows:

- Promote the use of EBP among advanced practice nurses (APNs) and nurses.
- Establish the network of clinicians who are supporting EBP.
- Obtain funding for ARCC.
- Disseminate the best evidence.
- Conduct an annual conference on EBP.
- Conduct studies to evaluate effectiveness of the ARCC model on process and outcomes of clinical care (Melnyk & Fineout-Overholt, 2005).

This model was originally developed to create a link between a college of nursing and a medical center. It is referred to as a *clinical scholar model* and relies on mentors with in-depth knowledge of EBP and expert clinical and group facilitation skills. The following are the five steps in the model:

Step 1: Asking the clinical question
Step 2: Searching for the best evidence

Step 3: Critically appraising the evidence

Step 4: Addressing the sufficiency of the evidence: To implement or not to implement

Step 5: Evaluating the outcome of evidence implementation

Melnyk and Fineout-Overholt (2005) conducted a pilot study to test the ARCC model at two acute-care sites. The pilot study examined what must be present for a successful implementation of EBP in the acute-care setting. These essentials include identifying EBP champions, redefining nurses' roles to include EBP activities, allocating time and money to the EBP process, and creating an organizational culture that fosters EBP. In addition, practical strategies for implementing EBP are presented to encourage implementation of EBP (Melnyk & Fineout-Overholt).

Veterans Administration's Quality Enhancement Research Initiative Model

The Quality Enhancement Research Initiative (QUERI) model (Figure 1.11) was developed by the Department of Veterans Affairs in 1998 to improve the quality of health care throughout the veterans system through the use of research-based best practices (Stetler, Mittman, & Francis, 2008). The program had a quality improvement focus and included a redesign of organizational structures and policies, and implementation of new information technology and a performance accountability system (Perrin & Stevens, 2004). The QUERI process model includes six steps:

1. Select conditions per patient population that are associated with a high risk of disease and/or disability and/or burden of illness for veterans.
2. Identify evidence-based guidelines, recommendations, and best practices.
3. Measure and diagnose the quality and performance gaps.
4. Implement improvement programs.

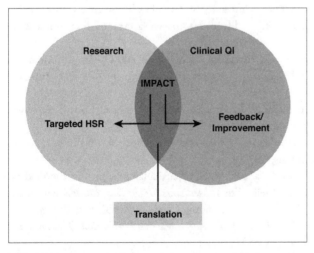

FIGURE 1.11   Quality enhancement research initiative model. Figure adapted from Feussner, J. R., Kizer, K. W., & Demakis, J. G. (2000). The Quality Enhancement Research Initiative (QUERI): From evidence to action. *Medical Care, 38*(6 Suppl. 1), 11–16.

5. Assess improvement program feasibility, implementation, and effects on patient, family, and health care system processes and outcomes.
6. Assess improvement program effects on HRQOL (Stetler et al., 2008).

The program has been implemented in a 4-phase pipeline framework that begins with pilot projects for improvement and feasibility, then advances to small clinical trials, moves to regional roll-outs, and, finally, the improvement based on research becomes a national effort (Department of Veterans Affairs, 2011a and Department of Veterans Affairs, 2011b). The QUERI model is highlighted graphically showing an intersection between research and practice, and showing that the translation of research is accomplished through clinical and quality improvement (QI) activities and enhanced by feedback in the system.

■ SUMMARY

Nursing has entered an important era in the profession's development. A key to making important contributions in today's complex health care environment is understanding the need to develop and sustain EBP. Health care systems need to implement the interventions that not only increase nurses' EBP knowledge and skills, but also strengthen their beliefs about the benefit of evidence-based care (Melnyk, Fineout-Overholt, Stone, & Ackerman, 2000). However, there is a lot to be learned about how those interventions are implemented and how evidence is translated into practice. The next two chapters in this book will present translation frameworks that can be used to guide the implementation of evidence into practice and explore the key interrelationships within organizations that drive or restrain the translation.

■ REFERENCES

Academic Center for Evidence-Based Practice, University of Texas Health Science Center at San Antonio. (n.d.). *The ACE Star model*. Retrieved from http://www.acestar.uthscsa.edu/acestar-model.asp

Balas, E. A., & Boren, S. A. (2000). Managing clinical knowledge for health care improvement. In J. van Bemmel & A. T. McCray (Eds.), *Yearbook of medical informatics* (pp. 65–70). Stuttgart, Germany: Schattauer.

Cumulative Index to Nursing and Allied Health Literature. (n.d.). Retrieved from http://www.ebscohost.com/academic/the-cinahl-database

Cochrane, A. L. (1972). *Effectiveness and efficiency: Random reflections on health services*. London, England: Nuffield Provincial Hospitals Trust.

Cochrane, A. L. (1979). 1931–1971: A critical review, with particular reference to the medical profession. In G. Teeling-Smith & N. Wells (Eds.), *Medicines for the year 2000: A symposium held at the Royal College of Physicians* (pp. 1–11). London: Office of Health Economics.

Crane, J., Pelz, D. C., & Horsley, J. A. (1977). *CURN. Project Research Utilization Questionnaire*. Michigan: School of Nursing, University of Michigan.

Davidoff, F., Haynes, B., Sackett, D., & Smith, R. (1995). Evidence-based medicine. *British Medical Journal, 310*(6987), 1085–1086.

Dearholt, S. L., White, K. M., Newhouse, R. P., Pugh, L. C., & Poe, S. (2008). Educational strategies to develop evidence-based practice mentors. *Journal for Nurses in Staff Development, 24*(2), 53–59.

Department of Veterans Affairs. (2011a). Retrieved from http://www.queri.research.va.gov/implementation/

Department of Veterans Affairs. (2011b). *Quality Enhancement Research Initiative* [Brochure]. Retrieved from http://www.queri.research.va.gov/queribrochure2010.pdf

DiCenso, A., Virani, T., Bajnok, I., Borycki, E., Davies, B., Graham, I., . . . Scott, J. (2002). A toolkit to facilitate the implementation of clinical practice guidelines in healthcare settings. *Hospital Quarterly, 5*(3), 55–60.

Dobbins, M., Ciliska, D., Cockerill, R., Barnsley, J., & DiCenso, A. (2002). A framework for the dissemination and utilization of research for health-care policy and practice. *The Online Journal of Knowledge Synthesis for Nursing, 9,7*.

Dobbins, M., Cockerill, R., & Barnsley, J. (2001). Factors affecting the utilization of systematic reviews: A study of public health decision makers. *International Journal of Technology Assessment in Health Care, 17*(2): 203–214. doi: 10.1017/S0266462300105069.

Evidence-Based Medicine Working Group. (1992). Evidence-based medicine: A new approach to teaching the practice of medicine. *The Journal of the American Medical Association, 268*(17), 2420–2425.

Feussner, J. R., Kizer, K. W., & Demakis, J. G. (2000). The Quality Enhancement Research Initiative (QUERI): From evidence to action. *Medical Care, 38*(6 Suppl. 1), I1–I6.

Fineout-Overholt, E., Melnyk, B. M., & Schultz, A. (2005). Transforming health care from the inside out: Advancing evidence-based practice in the 21st century. *Journal of Professional Nursing, 21*(6), 335–344.

Foxcroft, D. R., & Cole, N. (2006). Organisational infrastructures to promote evidence-based nursing practice. *Cochrane Database of Systematic Reviews, 3*, CD002212. doi:10.1002/14651858.CD002212.

Funk, S. G., Champagne, M. T., Wiese, R. A., & Tornquist, E. M. (1991). BARRIERS: The barriers to research utilization scale. *Applied Nursing Research, 4*(1), 39–45.

Funk, S. G., Tournquist, E. M., & Champagne, M. T. (1989). A model for the dissemination of nursing research. *Western Journal of Nursing Research, 11*(3), 361–372.

Funk, S. G., Tornquist, E. M., & Champagne, M. T. (1995). Barriers and facilitators of research utilization: An integrative review. *Nursing Clinics of North America, 30*, 395–407.

Gawlinski, A., & Rutledge, D. (2008). Selecting a model for evidence-based practice changes: A practical approach. *AACN Advanced Critical Care, 19*(3): 291–300.

Larrabee, J. H. (2009). *Nurse to nurse: Evidence-based practice* (p. 22). New York: McGraw-Hill.

Leasure, A. R., Stirlen, J., & Thompson, C. (2008). Barriers and facilitators to the use of evidence-based best practices. *Dimensions of Critical Care Nursing, 27*(2), 74–82.

Melnyk, B. M., & Fineout-Overholt, E., (Eds.). (2005). *Evidence-based practice in nursing and healthcare: A guide to best practice* (pp. 185–219). Philadelphia, PA: Lippincott Williams & Wilkins; 185–219.

Melnyk, B. M., Fineout-Overholt, E., Giggleman, M., & Cruz, R. (2010). Correlates among cognitive beliefs, EBP implementation, organizational culture, cohesion and job satisfaction in evidence-based practice mentors from a community hospital system. *Nursing Outlook, 58*(6), 301–308.

Melnyk B. M., Fineout-Overholt, E., Stone, P., & Ackerman, M. (2000). Evidence-based practice: The past, the present, and recommendations for the millennium. *Pediatric Nursing. 26*(1), 77–80.

Mitchell, A., Janzen, K., Pask, E., & Southwell, D. (1995). Assessment of nursing research utilization needs in Ontario heatlh agencies. *Canadian Journal of Nursing Administration, 8*(1), 77–91.

National Library of Medicine. MEDLINE. Retrieved from http://www.nlm.nih.gov/bsd/num_ titles.html

Newhouse, R. P., Dearholt, S. L., Poe, S. S., Pugh, L. C., & White, K. M. (2005). Evidence-based practice: A practical approach to implementation. *The Journal of Nursing Administration*, *35*(1), 35–40.

Newhouse, R. P., Dearholt, S. L., Poe, S. S., Pugh, L. C., & White, K. (2007). *Johns Hopkins Nursing evidenced-based practice model and guidelines*. Indianapolis, IN: Sigma Theta Tau International.

Parahoo, K. (2000). Barriers to, and facilitators of, research utilization among nurses in Northern Ireland. *Journal of Advanced Nursing*, *31*(1), 89–98. doi: 10.1046/j.1365-2648.2000.01256.x.

Perrin, R., & Stevens, J. (2004). Information technology: Facilitating the translation of research into practice. *QUERI Quarterly*, *6*(1), 1–4.

Pravikoff, D. S., Tanner, A. B., & Pierce, S. T. (2005). Readiness of U.S. nurses for evidence-based practice. *American Journal of Nursing*, *105*(9), 40–51.

Registered Nurses Association of Ontario. (2002). *Toolkit: Implementation of clinical practice guidelines*. Retrieved from http://www.rnao.org/Page.asp?PageID=924&ContentID=823

Richardson, W. S., Wilson, M. C., Nishikawa, J., & Hayward, R. S. (1995). The well-built clinical question: A key to evidence-based decision. *ACP Journal Club*, *123*(3), A12–A13.

Rosswurm, M. A., & Larrabee, J. H. (1999). A model for change to evidence-based practice. *Image—The Journal of Nursing Scholarship*, *31*(4), 317–322.

Stetler, C. B. (2001). Updating the Stetler Model of research utilization to facilitate evidence-based practice. *Nursing Outlook*, *49*(6), 272–279.

Stetler, C. B. (1985). Research utilization: Defining the concept. *Journal of Nursing Scholarship*, *17*(2), 40–44.

Stetler, C., Brunell, M., Giulano, K., Morsi, D., Prince, L., & Newell-Stokes, V. (1998). Evidence-based practice and the role of nursing leadership. *Journal of Nursing Administration*, *28*(7–8), 45–53.

Stetler, C. B., & Marram, G. (1976). Evaluating research findings for applicability in practice. *Nursing Outlook*, *24*(9), 559–563.

Stetler, C. B., Mittman, B. S., & Francis, J. (2008). Overview of the VA quality enhancement research initiative (QUERI) and QUERI theme articles: QUERI series. *Implementation Science*, *3*, 8.

Stevens, K. R. (2004). *ACE Star model of EBP: Knowledge transformation*. Academic Center for Evidence-Based Practice, The University of Texas Health Science Center at San Antonio. Retrieved from http:// www.acestar.uthscsa.edu

Titler, M. G., Kleiber, C., Steelman, V. J., Rakel, B. A., Budreau, G., Everett, L. Q., . . . Goode, C. J. (2001). The Iowa model of evidence-based practice to promote quality care. *Critical Care Nursing Clinics of North America*, *13*(4), 497–509.

CHAPTER TWO

The Science of Translation and Major Frameworks

Kathleen M. White

"Research is only a beginning, and not an end in itself."
—Carolyn Clancy, Director, AHRQ

■ THE DEVELOPMENT OF THE SCIENCE OF TRANSLATION

The challenge to clinicians and health care organizations to translate research findings into routine practice, often taking 17 or more years (Balas & Boren, 2000), is a major challenge to the U.S. health care system. The ability to translate evidence into routine clinical practice in health care is fundamental in ensuring quality of health care delivery. Despite the large numbers of well-designed clinical intervention studies in health care today, it is widely recognized that findings from these studies are not being implemented in clinical practice settings. For example, a 1998 review of published studies on the quality of care received by Americans found that some people are receiving more care than they actually need, whereas some are receiving less. The findings showed that taking simple averages from many studies indicate that 70% of people receive recommended acute care; 60% receive recommended chronic care; 50% receive recommended preventive care; 30% receive contraindicated acute care; and 20% receive contraindicated chronic care (Schuster, McGlynn, & Brook, 1998).

The Agency for Healthcare Research and Quality (AHRQ) identified that this translational hurdle exists despite a wide range of strategies for implementing research in practice that includes provider reminder systems, use of local opinion leaders, new computer decision support systems, and even financial incentives (AHRQ, 2001).

To decrease the time from discovery to translation of evidence at the bedside, AHRQ began a program in 1999 called Translating Research Into Practice (TRIP) to evaluate different strategies for translating research findings into clinical practice, primarily using randomized controlled trials. Fourteen projects were funded in the TRIP-I program. The purpose was to generate new knowledge about approaches that promoted the utilization of rigorously derived evidence to improve patient care and to enhance the use of research findings, tools, and scientific information that would work in diverse practice settings, among diverse populations, and under diverse payment systems (AHRQ, 2001).

The following year, AHRQ funded 13 more projects as part of TRIP-II, which continued building on the first program and then focused on implementation techniques and factors, such as organizational and clinical characteristics, which were associated with successfully translating research findings into diverse applied settings. The TRIP-II program was aimed at applying and assessing strategies and methods that were developed in idealized practice settings or that are in current use but have not been previously or rigorously evaluated. The aim of these 3-year cooperative agreements was to identify sustainable and reproducible strategies to accelerate the impact of health services research on direct patient care and improve the outcomes, quality, effectiveness, efficiency, and/ or cost-effectiveness of care through partnerships between health care organizations and researchers (AHRQ, 2001).

Special areas of interest included reducing disparities, such as diabetes and cardiovascular disease, that disproportionately affect minority populations, and using information technology to accelerate more rapidly the implementation of research throughout organizations and to evaluate how computer-based interventions contribute to translating research findings into health care improvements and health policy.

Farquhar, Stryer, and Slutsky (2002) studied the 27 TRIP projects funded by AHRQ and looked at several dimensions for successful programs, including provider focus, patient population, vulnerable populations, methodologies, interventions for change, outcomes measured, and conceptual framework used. They found that the most common TRIP intervention that was used for translation was educational and that the most common frameworks that were used to organize for the translation were either adult learning theory or organizational theory. Other implementation strategies that were used in the projects were continuing education, self-instructed learning, academic detailing, audit and feedback, provider reminder systems, incentives, local opinion leaders, outreach visits, continuous quality improvement, clinical information systems, computer decision support systems. Farquhar et al. (2002) concluded that the challenge for the TRIP projects was to find a balance between rigor and generalizability, because it was often necessary to make trade-offs between optimal study design to maintain internal validity and the need for relevance. However, even noting this challenge, most TRIP projects used randomized controlled designs. Kirchhoff (2004) reported that nursing investigators responded to this review of the TRIP projects, but noted that questions remain about the reproducibility of the intervention, the dependent variable selection and measurement, and how the intervention interacts with the environment.

In 2005, as part of the National Institutes of Health (NIH) Roadmap for Medical Research, three themes emerged (Westfall, Mold, & Fagnan, 2007). The third theme resulted in the development of a program of translational research that created the Institutional Clinical and Translational Science Awards (CTSAs) program, designed to support the clinical and translational science at the academic health centers (Zerhouni, 2005). NIH defined translational research in two ways along the research continuum. The first, or Type I Translational Research, is the process of applying discoveries made in the laboratory, testing them in animals, and then developing trials and studies for humans for treatment and prevention approaches. The second, or Type II Translational Research, is research aimed at enhancing the

adoption of best treatment practices into the medical community with a goal of institutionalizing effective programs, products, and services. The goals of these NIH TRIP-II translational
research studies are to (a) identify community, patient, physician, and organizational factors that serve as barriers and facilitators to translation; (b) develop novel intervention and
implementation strategies to increase translation, such as quality improvement programs or
policies; and (c) evaluate the impact of strategies to increase translation of relevant healthy
behaviors and processes of care (NIH, 2005).

There remain major challenges to adopting and integrating new evidence into practice
with little understanding of how this adoption takes place (Green & Siefert, 2005). How
do health care practitioners translate new knowledge into their specific actions that they put
into practice? Why do health care practitioners and organizations not incorporate new evidence or best practices quickly and reliably into their work (Berwick, 2003)? As the Institute
of Medicine's (IOM) report "Crossing the Quality Chasm" stated, "Between the health care
we have and the care we could have lies not just a gap, but a chasm" (IOM, 2001, p. 1).
This failure to use new knowledge and evidence is costly, harmful, inefficient, and results in
ineffective care being delivered to the American public. There is a critical need to understand
the process of translating or integrating the new evidence into the existing organization or
practice delivery.

Green and Siefert (2005), in an article called with a very apropos title, "Translation
of Research: Why We Can't 'Just Do It'?" suggested that translation of research to practice
happens in three stages: (1) awareness, (2) acceptance, and (3) adoption. However, they
further describe that most efforts have focused on awareness and acceptance by the clinicians and organizations and that very little attention is paid to the adoption stage. There
has been research in identifying the factors that affect adoption, which are the first two
stages, specifically how to increase and foster awareness and acceptance, but not much
on understanding how the adoption takes place and how to make it more effective. Their
work embraces cognitive skill learning research that suggests that the clinician must move
from awareness and acceptance, where the new knowledge is acquired, to the adoption
stage where the knowledge becomes a part of the clinician's routine procedures in practice.
Critical to this change is the implementation of strategies that support clinician learning
and disrupt well-practiced procedures and rules in order to incorporate the new knowledge
(Green & Siefert, 2005).

Key to this learning and adoption of new knowledge is the use of appropriate implementation strategies. Glasgow and Emmons (2007) conducted a systematic review of the
literature on interventions that promote the translation of research findings into practice and
found four factors that serve as barriers to the translation of new knowledge: the characteristics of the intervention, the current target setting or environment, the research or evaluation
design, and the interaction among the first three factors. This attention to the connectedness
of the factors is particularly important for complex interventions and multifaceted programs.
They posit that the implementation will be more successful when integrated and delivered in
a coordinated way that reinforces all the factors, as opposed to strategies happening in separate "silos" of unrelated activities (Figure 2.1).

A systematic approach to the translation of new knowledge into practice, guided by a
framework or model, will increase the chances of a successful implementation. This chapter
will present an array of different translation models from the current literature.

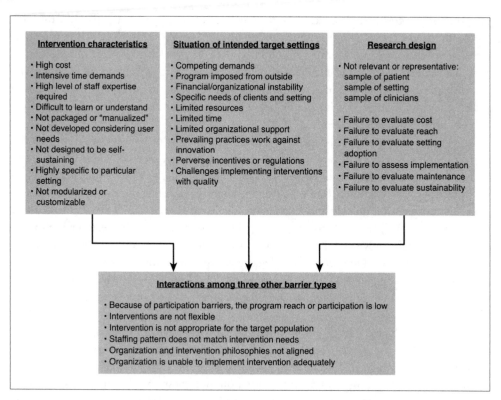

FIGURE 2.1   Glasglow and Emmons implementation model. From Glasglow, R. E., & Emmons, K. M. (2007). How can we increase translation of research into practice? Types of evidence needed. *Annual Review of Public Health, 28,* 413–433. Copyright by Annual Reviews. Republished with permission.

Definitions of Key Translation Science Words

Knowledge Translation

Knowledge translation is the exchange, synthesis, and ethically sound application of knowledge—within a complex system of interactions among researchers and users—to accelerate the capture of the benefits of research . . . through improved health, more effective services and products, and a strengthened health care system. The collaborative and systematic review, assessment, identification, aggregation, and practical application of high-quality research by key stakeholders (e.g., consumers, researchers, practitioners, policy makers) have the purpose of improving the lives and health of individuals (Canadian Institutes of Health Research, 2010).

Knowledge Transfer

Knowledge transfer is a systematic approach to capture, collect, and share tacit knowledge in order for it to become explicit knowledge. By doing so, this process allows for individuals and/or organizations to access and use essential information, which previously was known intrinsically to only one or a small group of people (Graham et al., 2006).

Knowledge Exchange

Knowledge exchange is a collaborative problem solving between researchers and decision makers that happens through linkage and exchange. Effective knowledge exchange involves interaction between decision makers and researchers that results in mutual learning through the process of planning, producing, disseminating, and applying existing or new research in decision making (Canadian Health Services Research Foundation).

Synthesis

Synthesis, in this context, means the contextualization and integration of research findings of individual research studies within the larger body of knowledge on the topic. A synthesis must be reproducible and transparent in its methods, using quantitative and/or qualitative methods. It could take the form of a systematic review (follow the methods developed by the Cochrane Collaboration), result from a consensus conference or expert panel, or synthesize qualitative or quantitative results. Realist syntheses, narrative syntheses, meta-analyses, meta-syntheses, and practice guidelines are all forms of synthesis (Canadian Institutes of Health Research, 2010).

Research Utilization

Research utilization is the process by which specific research-based knowledge (science) is implemented in practice (Stetler, Corrigan, Sander-Buscemi, & Burns, 1999).

Implementation

Implementation is the execution of the adoption decision, that is, the innovation or the research is put into practice (Titler, 2008).

Dissemination

Dissemination is the spreading of knowledge or research, such as is done in scientific journals and at scientific conferences. Dissemination involves identifying the appropriate audience and tailoring the message and medium to the audience. Dissemination activities can include summaries for/briefings to stakeholders; educational sessions with patients, practitioners, and/or policy makers; engaging knowledge users in developing and executing dissemination/implementation plan; tools creation; and media engagement (Canadian Institutes of Health Research, 2010).

Diffusion

Diffusion is the process by which an innovation is communicated through certain channels over time among members of a social system (Rogers, 2003).

Websites for Knowledge Translation
http://www.ktclearinghouse.ca/knowledgebase/modelsandtheories

- **AHRQ's Translating Research Into Practice (TRIP) program:** An initiative focusing on the implementation techniques and factors associated with successfully translating research findings into diverse applied settings (http://www.ahrq.gov/research/trip2fac.htm).

- **Campbell Collaboration (C2):** An international organization that conducts systematic reviews of education, social welfare, and social science research (http://www.campbellcollaboration.org).

- **Canadian Institutes for Health Research (CIHR):** The major federal agency that is responsible for funding health research in Canada that has established charges for Knowledge Translation research, development, and dissemination (http://www.cihr-irsc.gc.ca/e/29529.html).

- **Cochrane Collaboration:** An international organization that conducts systematic reviews of health and medical research (http://www.cochrane.org).

- **Knowledge Translation Program (KTP) at the University of Toronto, Canada:** A multidisciplinary academic program that is developed to address the gap between research evidence and clinical practice and the need to focus on the processes through which knowledge is effectively translated into changed practices (http://www.stmichaelshospital.com/research/kt.php).

- **Knowledge Utilization Studies Program at the University of Alberta, Canada:** A health research program focusing on nursing, social sciences, and research utilization in the nursing profession (http://www.nursing.ualberta.ca/kusp/).

- **National Health Service (NHS) Centre for Reviews and Dissemination at the University of York:** An organization that conducts systematic reviews of research and disseminates research-based information about the effects of interventions used in health and social care in the United Kingdom (http://www.york.ac.uk/inst/crd/welcome.htm).

- **What Works Clearinghouse (WWC):** A clearinghouse established by the U.S. Department of Education's (ED) Institute of Education Sciences to provide educators, policy makers, and the public with a central, independent, and trusted source of scientific evidence of what works in education (http://ies.ed.gov/ncee/wwc/).

■ TRANSLATION THEORY AND FRAMEWORKS

Translation theory and frameworks focus on the interrelationships and complex organizational dimensions that are relevant to translation of research or new knowledge into practice. Common among the theories are discussions of the ongoing and iterative nature of the processes; the need to determine the strength and quality of the new knowledge; the inclusion of many stakeholders; the importance of context including culture, leadership styles, and decision making; and organizational structures.

Knowledge translation theories are needed to guide implementation of research-based interventions into practice. To this end, Estabrooks, Thompson, Lovely, and Hofmeyer (2006) provided an overview of perspectives that are useful for understanding the basis of knowledge translation theory that includes various perspectives that come from different disciplines. As described in the first chapter of this book, they begin by looking at the models of research utilization and evidence-based practice from the nursing literature. Additionally, they describe adjuvant theories considered as complements, such as theory on organizations, including the change process and decision making; social science theory on problem solving; political and tactical theory; and finally, behavioral and health promotion theory from the health sciences.

The development of translation models or frameworks has been slow but includes many and varied approaches for introducing evidence and changing behavior and performance, which are all based on different assumptions about change. The discussion will begin in the early 1990s and proceed through the development of today's latest models.

Coordinated Implementation Model

In 1993, Lomas, Sisk, and Stocking, in an overview of a journal issue on translation of knowledge into practice, questioned the putting of effort into translation of knowledge before targeting efforts to implement science and "validated truths" (p. 405) in medicine. They argued that there is too much use of untruths and invalid facts in medicine and that the profession had an ethical obligation to move toward appraising and using valid research in practice.

Lomas (1993) proposed an active model of dissemination, replacing the previously used diffusion models that were passive, that explores "sufficient conditions" for research translation into the practice environment. His coordinated implementation model involves the careful evaluation of (a) the research information including synthesis, distillation, and appraisal of that research evidence for use; (b) adoption by a credible body using active dissemination strategies; (c) consideration of the competing factors in the overall practice environment; and (d) the need for coordination among external audiences including patients, clinical policy makers, community groups, administrators, and public policy makers (Lomas, 1993). Lomas uses the Effective Care in Pregnancy and Childbirth program as a case study to present the model (Figure 2.2).

Haines and Jones's Translation Model

One of the earliest translation models was described by Haines and Jones (1994), citing unacceptable delays in implementing the findings of research into practice resulting in suboptimal patient care. They acknowledged that the top-down administrative, traditional

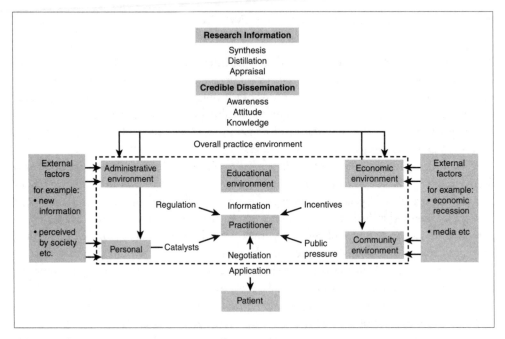

FIGURE 2.2   Lomas's coordinated implementation model. Adapted from Lomas, J., Sisk, J. E., & Stocking, B. (1993). From evidence to practice in the United States, the United Kingdom, and Canada. *Milbank Quarterly, 71*(3), 405–410.

education and economic strategies to contain cost have not been sufficient to promote change and that the strategies for implementation must be sustainable and dynamic, taking into account the changing evidence about effectiveness. They proposed that an integrated approach using several types of dissemination strategies, the critical appraisal and use of systematic reviews and clinical practice guidelines, along with adequate resources and culture change, when taken together, can speed up and increase successful implementation of research into practice (Figure 2.3).

Rogers's Theory of Diffusion of Innovations

Although not developed specifically for health care, the foundation for many translation models is Everett Rogers's theory of diffusion of innovations (Rogers, 2003). Rogers discusses that change is caused by an introduction of innovation and, for translation science, this is the new knowledge or evidence. He defines *innovation* as an idea, practice, or object that is perceived as new by an individual or other unit of adoption. Time is not important to the *newness*; it is not whether the innovation is objectively newly measured by the lapse of time since its first use or discovery, but by the perceived newness of the idea for the individual. This perceived newness is what determines a person's reaction to the innovation. If the idea seems new to the individual, it is considered as an innovation by the individual.

Rogers described five groups based on the characteristics of individuals on how they adopt to the introduction of an innovation. First are the *innovators* who are venturesome,

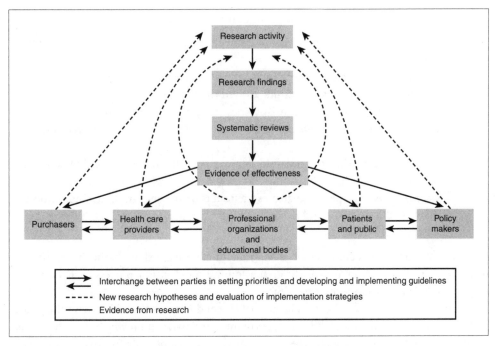

FIGURE 2.3   Haines and Jones translation model. From Haines, A., & Jones, R. (1994). Implementing findings of research. BMJ, 308(6942), 1488–1492. Copyright by BMJ Publishing Group. Republished with permission.

tolerant of risks, and like new ideas. These are estimated to be only about 2.5% of those involved with a change. The second group is the *early adopters*. The early adopters are usually the opinion leaders in an organization and are locally well connected; they focus on and select ideas that they like; and they like to associate with the innovators to learn, maintain, and connect to the outside. Rogers estimates that 13.5% of those involved with change are early adopters. The third group is the *early majority* who are local in their perspective, learn from people they know, rely on familiarity rather than science, and are risk averse. This is 34% or one-third of the group that is involved with change. Another one-third or 34% are called the *late majority*. The late majority will adopt an innovation when it finally appears to be status quo in an organization. They require and watch for local proof that the change is really going to work and stick around. The last group that Rogers identifies is the *laggards*. For this group, the point of reference is the past. They are the traditionalists in an organization and like the tried and true, not something that involves change. Unfortunately, Rogers's work shows that these account for 16% of our work group. Each of these groups of people must be planned for and included in the change process.

The second concept that is important to the Rogers's theory is the *diffusion*, defined as the process by which an innovation is communicated through certain channels over time among the members of an organization. Rogers calls his model an innovation–decision process that includes information and uncertainty, views change as dynamic, and stresses the importance of commitment and maintenance to any change.

Rogers's theory describes a five-step innovation–decision process:

1. *Knowledge.* The person becomes aware of an innovation and has some idea of how it functions.
2. *Persuasion.* The person actively seeks information about the innovation and forms a favorable or unfavorable attitude toward the innovation.
3. *Decision.* The person engages in activities that lead to a choice, benefit, or risk to adopting the innovation and makes a choice whether to accept or reject the innovation.
4. *Implementation.* The person considers the uses of the innovation and puts the innovation into practice.
5. *Confirmation.* The person evaluates the results of an innovation–decision process that was already made and makes a decision whether to continue to use the innovation or not.

The personal characteristics of those individuals involved with the innovation, as described previously, affect how early in the innovation–decision process each individual engages and begins to adopt the new idea.

Oxman, Thomson, Davis, and Haynes (1995) conducted a systematic review of methods to determine the effectiveness of different types of interventions in improving health professional performance and health outcomes. They found that dissemination-only strategies, such as conferences or the mailing of unsolicited materials, demonstrated little or no changes in the behavior of health professionals when used alone, and that more complex interventions, such as the use of outreach visits or local opinion leaders, were only moderately effective but ranged from 20% to 50% in reducing the incidence of inappropriate performance. They concluded that there were no "magic bullets" to improve a professional's practice and resulting patient outcomes.

Following up on this study, Bero et al. (1998) found that providing systematic reviews of rigorous research is helpful, but the passive dissemination of information was generally ineffective. They categorized interventions that promote behavioral changes among health professionals:

- Consistently effective interventions were reminders (manual or computerized), multifaceted interventions (a combination that includes two or more of the following: audit and feedback, reminders, local consensus processes, or marketing), and interactive educational meetings (participation of health care providers in workshops that include discussion or practice).
- Interventions of variable effectiveness were audit and feedback (or any summary of clinical performance), use of local opinion leaders (practitioners identified by their colleagues as influential), local consensus processes (inclusion of participating practitioners in discussions to ensure that they agree that the chosen clinical problem is important and that the approach to managing the problem is appropriate), and patient-mediated interventions (any intervention aimed at changing the performance of health care providers for which specific information was sought from or given to patients).
- Interventions that have little or no effect included distributing educational materials (distribution of recommendations for clinical care, including clinical practice guidelines, audiovisual materials, and electronic publications) and didactic educational meetings (such as lectures).

This early research lays the foundation for subsequent translation discussions and modeling to emphasize the active participation and involvement of those needing to translate new knowledge into practice.

Framework for Changing Behavior

Grol and Grimshaw (1999) described lessons for the implementation of evidence into practice from reviewing strategies to implement change. They reviewed change approaches from seven theoretical perspectives and concluded that the change approach determines the implementation plan. The seven approaches (Grol & Grimshaw, 1999) are as follows with considerations for each:

1. *Educational.* Assumes that an internal motivation to improve exists, so the strategy must convey ownership of the change process
2. *Epidemiological.* Assumes the presence of sound and convincing evidence and rigorous procedures, so the strategy must include strength and quality of the evidence
3. *Marketing.* Assumes providing an attractive message, so the strategy must adapt the message to the needs of the target group
4. *Behavioral.* Assumes that human behavior can be influenced, so the strategy would include providing feedback and incentives or sanctions
5. *Social influence.* Assumes that learning and changing are part of a social network, so the strategy would be to include opinion leaders and champions
6. *Organizational.* Assumes a focus on creating conditions for change, so the strategy would be to identify areas of failure that need improvement
7. *Coercive.* Assumes that controls are needed, so the strategy would be to develop laws, regulations, policies, and procedures

They expanded their work and emphasized the importance of clinicians' decision making using knowledge of the medical evidence, the patient-specific or social context of care, and the organizational and policy evidence, including efficiency, equity, and rationing (Grol & Grimshaw, 2003). They suggest to analyze the target setting and the target group and identify obstacles to change; link the interventions to the needs, facilitators, and obstacles to change; know the critical importance of developing a plan for change in clinical practice; implement and, finally, evaluate the progress toward change.

Greenhalgh's Diffusion of Innovations in Service Organizations

Following on Rogers's work, Greenhalgh, Robert, McFarlane, Bate, and Kyriakidou (2004) conducted a modified systematic review of the health care research literature to answer the question, "How can health service organizations spread and sustain innovations?" The review considered both the process and how to measure the diffusion of innovations in service organizations. Innovation in service delivery and organization was defined as "a novel set of behaviors, routines, and ways of working that are directed at improving health outcomes, administrative efficiency, cost effectiveness, or users' experience and that are implemented by planned and coordinated actions" (Greenhalgh et al., 2004, p. 582). They tried to distinguish among diffusion, dissemination, implementation, and sustainability.

The final review had 495 sources, including 213 empirical studies and 282 nonempirical references. Thirteen research areas relevant to diffusion of innovations in health care organizations were identified. The first four areas were considered early diffusion research and included: (a) rural sociology, from which Rogers first developed the concept of diffusion of innovations and the research that dealt with social networks and adoption decisions; (b) medical sociology that studied physician clinical behavior and set a foundation for network analysis; (c) communication studies with research that measured the speed and direction of spread of new information; and (d) marketing research that studied the rational analysis of costs and benefits (Greenhalgh et al., 2004). Next, the review identified the research areas that emerged as developments from this early research and included the following:

- *Development studies.* Expanded the spread of innovations to include political, technological, and ideological contexts of innovation
- *Health promotion research.* Traditionally used as a social marketing of good ideas but expanded to models of partnership and community development
- *Evidence-based medicine.* Research described a linear process until recently, when new developments suggested that planning had to include local context and priorities (Greenhalgh et al., 2004).

Finally, the review found relevant research in the organization and management literature including studies that focused on the structural determinants of organizational innovativeness; organizational process, context, and culture; interorganizational studies; knowledge-based approaches to innovation in organizations; narrative organizational studies; and complexity studies focusing on adaptation (Greenhalgh et al., 2004).

Greenhalgh et al. (2004) developed a unifying conceptual model from the synthesis of their work to serve as a "memory aid for considering the different aspects of a complex situation and their many interactions" (p. 594). This quote sums up the main purpose for writing this book and proposing that a systematic approach, using a model or framework to translate research into practice, is the basis for the science of translation. The model of diffusion in service organizations includes nine components but, because it was synthesized from the literature, it does not necessarily include all the components that must be considered in a diffusion of innovation: (a) innovation characteristics; (b) adoption by individuals; (c) assimilation by the system (system planning and decision making); (d) diffusion and dissemination (use of opinion leaders, champions, and type of program); (e) system antecedents for innovation (structure and culture); (f) system readiness for innovation including tension, fit, support and advocacy, and time resources; (g) the outer context: interorganizational networks and collaborations; (h) implementation and routinization (leadership and management); and (i) the linkages among components of the model (Figure 2.4).

Agency for Healthcare Research and Quality: Knowledge Transfer

AHRQ continued its work to improve the translation of research into practice as it focused its efforts on the agency's patient safety initiative. The AHRQ Patient Safety Research Coordinating Center (PSRCC) and its steering committee developed a conceptual model to accelerate the transfer of research results from its portfolio to organizations that could benefit from the findings (Nieva et al., 2005). The AHRQ model includes three phases for knowledge transfer into practice. The first phase of the model is *knowledge creation and distillation* and includes the conducting of

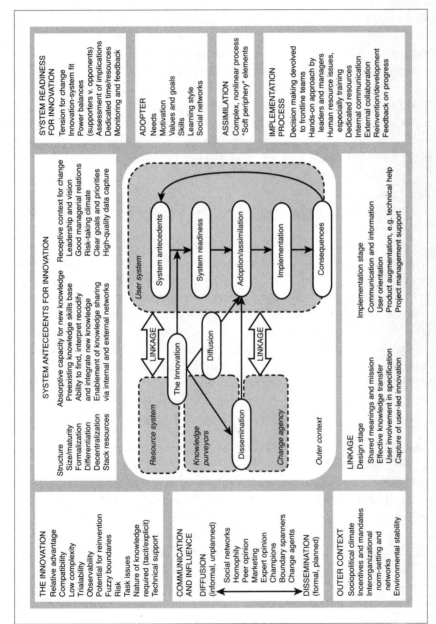

FIGURE 2.4 Conceptual model for considering the determinants of diffusion, dissemination, and innovation of implementations in Health Services Delivery and Organization, based on a systematic review of empirical research studies. Adapted from Agency for Healthcare Research and Quality. (2001). Translating research into practice (TRIP)-II. Fact Sheet. Retrieved from http://www.ahrq.gov/research/trip2fac.htm

the research, followed by a process of sifting through the research results to package them in ways that will be meaningful to potential users to increase the likelihood that the research evidence will find its way into practice. This sifting process has been labeled *knowledge distillation* (Nieva et al, 2005). The knowledge distillation process must identify a broad range of users and be informed and guided by these end users of the research findings in order for the results to be implemented in care delivery. In addition to the perspectives of the end users, the criteria used in knowledge distillation should include consideration of the transportability to the real-world health care setting, the feasibility of translation, the volume of evidence needed by health care organizations and clinicians, and strength and generalizability of the evidence (Nieva et al., 2005).

The second phase is *diffusion and dissemination*, whereby efforts aimed at marketing, selecting media, and appropriate messaging are used to "get the word out" about the new knowledge in an effort to raise awareness and to garner interest in translation and replication. This phase stresses the creation of interprofessional dissemination partnerships and knowledge transfer teams in health care organizations to disseminate knowledge that can form the basis of action, linking researchers with intermediaries that can connect to the practitioners, health care delivery organizations, and professional organizations. In addition, mass diffusion efforts and targeted dissemination efforts to reach end users using specific messages to particular audiences are used (Nieva et al., 2005). This push-pull of information for diffusion and dissemination should increase the effectiveness of the efforts.

The final phase is the *end-user adoption, implementation, and institutionalization*. To facilitate implementation, careful assessment of and attention to the complex interrelationships among the innovation itself, organizational structures and values, the external environment, and the individual clinicians is necessary (Nieva et al., 2005). The model focuses on the importance of the development of the intervention and recognition that changing practice takes time and considerable effort to sustain the change. Activities to increase adoption, successful implementation, and communication of the results of the implementation are identified to improve the likelihood that the innovation becomes a standard of care or "institutionalized" (Nieva et al., 2005; see Figure 2.5).

Knowledge to Action Model

The CIHR has been at the forefront of evidence-based practice and knowledge translation efforts and are often cited as the best source of definitions to clarify confusion about the concepts of knowledge translation, knowledge transfer, knowledge exchange, research implementation, diffusion, and dissemination. Dr. Ian Graham and colleagues at the University of Ottawa developed the Knowledge to Action (KTA) model as an integration of knowledge creation and knowledge application (Graham, Tetroe, & KT Theories and Research Group, 2007). The KTA process uses the word *action* rather than *practice*, because it is intended to be used by a wider range of users of knowledge and not just clinicians. The model visually conceptualizes the translation process or KTA as being similar to a *funnel*, where new knowledge moves through the stages until it is adopted and used. Knowledge, at the wide mouth of the funnel, includes the broad stage of inquiry and primary research. As knowledge proceeds through the funnel, it is synthesized, and finally, tools or products that are needed to present the new knowledge are developed so that those most likely to benefit can easily apply the knowledge. At each step in the knowledge creation process, the producer of the knowledge has the ability to tailor activities to meet specific research questions or end-user needs. The action cycle of the KTA process

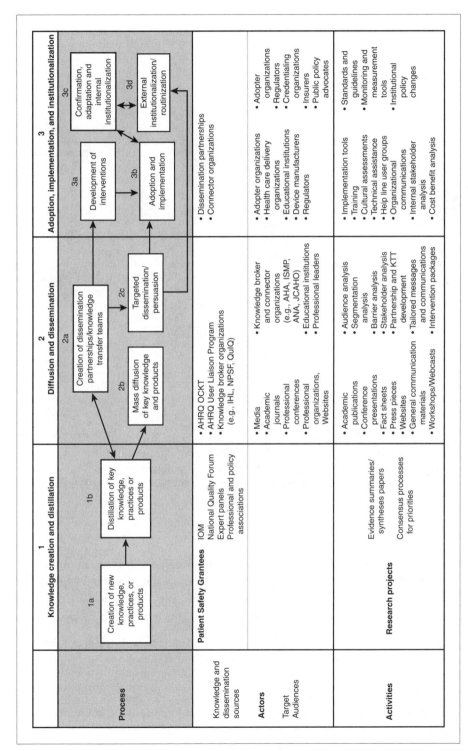

FIGURE 2.5 Knowledge transfer framework for AHRQ patient safety portfolio and patient safety grantees. Adapted from Agency for Healthcare Research and Quality. Translating research into practice (TRIP)-II. Fact Sheet. Retrieved from http://www.ahrq.gov/research/trip2fac.htm

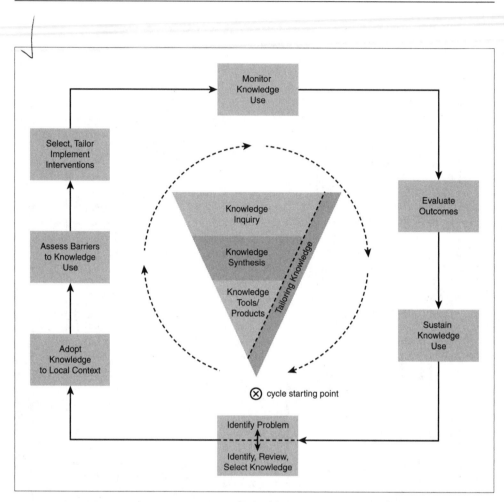

FIGURE 2.6   The knowledge to action cycle. From Graham, I. D., Tetroe, J., & the KT Theories Research Group. (2007). Some theoretical underpinnings of knowledge translation. *Academic Emergency Medicine, 14*(11), 936–941. Copyright by Hanley & Belfus, Inc. Reprinted with permission.

represents the activities that implement or apply the knowledge. Planned action theories are used to develop deliberate activities that facilitate change. Feedback exists among all phases and between both the knowledge creation and the action cycles. The KTA cycle is a synthesis of work that maps commonalities in the translation process and has seven phases (Figure 2.6):

1. Identify a problem that needs to be addressed and/or reviewed, and select the knowledge or research relevant to the problem
2. Adapt the knowledge use to the local context
3. Assess barriers to knowledge use
4. Select, tailor, and implement interventions to promote use of the knowledge
5. Monitor knowledge use
6. Evaluate outcomes of knowledge use
7. Sustain knowledge use

Ottawa Model of Research Use

The Ottawa Model of Research, developed by Logan and Graham (1998), views research as a dynamic process of decisions and actions that are interrelated and focuses implementation efforts on existing knowledge that is ready to be shared. The latest revision of the model (Graham & Logan, 2004) describes three phases and six primary elements necessary to consider when implementing research into practice. The first phase of the model is to assess the barriers and supports to the translation of the research into practice and must consider the first three elements: (a) the evidence-based innovation; (b) characteristics of potential adopters (from Everett Rogers' work); and (c) the structure and social context of the practice environment. The second phase of the model is to monitor the intervention and the degree of use, considering two more elements: implementation of interventions (considering diffusion, dissemination, and transfer strategies) and the adoption of the innovation. The final phase is the evaluation and monitoring of outcomes of the translation including patient, practitioner, and system outcomes (Figure 2.7).

Promoting Action on Research Implementation in Health Services Model

The Promoting Action on Research Implementation in Health Services (PARIHS) model was developed to represent essential determinants of successful implementation of research

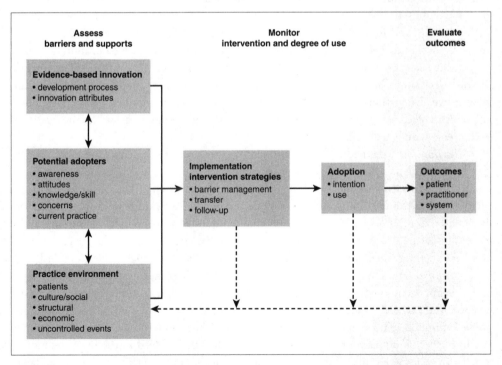

FIGURE 2.7   Ottawa model of research. From Graham, K., & Logan, J. (2004). Using the Ottawa model of research use to implement a skin care program. *Journal of Nursing Care Quality, 19*(1), 18–24. Copyright by Lippincott Williams & Wilkins. Reprinted with permission.

into clinical practice, a framework to enable implementation of evidence-based practice (Kitson, Harvey, & McCormack, 1998). Kitson and colleagues were dissatisfied with the lack of attention to rational decision making, linear processes, and failure to include the influence of context in research translation into practice (McCormack et al., 2002). The PARIHS framework posits that successful implementation is a function of three core elements: (1) the importance of clarity about the nature of the evidence being used, (2) the quality of the context, and (3) the type of facilitation needed to ensure a successful change process. Each of the three core elements has many components to consider.

Evidence is the knowledge that is derived from various sources and includes the strength and nature of the evidence as perceived by multiple stakeholders. It is the information that needs to be combined to be used in clinical decision making and includes four components, corresponding to different sources of evidence: (a) research evidence from published sources or participation in formal experiments; (b) evidence from clinical experience or professional knowledge; (c) evidence from patient preferences or based on patient experiences, including those of caregivers and family; and (d) routine information derived from local practice context, which differs from professional experience, in that it is the domain of the collective environment and not the individual (Kitson et al., 2008; Rycroft-Malone et al., 2004a, 2004b). Although research evidence is often treated as the most heavily weighted form, the PARIHS framers emphasize that all four forms have meaning and constitute evidence from the perspective of users.

The concept of *context* is defined as the environment or setting in which the proposed change or translation of research is to be implemented. This concept comes from the literature on learning organizations and comprises three components: (a) organizational culture, (b) leadership, and (c) evaluation (Kitson et al., 2008; McCormack et al., 2002). Culture refers to the values, beliefs, and attitudes shared by members of the organization, and may vary at different levels of the organization. Leadership includes the elements of teamwork, control, decision making, effectiveness of organizational structures, and issues related to empowerment. Evaluation relates to how the organization measures its performance, and how (or whether) feedback is provided to people within the organization, as well as the quality of measurement and feedback.

Facilitation is defined as "the technique by which one person makes things easier for others, help others towards achieving particular goals, encourage others and promote action (distinguish from opinion leader)," which is achieved through "support to help people change their attitudes, habits, skills, ways of thinking, and working" (Kitson et al., 1998). Facilitation is necessary to help those individuals and teams who are involved in the translation to understand what they have to change and how they are going to change it to achieve desired outcomes. Facilitation can include both internal and external facilitation. Although most prior work on the PARIHS framework focused on external facilitation, internal facilitation is important, because it is a function of the organization and is therefore a constant, whereas the external facilitation can be designed or developed according to the needs of the organization (Kitson et al., 2008; Harvey et al., 2002). Internal facilitators are local to the implementation team or organization and are directly involved in the implementation, usually in an assigned role. They can serve as a major point of interface with external facilitators (Stetler et al., 2007). Facilitation involves personal characteristics of those involved and styles of leadership, including openness, supportiveness, approachability, reliability, self-confidence, and the ability to think laterally and nonjudgmentally.

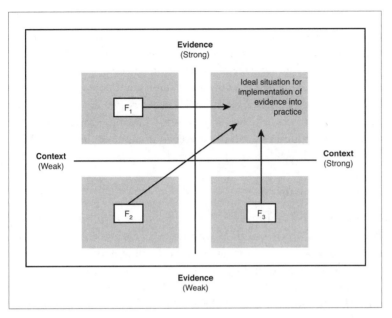

FIGURE 2.8   Promoting Action on Research Implementation in Health Services
(PARIHS) diagnostic and evaluative grid. Adapted from Kitson, A., Harvey, G.,
& McCormack, B. (1998). Enabling the implementation of evidence-based
practice: A conceptual framework. *Quality in Health Care, 7*(3), 149–158.

The PARIHS model visually depicts the relationship between evidence, context, and
facilitation in four positions called the PARIHS diagnostic and evaluative grid (Figure 2.8).

The team has continued to define and clarify the model, performing concept analysis
of each of the dimensions and studying content validity. They have hypothesized that the
PARIHS framework could be applied by practitioners not only as a diagnostic and evaluative
tool to successfully implement evidence into practice, but also used by practitioners and researchers to evaluate such activity (Kitson et al., 2008). There are challenges of measurement
to this; however, their work continues.

Pathman's Pipeline

Donald Pathman, a pediatrician, along with Konrad, Freed, Freeman, and Koch (1996),
studied vaccine compliance and designed a multistage model for moving from evidence to
practice involving clinician uptake of the evidence, incorporation into routine practice, and
patient compliance with the clinician's recommendation for the vaccine. The study concluded that the model was useful in identifying factors underlying adherence; however, they
postulated that each situation where the model is applied would have its own complexities
and need to be individualized. Pathman's work was tested and expanded upon, and a visual
depiction was created, showing a water pipeline with faucets and leaks that represent the process of moving evidence to bedside practice. There are seven faucets or stages from evidence to
action: awareness, acceptance, applicable, able, act on/adopt, agree, and adhere (Diner et al.,

2007; Glasziou & Haynes, 2005). The "leaks" or barriers to implementation of new knowledge can occur at any one of the seven steps in the process (Glasziou & Haynes, 2005). Diner et al. (2007) used the Pathman Pipeline Model at a graduate medical education consensus conference to discuss the study resident's uptake of research into practice. They focused on only four of the seven As (faucets): acceptance, application, ability, and remembering to act on the existing evidence. However, the discussion quickly went to recommendations for identifying barriers for the uptake of the evidence, how to break down the barriers, how can this be incorporated into medical education, and the strategies to monitor the sustainability of implementation efforts (Figure 2.9).

Framework for Knowledge Transfer

Lavis, Robertson, Woodside, McLeod, and Abelson (2003) provide an organizing framework for knowledge transfer in the form of five questions with four specific audiences to consider. The four audiences are the general public, such as patients, families, citizens, and clients; service providers or the clinicians; managerial decision makers, such as managers in hospitals, community settings, and businesses; and policy makers at federal, state, and local levels. The five questions that are the basis for the framework should be considered for each unique situation:

1. What should be transferred to the decision makers (the message)?
2. To whom should research knowledge be transferred (the target audience)?
3. By whom should research knowledge be transferred (the messenger)?
4. How should research knowledge be transferred (the KT process and support system)?
5. With what effect should research knowledge be transferred (evaluation)?

The research on this framework will be discussed in Chapter 8, Translation of Evidence for Health Policy.

Re-AIM Model

The RE-AIM model was originally developed (Glasgow, Vogt, & Boles, 1999) as a framework to report research results and later to organize reviews of the health promotion and disease management literature. The acronym stands for reach, effectiveness, adoption, implementation, and maintenance. The goal of the RE-AIM model is to encourage planners, evaluators, funders, and policy makers to pay close attention to essential program elements, including external validity, to improve the implementation and sustainable adoption of generalizable evidence-based interventions (RE-AIM, n.d.). There have been more than 100 publications since the development of the model, using the model as a guide to implement new knowledge into practice in many different health care conditions: aging, cancer, dietary and weight loss, medication adherence, environmental change, chronic illness self-management, well-child care, eHealth, women's health, smoking cessation, and diabetes prevention. The five steps in the RE-AIM translation model are as follows:

- **Reach** the target population (How do I reach the target population?)
- **Effectiveness** of efficacy (How do I know if my intervention is effective?)
- **Adoption** by target settings or institutions (How do I develop organizational support to deliver my intervention?)

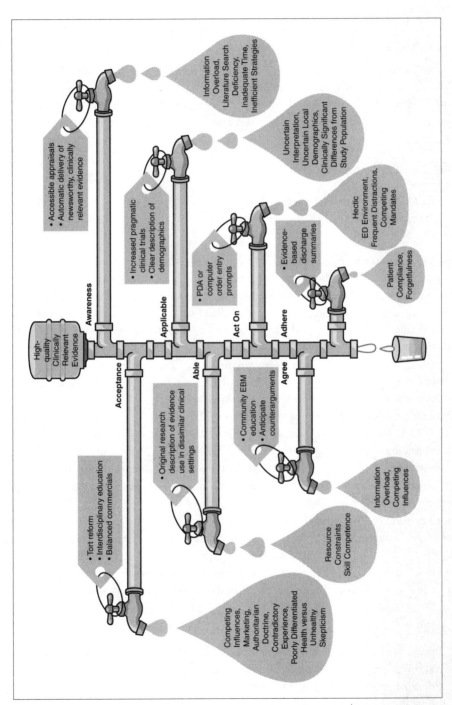

FIGURE 2.9   Pathman Pipeline Model. From Diner, B. M., Carpenter, C. R., O'Connell, T., Pang, P., Brown, M. D., Seupaul, R. A., . . . Mayer, D. (2007). Graduate medical education and knowledge translation: Role models, information pipelines, and practice change thresholds. *Academic Emergency Medicine, 14*(11), 1008–1014. Copyright by Hanley & Belfus, Inc. Reprinted with permission.

- **Implementation** consistency of the delivery of intervention (How do I ensure that the intervention is delivered properly?)
- **Maintenance** of intervention effects in individuals and setting over time (How do I incorporate the intervention so that it is delivered over the long term?)

The model stresses the importance of both the impact and importance of attention to the individual and institutional levels. Reach and efficacy are the first steps in the model and are more individual in impact; however, adoption and implementation are institutional levels of impact. Maintenance is seen as important for both levels (RE-AIM, n.d.).

■ TRANSLATING EVIDENCE INTO PRACTICE: A MODEL FOR LARGE-SCALE KNOWLEDGE TRANSLATION

Pronovost, Berenholtz, and Needham (2008) proposed a collaborative model for large-scale knowledge translation that has been shown to improve the reliability of care associated with substantial and sustained reductions in bloodstream infections associated with central lines (Pronovost et al., 2006). The integrated approach has five key components: (a) a focus on systems rather than the care of individual patients, (b) engagement of local interdisciplinary teams to assume ownership of the improvement project, (c) creation of centralized support for the technical work, (d) encouraging local adaptation of the intervention, and (e) creating a collaborative culture within the local unit of implementation and the larger system. This approach has matured into the Johns Hopkins Quality and Safety Research Group translating evidence into practice model; it has four phases and is intended for large-scale collaborative projects aimed at organizational change. The first phase is to summarize the evidence for improving a specific outcome. An assembled interdisciplinary team, specific to the problem, should review the evidence using standard criteria for evidence review and identify the interventions with the greatest benefit. The second phase of the model is to identify local barriers to implementation and assess the current processes and context of work, paying close attention to culture, teamwork, and communication. The third phase is to identify rigorous outcomes of the implementation and measure performance and engage in an iterative process of evaluation. The final phase is to ensure that all patients reliably receive the intervention. This is the most complex phase and must fit the organization. The model includes a "four Es" approach to improve this reliability of intervention that recognizes the importance of culture change, contextual factors, and engaging staff (Pronovost et al., 2008). The four Es are as follows (Figure 2.10):

1. *Engage* by sharing patient stories and providing an estimate of the harm that could result if the intervention is not implemented.
2. *Educate* by summarizing the scientific evidence supporting the intervention and providing the education to the staff.
3. *Execute* the intervention by standardizing care processes, creating independent checks (or checklists), and learning from the mistakes.

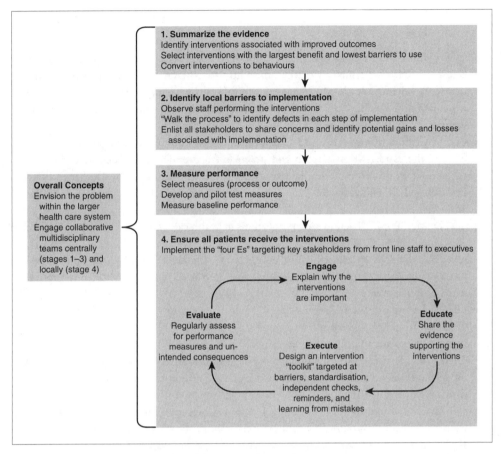

FIGURE 2.10   Strategy for translating evidence into practice. From Pronovost, P. J., Berenholtz, S. M., & Needham, D. N. (2008). Translating evidence into practice: A model for large scale knowledge translation. *BMJ, 337,* a1714. Copyright by BMJ Publishing Group Ltd. Reprinted with permission.

4.   *Evaluate* the intervention by comparing baseline data against the outcomes identified to measure successful implementation.

■   SUMMARY

This chapter has presented the key developments in translation theory and models over the last 15 years. With the subsequent development of each model, additional concepts were posited for consideration in the translation process. Agreed-upon themes are the criticality that active coordination, implementation, and dissemination of new knowledge must be guided by the evidence; the clinicians involved; the characteristics of the organization; consideration of facilitators and barriers; and the need for evaluation, monitoring, and sustainability of the implementation. The importance of planning and attention to principles of the change process for translation of research into practice were highlighted.

■ REFERENCES

Agency for Healthcare Research and Quality (2001). Translating research into practice (TRIP)-II fact sheet. Retrieved January 15, 2011, from http://www.ahrq.gov/research/trip2fac.htm

Balas, E. A., & Boren, S. A. (2000). Managing clinical knowledge for health care improvement. In J. van Bemmel & A. T. McCray (Eds.), *Yearbook of medical informatics* (pp. 65–70). Stuttgart, Germany: Schattauer Publishing.

Bero, L. A., Grilli, R., Grimshaw, J. M., Harvey, E., Oxman, A. D., & Thomson, M. A. (1998). Closing the gap between research and practice: An overview of systematic reviews of interventions to promote the implementation of research findings. The Cochrane Effective Practice and Organization of Care Review Group. *British Medical Journal, 317*(7156), 465–468.

Berwick, D. M. (2003). Disseminating innovations in health care. *Journal of the American Medical Association, 289*(15), 1969–1975.

Canadian Health Services Research Foundation. (2011). *Glossary of knowledge exchange terms used by Canadian Health Services Research Foundation.* Retrieved June 20, 2011, from http://www.chsrf.ca/home_e.php

Canadian Institutes of Health Research. (2010). *About knowledge translation.* Retrieved January 15, 2011, from http://www.cihr-irsc.gc.ca/e/29418.html

Diner, B. M., Carpenter, C. R., O'Connell, T., Pang, P., Brown, M. D., Seupaul, R., . . . KT-CC Theme Illa Members. (2007). Graduate medical education and knowledge translation: Role models, information pipelines, and practice change thresholds. *Academic Emergency Medicine, 14*(11), 1008–1014.

Estabrooks, C. A., Thompson, D. S., Lovely, J. J., & Hofmeyer, A. (2006). A guide to knowledge translation theory. *Journal of Continuing Education in the Health Professions, 26*(1): 25–36. Retrieved from http://www.jcehp.com/vol26/2601_estabrooks.asp

Farquhar, C. M., Stryer, D., & Slutsky, J. (2002). Translating research into practice: The future ahead. *International Journal for Quality in Health Care, 14*(3), 233–249.

Glasgow, R. E., & Emmons, K. M. (2007). How can we increase translation of research into practice? Types of evidence needed. *Annual Review of Public Health, 28*, 413–433.

Glasgow, R. E., Vogt, T. M., & Boles, S. M. (1999). Evaluating the public health impact of health promotion interventions: The RE-AIM framework. *American Journal of Public Health, 89*(9), 1322–1327.

Glasziou, P., & Haynes, B. (2005). The paths from research to improved health outcomes. *ACP Journal Club, 142*(2), A8–A10.

Graham, I. D., Logan, J., Harrison, M. B., Straus, S. E., Tetroe, J., Caswell, W., & Robinson, N. (2006). Lost in knowledge translation: Time for a map? *Journal of Continuing Education in the Health Professions, 26*(1), 13–24.

Graham, I. D., Tetroe, J., & KT Theories Research Group (2007). Some theoretical underpinnings of knowledge translation. *Academic Emergency Medicine, 14*(11), 936–941.

Graham, K., & Logan, J. (2004).Using the Ottawa model of research use to implement a skin care program. *Journal of Nursing Care Quality, 19*(1), 18–24.

Green, L. A., & Siefert, C. M. (2005). Translation of research into practice: Why we can't "just do it". *Journal of the American Board of Family Practice, 18*(6):541–545.

Greenhalgh, T., Robert, G., MacFarlane, F., Bate, P., & Kyriakidou, O. (2004). Diffusion of innovations in service organizations: Systematic review and recommendations. *The Milbank*

Quarterly, 82(4), 581–629. Retrieved from http://www3.interscience.wiley.com/cgi-bin/fulltext/118784115/PDFSTART

Grol, R., & Grimshaw, J. (1999). Evidence-based implementation of evidence-based medicine. *Joint Commission Journal on Quality Improvement, 25*(10), 503–513.

Grol, R., & Grimshaw, J. (2003). From best evidence to best practice: Effective implementation of change in patients' care. *Lancet, 362*(9391), 1225–1230.

Haines, A., & Jones, R. (1994). Implementing findings of research. *British Medical Journal, 308*(6942), 1488–1492.

Harvey, G., Loftus-Hills, A., Rycroft-Malone, J., Titchen, A., Kitson, A., McCormack, B., & Seers, K. (2002). Getting evidence into practice: The role and function of facilitation. *Journal of Advanced Nursing, 37*(6), 577–588.

Institute of Medicine. (2001). *Crossing the quality chasm: A new health system for the 21st century.* Washington, DC: National Academy Press.

Kirchhoff, K. T. (2004). State of the science of translational research: From demonstration projects to intervention testing. *Worldviews on Evidence-Based Nursing. 1*(Suppl 1): S6–S12.

Kitson, A., Harvey, G., & McCormack, B. (1998). Enabling the implementation of evidence based practice: A conceptual framework. *Quality in Health Care, 7*(3), 149–158.

Kitson, A. L., Rycroft-Malone, J., Harvey, G., McCormack, B., Seers, K., & Titchen, A. (2008). Evaluating the successful implementation of evidence into practice using the PARiHS framework: Theoretical and practical challenges. *Implementation Science, 3*, 1. Retrieved from http://www.implementationscience.com/content/pdf/1748-5908-3-1.pdf

Lavis, J. N., Robertson, D., Woodside, J. M., McLeod, C. B., & Abelson, J. (2003). How can research organization more effectively transfer research knowledge to decision makers? *The Milbank Quarterly, 81*(2), 221–248.

Logan, J., & Graham, I. D. (1998). Toward a comprehensive interdisciplinary model of health care research use. *Science Communication, 20*(2), 227–246.

Lomas, J. (1993). Retailing research: Increasing the role of evidence in clinical services for childbirth. *The Milbank Quarterly, 71*(3), 439–475.

Lomas, J., Sisk, J. E., & Stocking, B. (1993). From evidence to practice in the United States, the United Kingdom, and Canada. *The Milbank Quarterly, 71*(3), 405–410.

McCormack, B., Kitson, A., Harvey, G., Rycroft-Malone, J., Titchen, A., & Seers, K. (2002). Getting evidence into practice: The meaning of 'context'. *Journal of Advanced Nursing, 38*(1), 94–104.

National Institutes of Health (2005). *Fact sheet: NIH Clinical and Translational Science Awards (CTSA).* Retrieved from http://www.nih.gov/news/pr/oct2005/FactSheetCTSAclearance.pdf

Nieva, V., Murphy, R., Ridley, N., Donaldson, N., Combes, J., Mitchell, P., . . . Carpenter, D. (2005). From science to service: A framework for the transfer of patient safety research into practice. In K. Henriksen, J. B. Battles, & E. S. Marks (Eds.), *Advanced in patient safety: From research to implementation* (Vol. 2, pp. 441–453). Rockville, MD: Agency for Healthcare Research and Quality.

Oxman, A. D., Thomson, M. A., Davis, D. A., & Haynes, R. B. (1995). No magic bullets: A systematic review of 102 trials of interventions to improve professional practice. *Canadian Medical Association Journal, 153*(10), 1423–1431.

Pathman, D. E., Konrad, T. R., Freed, G. L., Freeman, V. A., & Koch, G. G. (1996). The awareness-to-adherence model of the steps to clinical guideline compliance: The case of pediatric vaccine recommendations. *Medical Care, 34*(9), 873–889.

Pronovost, P., Needham, D., Berenholtz, S., Sinopoli, D., Chu, H., Cosgrove, S., . . . Goeschel, C., (2006). An intervention to decrease catheter-related bloodstream infections in the ICU. *New England Journal of Medicine, 355*(26), 2725–2732.

Pronovost, P. J., Berenholtz, S. M., & Needham, D. M. (2008). Translating evidence into practice: A model for large scale knowledge translation. *British Medical Journal, 337*, a1714.

RE-AIM. (n.d.). What is RE-AIM? Retrieved January 15, 2011, from http://www.re-aim.org/about-re-aim/what-is-re-aim.aspx

Rogers, E. M. (2003). *Diffusion of innovations* (5th ed.). New York, NY: Free Press.

Rycroft-Malone, J., Harvey, G., Seers, K., Kitson, A., McCormack, B., & Titchen, A. (2004a). An exploration of the factors that influence the implementation of evidence into practice. *Journal of Clinical Nursing, 13*(8), 913–924.

Rycroft-Malone, J., Kitson, A., Harvey, G., McCormack, B., Seers, K., Titchen, A., & Estabrooks, C. (2002). Ingredients for change: Revisiting a conceptual framework. *Quality and Safety in Health Care, 11*(2), 174–180.

Rycroft-Malone, J., Seers, K., Titchen, A., Harvey, G., Kitson, A., & McCormack, B. (2004b). What counts as evidence in evidence-based practice. *Journal of Advanced Nursing, 47*(1), 81–90.

Schuster, M. A., McGlynn, E. A., & Brook, R. H. (1998). How good is the quality of health care in the United States? *The Milbank Quarterly, 76*(4), 517–563.

Stetler, C. B., Corrigan, B., Sander-Buscemi, K., & Burns, M. (1999). Integration of evidence into practice and the change process: Fall prevention program as a model. *Outcomes Management for Nursing Practice, 3*(3), 102–111.

Stetler, C. B., Ritchie, J., Rycroft-Malone, J., Schultz, A., & Charns, M. (2007). Improving quality of care through routine, successful implementation of evidence-based practice at the bedside: An organizational case study protocol using the Pettigrew and Whipp model of strategic change. *Implementation Science, 2*, 3. Retrieved from http://www.implementationscience.com/content/pdf/1748-5908-2-3.pdf

Titler, M. G. (2008) The evidence for evidence-based practice implementation. In R. G. Hughes (Ed.), *Patient safety and quality: An evidence-based handbook for nursing* (pp. i113–i161). Rockville, MD: Agency for Healthcare Research and Quality.

Westfall, J. M., Mold, J., & Fagnan, L. (2007). Practice-based research—"Blue highways" on the NIH Roadmap. *Journal of the American Medical Association, 297*(4), 403–406.

Zerhouni, E. A. (2005). Translational and clinical science—time for a new vision. *New England Journal of Medicine, 353*(15), 1621–1623.

C H A P T E R   THREE

Change Theory and Models: Framework for Translation

Kathleen M. White

Innovation is 1 percent inspiration and 99 percent perspiration.
> —Thomas A. Edison

Translation models, discussed in Chapter 2, are also models of change but have been designed to guide thinking and planning specifically about the translation of new knowledge into practice. It is also useful in the discussion of translation of research practice to consider change theory and models. The challenges to translation of research into practice are similar to the commonly described challenges to implementation of change in the literature, such as gaining internal support for the change, ensuring effective leadership, integrating with existing programs, organizational culture, maintaining momentum while changing, documenting and positively publicizing the outcomes of the change (Bradley, Schlesinger, Webster, Baker, & Inouye, 2004).

Change—the transformation of tasks, processes, methods, structures, and/or relationships—is necessary for organizational survival. Changes, such as the diffusion of evidence-based practice into an organization or, more specifically, the translation of new knowledge into practice, must be planned for, managed, and considered based on how the change affects the people of the organization. When planning for change, situations vary widely according to the impetus for the change, the type of change needed, the personnel and clients involved, and many characteristics of the organization, agency, or practice where the change is necessary. The planning and management of change determines whether the change will be a success or a failure (Crow, 2006).

McConnell (2010) identified two major categories of resistance to change that must be planned for and managed as the change process is implemented. The principal cause of most resistances to change is the disturbance to the status quo or as he describes, "equilibrium," especially if the disturbance or direction for change leads into unfamiliar territory. Secondary causes of resistance are intellectual shortcomings, or the inability to conceive of certain possibilities or to think beyond the boundaries of what is presently known or believed. Both of these causes of resistance to change are rooted in the evidence-based practice movement. Assessment of these causes of resistance and the development of strategies that anticipate and manage the resistance will enhance the adoption of or translation of new knowledge into practice.

Change has traditionally been viewed as a continual and sequential process, affected by a complex set of interacting factors. Rational change theory, with roots in economics, assumes those involved in the change will have full information, act reasonably and sensibly, use sound judgment, and good sense, and that the change process is predictable, linear, and static. Behavioral change theory considers that organizations and their people are goal-oriented, focused on purpose, and problem-driven and that they have activities, patterns, and routines that they follow as long as they work. When those patterns and activities prove insufficient, they seek to change.

Change theory has developed over the last 50 years but much can still be learned by considering the assumptions of the classic change theories originally developed by Lewin, Lippitt, and Havelock. This chapter will discuss change theories and how they can be used to translate new knowledge into practice.

■ ORGANIZATIONAL THEORIES OF CHANGE

Lewin's Force Field Analysis

Kurt Lewin's (1951) classic theory of change is a three-phase change model that views change as a dynamic balance of forces (driving and restraining) working in opposite directions within an organization or *field* (Figure 3.1). The driving forces promote or move individuals toward the change direction, and the restraining forces inhibit or move individuals away from the change. Lewin's theory of change was developed after World War II when he carried out research exploring how individuals change their dietary habits. He discovered that if the individual is involved in the discussion about the change and issues surrounding the change,

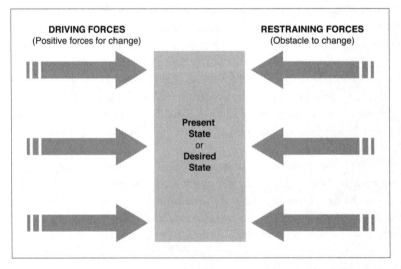

FIGURE 3.1 Lewin's force field analysis. From Lewin, K. (1947). Frontiers in group dynamics: Concept, method, and reality in social science; social equilibria and social change. *Human Relations, 1*(1), 5–41. Copyright by Sage Publications Ltd. Republished with permission.

they are able to make their own decisions to change their behavior (Lewin, 1947). The first phase of the change process is to *unfreeze* the current situation by increasing the driving forces or decreasing the restraining forces toward change. *Moving or changing* is the second phase where the organization is moved toward a new equilibrium of driving and restraining forces. The final phase is *refreezing* that must occur after the change is implemented to sustain the change within the organization. Assessment of the forces, both driving and restraining, throughout the change process is necessary to recognize the power of the forces and to involve the individuals in the organization, build trust, encourage a new view, and to integrate new ideas into the organization.

Lippitt's Model of Change

Lippitt, Watson, and Westley (1958) built on the work of Lewin and developed a seven-step model of change that concentrated on the role of the leader in the change process and added the change agent role (Figure 3.2). The seven steps are:

1. Develop need for change by diagnosing the change.
2. Establish change relationship and assess the motivation and capacity to change.
3. Clarify assessment for change and determine resources.
4. Establish goals and intentions for an action plan.
5. Examine alternatives.

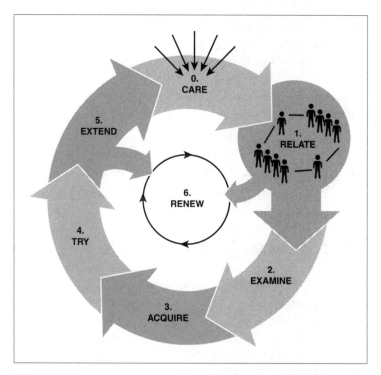

FIGURE 3.2   Lippitt's stages of planned change. From Lippit, R., Watson, J., & Westley, B. (1958). *The Dynamics of Planned Change*. New York, NY: Harcourt, Brace & World, Inc.

6. Transform intentions into actual change and maintain the change.
7. Generalize and stabilize change and end the helping relationship of the change agent.

Havelock's Theory of Planned Change

Havelock (1976) further modified Lewin's theory of change and created a process for change agents to organize their work and to implement innovation in the work environment. They postulated that change is made up of cycles of action that are repeated as change advances and that the change agent must pay attention to the steps. They described six steps, but the visual of the model includes a stage 0 called *Care*, where a concern for needed change first occurs:

Care—attention to the need for change
Relate—build a relationship
Examine—diagnose the problem
Acquire—acquire the relevant sources
Try—choose the solution
Extend—disseminate, diffuse, and gain acceptance
Renew—stabilize and sustain capacity

Havelock, with colleague Zlotolow (1995), created a visual of the model for change agents to use and to guide the change process.

Framework for Guiding the Process of Implementation

Howes and Quinn (1978) summarized the organizational change literature on factors related to the successful implementation of change with a "how to" list for managers to implement change. They described two phases and 12 levers or guidelines for change, six levers in each phase.

The first phase is to *set up an adequate orientation environment* to prepare and positively influence the change by the following:

- Set aside enough time for adequate introduction to the change.
- Make the relative advantage of the change easily visible.
- Show organization members (users) that their efforts will be supported.
- Show users that it will be easy to institutionalize the change and that it will be relatively nonthreatening afterward.
- Show that immediate superiors accept and support the change.

Clearly identify the roles and responsibilities of all who will be involved in the change process. The perceived characteristics of the change, such as the relative advantage of and compatibility of the change with the present way of doing things, and its simplicity, ease of understanding, and trial ability are critically important to the user in this first phase of a change.

The second phase, to *set up adequate support networks for the implementation effort*, includes the six levers that assist the change to happen and focus on the climate within the organization to facilitate the change:

- Produce and make supportive services available.
- Set up formal training programs to develop members' roles.

- Encourage and reward the use of horizontal and vertical communication channels.
- Relax standard operating procedures in affected (changing) units.
- Integrate change agents, managers and users.
- Make sure users feel adequately involved.

Pettigrew and Whipp's Model of Strategic Management of Change

Pettigrew and Whipp (1991) developed a strategic model of change that involves the interaction of three essential dimensions of strategic change: context, content, and process. They also described the importance of historical, cultural, and political factors in the interaction of the essential elements. The *context* includes both external and internal factors and events that are driving the change, the *why* of change, including the organization's culture, leadership, type of clinical setting, and the characteristics of the organization. The *content* dimension describes the activities to be transformed or the *what* of change. In translation of research into practice efforts, these are the key organizational elements in the system focused on to enhance or to support the use of evidence. The third dimension, the *process* or *how* of change, includes the methods, strategies, and actions and interactions that will be used to make the change happen and enable the use of the new evidence (Stetler, Ritchie, Rycroft-Malone, Schultz, & Charns, 2007). The model stresses the continuous, iterative, dynamic, and uncertain nature of the change management process.

Ferlie and Shortell: Framework for Change

Ferlie and Shortell's (2001) work is similar and proposes a model for implementing change for quality improvement in health care. The model focuses on the importance of context in change and describes four levels of change: (a) the individual health care practitioner, (b) the health care team, (c) the overall organization, and (d) the cultural environment of the organization.

Contemporary Change Theory

John Kotter's (1996) view of contemporary change sets up eight steps toward leading change in organizations: (a) establish a sense of urgency, (b) create the guiding coalition, (c) develop a vision and strategy, (d) communicate the change vision, (e) introduce the change and empower a broad base of people to take action, (f) generate short-term wins, (g) consolidate gains and the production of even more change, and (h) institutionalize new approaches in the corporate culture to ground the changes in the culture and make them stick.

Kotter (1995) also describes why change efforts fail:

- Allowing too much complacency
- Failing to create a sufficiently powerful guiding coalition
- Underestimating the power of vision
- Undercommunicating the vision
- Permitting obstacles to block the vision
- Failing to create short-term wins
- Declaring victory too soon
- Neglecting to anchor changes firmly in the corporate culture

This contemporary view on leading change for translation of new knowledge to practice efforts stresses the importance of the people involved in the change; their reactions to all aspects of the change, linking to context, content, and processes/facilitation; and the bigger picture or fit of the change for the organization (Kotter, 1999).

Behavioral Theories of Change

Social Cognitive Theory

Social cognitive theory posits that individuals learn by direct experiences, human dialogue and interaction, and observation. It began as social learning theory developed by Albert Bandura and was renamed social cognitive theory. Bandura (1986) described that the purpose of the theory is to understand and predict individual and group behavior, identify methods in which behavior can be modified or changed, and to test interventions aimed at personality development, behavior pathology, and health promotion. This theory of change proposes that behavior change is affected by personal factors, attributes of the behavior itself, and environmental influences (Robbins, 2003). The individual must believe in their capability to change and possess the self-efficacy to change. Additionally, they must perceive that there is an incentive to change, which in social learning theory is referred as operant conditioning, with the positive expectations outweighing the negative consequences. Social cognitive theory is particularly useful when dealing with educational programs aimed at changing behavior, such as implementing new knowledge into practice.

Stages of Change Theory

Prochaska and DiClementi's model of change behavior (1986) was originally developed for use with individual patients to change health behaviors, specifically to study smokers in therapy to self-changers. The model had four stages and was considered linear in its original development. However, the model now has five stages (Figure 3.3) with an added stage for preparation for action and is now viewed as a cyclical process. The model's use has also

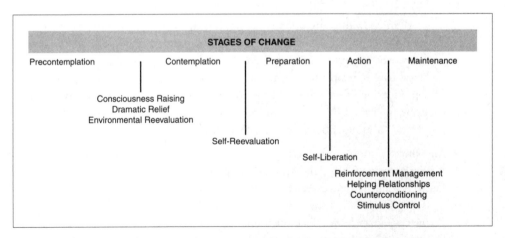

FIGURE 3.3   Stages of change theory. From Prochaska, J., DiClementi, C., & Norcross, J. (1992). In search of how people change: Applications to addictive behaviors. *American Psychologist, 47*(9), 1102–1114.

extended beyond the individual patient to other audiences over time. The model describes five stages that people pass through when change occurs:

1. Precontemplation—is when an individual is unaware of or does not acknowledge that a problem exists and that there is a need for change.
2. Contemplation—is the stage when the individual becomes aware of the issue/ problem and begins to think about changing behavior.
3. Preparation for action—is when the individual is ready to change and prepares to make a change. This preparation for action is defined within a 2-week decision to change period.
4. Action—is when the individual engages in change activities and increases coping behaviors to deal with the change.
5. Maintenance—is the final stage and may take up to 6 months. The change behaviors must be reinforced to sustain the change.

Prochaska, DiClementi, and Norcross (1992) described 10 processes that predict and motivate movement through the stages: (a) consciousness raising, (b) dramatic relief, (c) environmental reevaluation, (d) self reevaluation, (e) self-liberation, (f) social liberation, (g) reinforcement management, (h) helping relationships, (i) counter-conditioning, and (j) stimulus control. This model has been used successfully with HIV/AIDS and sexually transmitted diseases (STD) counseling (CDC, 1993). However, the influence of structure and environment are two key elements that are not specifically addressed in the model and are necessary components of planning for change or translation of new knowledge into the practice setting.

Theory of Reasoned Action

This theory was developed in the late 1960s and has been used to describe an individual's intention to perform certain behaviors. The theory assumes that individuals are rational and links the individual's behavior to beliefs, attitudes, and intentions (Ajzen & Fishbein, 1980). Fishbein, Middlestadt, and Hitchcock (1994) further defined the variables:

- *Behavior*—a specific behavior that should occur so that the individual understands the needed action, for whom, when, and where
- *Intention*—the best predictor that a behavior will occur and is influenced by attitude and norms (Family Health International, 2002)
- *Attitude*—the individual's positive or negative feelings toward performing the behavior
- *Norms*—the individual's perception of other's opinion of the behavior

These variables are interrelated and describe the individual's reasoned action or intention to change. The individual must have a positive attitude toward change, must feel that they have control over the change, and that changing is perceived as positive by their social group. The model describes a linear change process that posits that a change in behavior is dependent on behavioral and normative beliefs. This change model has been used successfully in behavior change for individuals and groups related to smoking cessation, condom use for prevention of STDs and HIV/AIDS nationally and internationally, dieting, exercise, seat belt and safety helmet use, and breastfeeding (Fishbein et al., 1994).

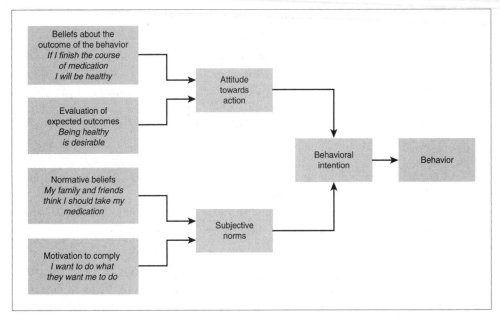

FIGURE 3.4   Theory of reasoned action. From Munro et al. (2007). A review of health behaviour theories: how useful are these for developing interventions to promote long-term medication adherence for TB and HIV/AIDS? *BMC Public Health 7*,104. doi: 10.1186/1471-2458-7-104. Copyright by Biomed Central, Ltd. Republished with permission.

Social Ecological Theory

The social ecological theory offers a model to guide translation efforts that integrates multiple perspectives into the planning of interventions for behavior change, addressing the interdependencies between socioeconomic, cultural, political, environmental, organizational, psychological, and biological determinants of health (Whittemore, Melkus, & Grey, 2004). The model proposes that any individual behavior is supported and influenced by numerous systems and groups, and that any lasting behavior change requires implementation of strategies at multiple levels of influence (Emmons, 2000). Whittemore, Melkus, and Grey (2004) described five levels of influence and the implementation strategies at each to expand diabetes prevention and management evidence:

- Intrapersonal level—includes individual beliefs, values, education level, skills, and other individual factors that affect the individual's ability to change
- Interpersonal level—the relationships between individuals, families, groups, and communities that are part of social support to promote behavioral change
- Institutional level—the influence that relevant institutions have on change activities
- Community level—the influence that communities have on the individual, the community attitudes, and the relationship among different institutions within communities
- Public policy level and the influence of policies and regulations that affect the change intervention, the participants, and the institutions in which they function

The Learning Organization

Peter Senge (2006), the leading expert on learning organizations, explained that the fundamental learning units of an organization are working teams or people who need one another to produce an outcome. He described five disciplines to becoming a learning organization. First is to develop *systems thinking* or the ability to see the big picture, to distinguish patterns instead of conceptualizing change as isolated events, and to feel interconnected to the whole (Senge, 2006). *Personal mastery* is to focus on becoming the best person possible, embrace lifelong learning, and to strive for a sense of commitment in our careers (Senge, 2006). The third discipline is to use *mental models.* Senge suggests that the process of using mental models begins with self-reflection, unearthing deeply held beliefs to understand how they influence the way we operate. He also believes that until there is a focus on openness, real change can never be implemented (Senge, 2006). Fourth, *building shared visions* is needed to bind an organization together and fosters long-term commitment (Senge, 2006). Finally, *team learning,* critically important to today's organization, is the process of bringing team members together, to develop in the team a desire to create results, to have a goal in mind, and to work together to attain it (Senge, 2006). The interaction of these five disciplines is to challenge the organization to look into their own resources and potentials, to build a collective will to learn, and to embrace change. The principles of a learning organization have great applicability to dissemination and translation of new knowledge to practice, with a focus on the team, what is necessary to implement a change, and the team's involvement in moving toward a desired new state.

Research on Change Interventions

Pascale, Millemann, and Gioja (1997) identified three concrete interventions that will "change the way people change": (a) incorporating employees into the process of dealing with work challenges, (b) leading from a different place to sharpen and maintain employee involvement, and (c) instilling mental discipline to make people behave differently and then to sustain that behavior. If done properly, their proposal will create an agile organization and will shift the organization's operations or culture by altering the way people experience their own power and identity and the way they deal with conflict and learning.

Thomas et al. (1999) performed a systematic review of the evidence to evaluate strategies for successful change, specifically, the introduction of guidelines into practice. Although the evidence was insufficient, the literature suggested that essential strategies for successful change in health care practices included: organizational commitment, active support from key stakeholders, recognition of the importance of change, a credible change agent, face-to-face contact with practitioners to promote enthusiasm, and ensuring targeted staff have ownership of the innovation and are empowered to change.

Gustafson et al. (2003) developed and tested a Bayesian model that used subjective probability estimates to predict outcomes of organization changes, specifically health care improvement projects. The model was developed with 18 factors that were identified by an expert panel that predict implementation success. The 18 factors included: (a) exploration of problem and customer needs; (b) change agent prestige, commitment, and customer focus; (c) source of ideas; (d) funding; (e) advantages to staff and customers; (f) radicalness of design; (g) flexibility of design; (h) mandate; (i) leader goals, involvement, and support; (j) supporters and opponents; (k) middle managers goals, involvement, and support; (l) tension for change;

(m) staff needs assessment, involvement, and support; (n) evidence of effectiveness; (o) complexity of implementation plan; (p) work environment; (q) monitoring and feedback; and (r) staff changes required. The model performed well on three definitions of success; however, there was no objective measure of success, only the opinions of people were involved. Identifying factors that predict success can lead to planning that increases attention to facilitators and removes barriers to the implementation of the desired change, which is similar to Lewin's classic description of the equilibrium of the force field in an organization.

Finally, Berwick (2003) studied innovations in health care specifically and summarized the literature, which he found to be mostly descriptive in two ways. The first was a focus on three areas of influence that correlate with the rate of spread of change: (a) perception of the innovation (i.e., the benefit of the change, which is compatible with values, beliefs, past history and current needs), and the complexity of innovation; (b) characteristics of the people who adopt the innovation or fail to do so; and (c) contextual factors, especially communication, incentives, leadership, and management. Second, he added that the research, although descriptive, offers seven guesses about what might help leaders to nurture good changes:

- Find sound innovations
- Find and support innovators
- Invest in early adopters
- Make early adopter activity observable
- Trust and enable reinvention
- Create slack for change
- Lead by example

A Final Issue to Consider in Translation of New Knowledge

A final issue that needs to be considered when designing the change to translate new knowledge into practice is fidelity of implementation. Fidelity refers to the degree in which program providers implement programs as intended by developers/researchers (Rohrbach, Dent, Skara, Sun, & Sussman, 2007). To make programs more acceptable for translation or for the change to be accepted, the implementers/change agents may try to adapt the new knowledge/research to achieve local buy-in. The users can also choose to modify the implementation to fit the needs or improve the fit of an intervention with local conditions. However, this makes fidelity difficult to achieve, and the research has shown that the fidelity with which an intervention is implemented affects how well it succeeds (Dusenbury, Brannigan, Falco, & Hansen, 2003; Elliott & Mihalic, 2004; Rohrbach et al., 2007).

■ SUMMARY

Translation of research into practice must be guided by the models and the frameworks that include the process of change and the identification of critical elements or variables in the organization that affect and determine whether the new knowledge fits the organization and will be feasible to implement. In addition to fit and feasibility, consideration must be given to the varied personnel, structures, environments, leadership styles, and the cultures of organizations, and their economic, ethical, and legal environments. Graham and Tetro (2007) caution against the "KT imperative," translating all new knowledge into practice at any cost, but suggested that each translation be judiciously evaluated for possible implementation, systematically planned, evaluated for success, and learning for future translation.

■ REFERENCES

Ajzen, I., & Fishbein, M. (1980). *Understanding attitudes and predicting social behavior.* Upper Saddle River, NJ: Prentice-Hall.

Bandura, A. (1986). *Social foundations of thought and action: A social cognitive theory.* Upper Saddle River, NJ: Prentice Hall.

Berwick, D. M. (2003). Disseminating innovations in health care. *The Journal of the American Medical Association, 289*(15), 1969–1975.

Bradley, E. H., Schlesinger, M., Webster, T. R., Baker, D., & Inouye, S. K. (2004). Translating research into clinical practice: Making change happen. *Journal of the American Geriatrics Society, 52*(11), 1875–1882.

Centers for Disease Control and Prevention. (1993). Distribution of STD clinic patients along a stages-of-behavioral-change continuum—selected sites, 1993. *Morbidity and Mortality Weekly Report, 42*(45), 880–883.

Crow, G. (2006). Diffusion of innovation: The leaders' role in creating the organizational context for evidence-based practice. *Nursing Administration Quarterly, 30*(3), 236–242.

Dusenbury, L., Brannigan, R., Falco, M., & Hansen, W. B. (2003). A review of research on fidelity of implementation: Implications for drug abuse prevention in school settings. *Health Education Research, 18*(2), 237–256.

Elliott, D. S., & Mihalic, S. (2004). Issues in disseminating and replicating effective prevention programs. *Prevention Science, 5*(1), 47–53.

Emmons, K. (2000). Health behaviors in a social context. In L. F. Berkman & I. Kawachi (Eds.), *Social epidemiology.* Oxford, England: Oxford University Press.

Family Health International. (2002). Behavior change: A summary of four major theories. Retrieved from http://www.fhi.org/en/index.htm

Fishbein, M., Middlestadt, S., & Hitchcock, P. (1994). Using information to change sexually transmitted disease-related behaviors. In R. DiClementi & J. Peterson (Eds.), *Preventing AIDS: Theories and methods of behavioral interventions.* New York, NY: Plenum Press.

Ferlie, E. B., & Shortell, S. M. (2001). Improving the quality of health care in the United Kingdom and the United States: A framework for change. *Milbank Quarterly, 79*(2), 281–315.

Graham, I. D., & Tetroe, J. (2007). Some theoretical underpinnings of knowledge translation. *Academic Emergency Medicine, 14*(11), 936–941.

Gustafson, D. H., Sainfort, F., Eichler, M., Adams, L., Bisognano, M., & Steudel, H. (2003). Developing and testing a model to predict outcomes of organizational change. *Health Services Research, 38*(2), 751–776.

Havelock, R. G. (1976). *Planning for innovation through dissemination and utilization of knowledge.* Ann Arbor, MI: University of Michigan, Center for Research on Utilization of Scientific Knowledge, Institute for Social Research.

Havelock, R. G., & Zlotolow, S. (1995). *The change agent's guide* (2nd ed.). Englewood Cliffs, NJ: Education Technology.

Howes, N. J., & Quinn, R. E. (1978). Implementing change: From research to a prescriptive framework. *Group & Organization Studies, 3*(1), 71–84.

Kotter, J. (1995). Leading change: Why transformation efforts fail. *Harvard Business Review*, *73*(2), 59–67.

Kotter, J. (1996). *Leading change.* Boston, MA: Harvard Business School Press.

Kotter, J. (1999). *What leaders really do.* Boston, MA: Harvard Business School Press.

Kritsonis, A. (2004). Comparison of change theories. *International Journal of Scholarly Academic Intellectual Diversity, 8*(1), 1–7.

Lewin, K. (1947). Frontiers in group dynamics. *Human Relations, 1*(1), 5–41.

Lewin, K. (1951). Field theory in social science. In D. Cartwright (Ed.), *Selected theoretical papers.* New York, NY: Harper & Row.

Lippitt, R., Watson, J., & Westley, B. (1958). *The dynamics of planned change.* New York, NY: Harcourt, Brace, and World.

McConnell, C. R. (2010). Change can work for you or against you: It's your choice. *The Health Care Manager, 29*(4), 365–374.

Pascale, R., Millemann, M., and Gioja, L. (1997). "Changing the Way We Change." *Harvard Business Review* 6:127–139.

Pettigrew, A., & Whipp, R. (1991). *Managing change for competitive success.* Oxford, England: Blackwell.

Prochaska, J. O., & DiClementi, C. C. (1986). Towards a comprehensive model of change. In W. R. Miller & N. Heather (Eds.), *Treating addictive behaviors.* New York, NY: Plenum Press.

Prochaska, J. O., DiClementi, C. C., & Norcross, J. C. (1992). In search of how people change— applications to addictive behaviors. *American Psychologist, 47*(9), 1102–1114.

Robbins, S. (2003). *Organizational behavior* (10th ed.). Upper Saddle River, NJ: Prentice Hall.

Rohrbach, L. A., Dent, C. W., Skara, S., Sun, P., & Sussman, S. (2007). Fidelity of implementation in project Towards No Drug abuse (TND): A comparison of classroom teachers and program specialists. *Prevention Science, 8*(2), 125–132.

Senge, P. M. (2006). *The fifth discipline: The art and practice of the learning organization.* New York, NY: Doubleday.

Stetler, C. B., Ritchie, J., Rycroft-Malone, J., Schultz, A., & Charns, M. (2007). Improving quality of care through routine, successful implementation of evidence-based practice at the bedside: An organizational case study protocol using the Pettigrew and Whipp model of strategic change. *Implementation Science, 2,* 3.

Thomas, L., Cullum, N., McColl, E., Rousseau, N., Soutter, J., & Steen, N. (1999). Guidelines in professions allied to medicine. (Cochrane Review) In: The Cochrane Library, Issue 3, Oxford: Update software.

Whittemore, R., Melkus, G. D., & Grey, M. (2004). Applying the social ecological theory to type 2 diabetes prevention and management. *Journal of Community Health Nursing, 21*(2), 87–99.

C H A P T E R   FOUR

Translation of Evidence to Improve Clinical Outcomes

Julie Stanik-Hutt

■ INTRODUCTION

Patient outcomes management and the application of evidence to practice are powerful tools that can improve quality of care (The Joint Commission, 2008). The application of these symbiotic processes is the responsibility of all nurses (Foster, 2001). Since Nightingale, the assessment of patient outcomes has been inextricably intertwined with nursing care. In fact, Nightingale's collection and analysis of data regarding morbidity and mortality rates of soldiers under her care in the Crimea contributed to changes in care and, ultimately, to improved patient outcomes. Its later publication led to public and political support for the profession of nursing.

The application of the nursing process involves the identification of desired patient outcomes. Desired patient outcomes are established to direct the application of selected care interventions. Nursing interventions, based on the biopsychosocial sciences, are developed and implemented with the intention of attaining the established desired outcome. Finally, results of nursing interventions are assessed and evaluated by comparing the patient's actual outcomes to the desired outcomes. By doing so, quality and effectiveness of the delivered care are assessed, and the need for continued or altered care is determined. The application of evidence-based care is one tool nurses use to improve patient outcomes. Evidence-based practice (EBP) processes can be used to improve care outcomes one patient at a time or can be used to create clinical practice guidelines (CPGs), which when applied in practice, can improve outcomes for groups or populations of patients.

■ CLINICAL OUTCOMES

In health care, quality is defined as the "degree to which health services for individuals and populations increase the likelihood of attaining desired health outcomes and are consistent with current professional knowledge" (Institute of Medicine [IOM], 1990, p. 21). Safety is also a component of quality. Safe care is unlikely to injure or harm the patient (IOM, 2001; Newhouse & Poe, 2005). In addition, the IOM asserts that in order for care to be considered high quality, it should also be patient centered, timely, efficient, and equitable (IOM, 2001). These characteristics clearly link patient preferences and care processes with quality (IOM, 1990). Donabedian, the "father" of health care quality, suggested that care quality could be improved by establishing standards for care structures and processes. Patient outcomes are the ultimate measures of quality as they incorporate the influence of both structures and processes of care (Donabedian, 2005; Van Driel, De Sutter, Christiaens, & De Maeseneer, 2005).

Clinical or patient outcomes are defined as the end results of care that can be attributed to services provided (treatments, interventions, and care). Donabedian (1985) referred to outcomes as "changes in the actual or potential health status of individual patients, groups, or communities" (p. 256). Clinical outcomes demonstrate the value and effectiveness of care and can be assessed for individuals, populations, and organizations (Hughes, 2008). Outcomes can be either desirable or undesirable (adverse). Outcomes are quantified or measured, through the use of indicators, sometimes also called a metric. Outcome indicators or metrics gauge how patients are affected by their care. Indicators must be valid and reliable measures that are related to the outcome.

For example, to measure the adequacy of blood glucose control in a patient with diabetes, you might measure the patient's finger stick blood glucose or glycosolated hemoglobin levels. In this case, the finger stick blood glucose or glycosolated hemoglobin is the indicator or metric used to measure the outcome of blood glucose control. Indicators or metrics that are reported are referred to as performance measures (Dennison & Hughes, 2009).

Structures that support care and processes, which are used to provide care, are also important to care quality and are additional sources of relevant health care outcomes (Donabedian, 2005; Hammermeister, Shroyer, Sethi, & Grover, 1995). Structure indicators assess the organization and delivery of nursing care. For example, the nurse-to-patient ratio and skill mix of staff providing care are structure indicators. Process indicators evaluate the nature and amount of care that nurses provide. For example, documentation of patient teaching or timely reassessment of a patient's pain after the administration of an analgesic is an indicator of care processes.

Some ask "what is the difference between goals, objectives, indicators, and outcomes?" Should they all be called "outcomes?" Outcomes are used to characterize the result (effect) of an intervention, treatment, or provider (cause). This is essentially a cause-and-effect relationship (Parse, 2006). "Goals and objectives are something to strive for; indicators are signs of progress toward achievement of something, whereas outcomes are predictors of end-performance" (Parse, p. 189).

■ LINKING OUTCOMES TO CARE

Assessing care outcomes is not the goal in and of itself. Instead, it is important to assess outcomes in relation to the care provided (Minnick, 2009). When outcomes data are linked to interventions, they provide patients, payers, and providers with information regarding the potential effect that a health care intervention or provider (individuals or agencies) can have on their life. It can help patients to make decisions regarding their health care (Brooks & Barrett, 1998). The data can also influence a payer's decision making regarding which services to cover or which providers to include in their network. For example, outcomes data can be used to compare one treatment for a condition with an alternative treatment, or to compare care provided by different health care providers and agencies (Dennison & Hughes, 2009). Outcomes data are useful to providers because they help them to better understand the effects of the services they provide on their patients. Outcomes can also be compared with standard levels of performance, the so-called benchmarks or norms, to determine whether a service or provider is performing at a level that meets the established norms.

Outcomes can be used by providers to evaluate and improve the care they deliver. The best care comes from providers who routinely evaluate care outcomes and use that data to make adjustments to the care they provide as part of a continuous quality improvement cycle (Mullins, Baldwin, & Perfetto, 1996). This is often called outcomes management. Outcomes management refers to the collection and analysis, in relation to the processes of care, of information that indicates effectiveness of care. It provides a "checks and balances" process in the provision of health care. It usually focuses on aggregated outcomes data on groups of patients with common characteristics—for example, patients with diabetes or asthma or some other health problem. By measuring and evaluating care outcomes of groups of patients, providers can identify areas of their practice that need improvement. Once problems are identified, providers can seek out evidence-based solutions to implement and evaluate. The effectiveness of the solution is judged by the new outcomes attained. In this way, outcomes measurement can be linked to EBP and both can become "complimentary, iterative processes which contribute to quality improvement" (Deaton, 2001, p. 83).

Minnick (2009) discusses challenges encountered in the design and implementation of evidence-based outcome improvement projects. She emphasizes that the first step is the identification of the overall outcome that a project is intended to address. A population, intervention, comparison, outcome (PICO) question or other formal purpose statement can be used to start the search for evidence, benchmarks, and other data related to the desired outcome. A PICO question allows one to explore and link knowledge related to the topic, with the patient population and setting involved, and outcome of interest. This information, as well as the necessary and available resources to carry out the outcome improvement project, should be verified and reviewed with project stakeholders. Subsequently, a design for implementing and assessing the effects of the project, specifically the outcomes to be measured, should be identified.

■ NURSING OUTCOMES

In the past, the "5-Ds"—death, disease, disability, discomfort, and dissatisfaction—were the most commonly monitored outcomes of health care quality (Lohr, 1988). They are outcomes that are easily measured and understood by the public and policy makers. Donabedian (2005) described the use of patient outcomes of "recovery, restoration of function and of survival" (p. 692) as indicators of care quality. However, these outcomes do not adequately represent quality and are not specific to nursing. The first challenge is to "describe what nurses do (nursing interventions) in response to what sort of patient conditions (nursing diagnoses) with what effect (nursing outcomes)" (Marek, 1997, p. 8). Researchers at the University of Iowa have provided leadership in this area by creating the Nursing Interventions Classification (NIC) and Nursing Outcomes Classification (NOC) that link nursing interventions to diagnoses and outcomes. These systems allow the evaluation of care provided by nurses and facilitate communication regarding the same.

In 2003, 15 nursing care outcomes were selected for national reporting on nursing care performance. They included measures of patient-centered outcomes (death among surgical inpatients with treatable serious complications, pressure ulcer prevalence, falls prevalence, falls with injury, restraint prevalence, catheter-related urinary tract infections, central line catheter-associated blood stream infection, and ventilator-associated pneumonia), as well as the nursing-centered intervention processes (smoking cessation counseling for acute myocardial infarction [AMI], heart failure [HF], and pneumonia), and system-centered structures and processes (skill mix, nursing care hours per patient day, Practice Environment Scale-Nursing Work Index, and voluntary turnover) (Kurtzman & Corrigan, 2007). In addition to their use in performance reporting, these measures can be used in research, quality improvement, and health care policy activities. For example, several of the measures are included in the Robert Wood Johnson Foundation's "Transforming Care at the Bedside" initiative.

There are various other outcomes that are of interest to and demonstrate the broader effects of nursing care (Mitchell, 2008). These broader categories of outcomes relevant to nursing would include physiologic, psychosocial, functional, behavioral, symptoms, quality of life, knowledge, and satisfaction. Physiologic outcomes would include pulse, blood pressure, blood sugar and lipid levels, peak expiratory flow rates, weight, skin condition, and many other parameters. Psychosocial outcomes could include the individual's mood, attitudes, and abilities to interact with others. An individual's mobility, physical independence, and ability to participate in desired activities of daily living are functional outcomes. For example, the ability of a patient with asthma to engage in physical activities such as walking, exercising, or doing housework is a functional outcome. Behavioral outcomes could include adequacy of coping with health care needs or a patient's ability to follow (adhere) to recommended care. Symptoms, such as pain, dyspnea, fatigue, and others, command attention independent from the diseases that cause them. Because symptoms interfere with a patient's physiologic, psychosocial, and functional status and their quality of life, nurses are especially interested in their control. Quality of life, another natural outcome of interest for nurses, is a patient's general perception of their physical and mental well-being that can be affected by many factors including disease and injury, stress and emotions, symptom control and functional status, as well as others. Knowledge level, the individual's understanding of health-related information, is another outcome of interest. For example, a patient's understanding of the causes of asthma and factors that can trigger and prevent exacerbations would be important to nurses because teaching patients and supporting their self-care management is a role of nursing. Although patient satisfaction is a quality indicator for all health care and health care providers, patient satisfaction with their nursing care would be relevant to nurses.

Outcomes of interest to nurses in advanced practice roles include these broad areas as well and would also include outcomes specific to their advanced practice roles. Oermann and Floyd (2002) categorize outcomes of advanced practice nurses into clinical, functional, cost, and satisfaction outcomes. For example, certified registered nurse anesthetists (CRNA) might be interested in complications of oral intubation or extubation failures, epidural catheter insertion site infections, or patient satisfaction with postoperative pain relief. Certified nurse midwives (CNM) might monitor perineal laceration rates, or newborn Apgar scores, and certified nurse practitioners (CNP) would be interested in missed diagnoses or prescribing patterns.

Identifying the outcomes that can be clearly attributed only to nursing is a challenge. Attribution requires a high level of confidence that the outcome is a direct result of the care provided (Dennison & Hughes, 2009). When many care providers interact with patients and contribute to the care, it is sometimes difficult to attribute the outcome in the patient to only one provider or treatment. For example, a diabetic patient is consistently having high fasting blood glucose levels. The nurse practitioner (NP) discusses the problem and alternative medication adjustments with the patient and then orders a new daily and sliding scale insulin dose. The registered nurse (RN) teaches the patient the correct technique for finger stick glucose monitoring. The registered dietitian (RD) reviews the recommended diet and helps the patient practice making better food selections. When the patient's mean fasting blood glucose levels fall to within the desired parameters, who will get the credit? To whom are these results attributed? Is it the NP, the RN, the RD, or the team?

Nurses affect patient safety outcomes by identifying and mitigating risks, monitoring patient status and communicating with others regarding changes in the patient's condition, and through surveillance activities that lead to systems improvement to enhance safety. On the micro level, nurses' effect on safety variables such as medication errors or patient falls might be possible. However, it is again difficult to quantify nursing's effect on safety outcomes because of the multidisciplinary nature and complexity of our current health care systems.

Finally, patients' utilization of health care services, both increased and decreased, can reflect the influence of nursing care. An increased utilization might derive from nurses teaching and coaching patients regarding when, where, and how to seek care. Conversely, if nursing care increases an individual's ability for self-care management, the need for unintended office and emergency department visits—decreased utilization—could be the outcome. Examples of utilization of service outcomes would be intended and unintended office visits, use of the emergency room, hospital admissions, and length of stay.

Theoretical frameworks can be used to identify and explore the factors that influence nursing's effect on patient outcomes. Joseph (2007) proposed a theoretical approach to the examination of the effect of nursing on patient and organizational outcomes. She proposed that six constructs influence outcomes, including the environment of the health facility, qualities of the nursing unit, individual nurse, and the patient, as well as nursing care. She proposed that nursing care is affected by qualities of the nursing unit where care is given, by the nurse providing the care, and by patient qualities associated with their needs. Joseph also proposes that the larger environment of the health facility also affects care by providing the context of care through its mission, organizational structure, and characteristics, as well as its leadership milieu. This framework is useful in identifying variables that may influence patient as well as organizational outcomes.

■ TRANSLATION OF EVIDENCE TO IMPROVE OUTCOMES

Research findings support the effect of research-based nursing on patient outcomes (Heater, Becker, & Olson, 1988). A meta-analysis was used to determine the contribution that research-based nursing practice makes to patient outcomes compared with routine, procedural nursing care. Eighty four studies (63 published, 21 unpublished) of independent nursing interventions from 1977 to 1984 were evaluated, and effect sizes were calculated. Outcomes were grouped into four content areas: behavioral, knowledge, physiological, and psychosocial. Results indicated that individuals who received research-based nursing care had better outcomes than 72% of subjects who received routine, procedural nursing care.

Unfortunately, health care providers frequently fail to integrate available evidence into day-to-day patient care (McGlynn et al., 2003). It is reported that the average time gap from discovery of knowledge to its application in practice is 17 years (IOM, 2001). Historically, care processes have been based on ritual, personal, and local institutional preferences (Ackerman, 1999; Kingston, Krumberger, & Peruzzi, 2000). For more than 25 years, attempts have been made to increase the linkage of empiric research results to practice and to narrow the "bench to bedside" gap to improve patient care. But very little progress has been made in synthesizing and applying results of research to improve patient care. To bridge the bench to bedside gap, evidence needs to be incorporated into care protocols that are easily implemented in practice.

Probably one of the earliest examples of the creation of an evidence-based approach to care was the development in the 1970s, of consistent expectations for the performance of cardiopulmonary resuscitation (CPR). These standards were used to train and test the competency of health care providers to perform external cardiac massage and rescue breathing for patients suffering from cardiopulmonary arrest. These standards were based on limited research data regarding CPR as well as expert opinion, but it standardized the process of CPR across the country and across disciplines.

Soon thereafter, many institutions developed standing orders (or order sets) to provide consistent care to specific patient populations. These documents were developed for use on one or perhaps two nursing units within an individual hospital. They simplified care by establishing one set of orders for the care of a highly selected group of patients—for example, only those admitted with specific diagnoses, usually surgical procedures. They were based on preferences and personal expertise of a single or small group of physicians. They sometimes underwent institutional vetting processes.

Critical pathways began to emerge in the 1980s and 1990s as payers and institutions responded to the demands for managed care. Managed care initiatives set expectations for the provision of timely, streamlined, evidence-based care to optimize patient outcomes (Rotter et al., 2009). Care pathways were usually created by a multidisciplinary team to establish a unified but detailed care plan for a set of specific patients, with clearly described patient outcomes and timelines that could be used to implement patient care and monitor progress. Variance from the path triggered analysis and intervention. Over time, these care pathways were more likely to reflect input from all care providers involved with the patient population, and were approved through consensus processes. These multidisciplinary teams included physicians in private practice. The pathways were used locally for all or most of the patients fitting the population and described the care they would receive and when they would receive care. They were also used in contracting with payers to provide specific services for their insured.

■ CLINICAL PRACTICE GUIDELINES

In 1994, the federal government became involved in the movement to translate research to practice. At that time, the Agency for Health Care Policy and Research (AHCPR), now the Agency for Healthcare Research and Quality (AHRQ), began to develop care recommendations for common problems (acute pain, cancer pain, pressure ulcers, etc.) and published them as CPGs. These documents were developed by teams comprised of experts from multiple health care professions, who completed exhaustive searches of the research literature related to the identified problem. The resulting body of research literature was subsequently reviewed, rated for quality, and synthesized into recommendations related to risk identification, problem assessment, prevention, and treatment. Larger groups of experts were asked to review and provide comments on the CPGs before revision and dissemination of the final versions. The CDC also got involved in establishing CPGs. For example, in 2003, they established guidelines for the prevention of health care–associated pneumonia (Tablan et al., 2004).

Today, demands from patients and families, insurers, business leaders, consumer groups (American Association for Retired Persons [AARP], American Lung Association, American Cancer Society, etc.), and professional organizations (American Association of Critical Care Nurses, American College of Chest Physicians, etc.) are promoting the increased integration of available research knowledge, practitioner expertise, and patient preferences to improve patient health care. This is called *evidence-based practice*. By using EBP to create clinical practice guidelines, the best available research evidence is translated into a clinically useful form that can be employed by providers in day-to-day practice to improve patient outcomes.

CPGs are official recommendations made by recognized authorities regarding the screening, diagnosis, treatment, and management of specific conditions. They are "systematically developed statements to assist practitioner and patient decisions about appropriate health care for specific clinical circumstances" (Lohr & Field, 1992, p. 27). Evidence-based CPGs may help bridge the gap between research and practice. In these CPGs, research provides the evidence that an intervention is efficacious (produces better outcomes). The CPG facilitates transfer of this intervention to every day practice, and subsequently allows the evaluation of its effect on outcomes in broader patient populations (effectiveness). In this way, EBP leads to the development of practice-based evidence (Greene, 2006). It allows the accumulation of evaluation data on both efficacy and effectiveness of the intervention.

■ FACTORS THAT AFFECT ADOPTION OF CLINICAL PRACTICE GUIDELINES

Various factors affect the adoption of CPGs. Qualities of CPGs, including ease of use, complexity, clear scientific basis, strong link between evidence and recommendations, and other factors influence the use of CPGs (Davis & Taylor-Vaisey, 1997; Sox, 1994). The existence of conflicting CPGs with differing recommendations regarding the same intervention or population, such as have recently been reported for several types of cancer screening, probably undermine their use. Characteristics of the health care professional also influence their use of CPGs. For example, personal involvement in CPG development, awareness of as well as agreement and familiarity with the CPG may influence their use (Cabana et al., 1999; Davis & Taylor-Vaisey, 1997; Haynes, 1993). Health care providers who perceive CPGs as "cookbook medicine" or as a threat to practitioner autonomy are not likely to follow a CPG (Sox). Patient-related factors, such as the ability to predict effect on the patient or multiple comorbid conditions, and even patient satisfaction with the CPG, have been reported to influence the use of CPGs (Sox). Characteristics of the practice setting, such as availability of time and personnel, work pressures, and even costs to the practice related to implementation of a CPG might influence their use.

An emerging issue that will affect provider use of CPGs, or at least their explanations of their application with patients, are consumers' understanding of and attitudes toward CPGs (Carman et al., 2010). Recent evidence reveals that patients do not understand that EBP and CPGs are meant to improve their health and the quality of health care delivered without increasing patient costs (Carman et al.). Instead, they believe that care, at least provided by their own physician, is optimal and that use of a CPG will restrict their access to desired care. Some also believe CPGs are used only to protect physicians from malpractice claims. These patient attitudes and beliefs could have a significant effect on their acceptance of CPG recommendations.

The federal government and some private payers are devising payment initiatives related to the use of CPGs. Although the evidence to support these plans is at best controversial, Medicare has implemented incentive programs to reward providers, hospitals, nursing homes, and home health agencies who demonstrate application of EBP, as well as patient outcomes monitoring (Tanenbaum, 2009). These programs reflect their desire to improve patient care and control costs through the use of patient outcomes monitoring combined with the application of research to practice. The Medicare Physician Quality Reporting Initiative (PQRI), also known as pay for performance (P4P), began in 2007. It allows providers (including nurse practitioners), who report satisfactory patient outcomes data related to covered professional services, to qualify to earn additional payments. Concerns have been expressed regarding the potential unexpected consequence of P4P, in that the need to meet patient outcomes benchmarks could cause provider avoidance of patients with comorbid or difficult to treat problems (cherry picking), which might dilute the providers' ability to show improved patient outcomes (Dennison & Hughes, 2009). Penalties to poor patient outcomes have also been adopted by Medicare. Since 2009, hospitals have not been reimbursed for services provided to treat nosocomial infections and other preventable conditions (e.g., catheter-related urinary tract infections, catheter-related blood stream infections, decubitus ulcers, air emboli, etc.). Although this may have reduced hospital reimbursement rates, it has also driven agencies to examine their patient outcomes and to search out and apply evidence-based solutions, often in the form of CPGs, to prevent these adverse patient outcomes.

CPG use has migrated into the health care regulatory arena, most notably via accreditation requirements of the Joint Commission. CPGs have also been used by groups responsible for provider credentialing and competency assessment (Anderson, 1993). In addition, Medicare, through their quality performance rating, publicly posts data regarding hospital performance on compliance with some CPGs. For example, hospital performance on recommendations such as time to antibiotic administration for patients with pneumonia, and prescription of aspirin and beta-blockers to patients discharged after myocardial infarction, are posted at the "Hospital Compare" website (http://www.hospitalcompare.hhs.gov; Dennison & Hughes, 2009). Additionally, some practice guidelines have been used to establish standards of care in medical malpractice claims (Mittman & Siu, 1992).

■ EVALUATING CLINICAL PRACTICE GUIDELINES

The development and expanded use of CPGs to facilitate the integration of evidence into practice is associated with several challenges. First, the development and use of CPGs encourage a critical scrutiny of the research literature. Optimally, recommendations included on the CPG should be supported by up-to-date systematic reviews. However, this is not always possible because of the limitations in the availability of adequate depth, breadth, and quality of research, as well as the availability of systematic reviews. This would logically lead to fuller discussion regarding the quality and meaning of evidence that should be considered in the development of a CPG. For example, if research evidence is not available, is there other empiric or experiential data that can be used to support recommendations? Questions also arise regarding whether CPGs developed in Western countries are useful and relevant to resource-poor, less developed countries. In addition, because of the evolving nature of knowledge, the knowledge and evidence basis for CPGs, and as a consequence the CPG as well, become out of date over time. In addition, as new research is completed, CPGs need to be updated or replaced.

It is important to understand the validity, quality, ease of use, and other characteristics of a CPG when deciding whether to apply it in practice (Kingston et al., 2000). Qualities of CPGs, including ease of use, complexity, clear scientific basis, a strong link between evidence and recommendations, and other factors influence the use of CPGs (Davis & Taylor-Vaisey, 1997; Sox, 1994). The Appraisal of Guidelines for Research and Evaluation (AGREE) Collaboration is an international group of researchers who have worked together to create an instrument that uses theoretically derived criteria to evaluate the quality and applicability of CPGs (http://www.agreecollaboration.org/pdf/agreeinstrumentfinal.pdf).

The AGREE instrument is meant to be used by developers of CPG, health care providers using CPG, educators who prepare future health care providers, and by policy makers who are considering and recommending the adoption of a CPG. It poses 23 questions related to six topical areas related to the guideline including: scope and purpose, stakeholder involvement, rigor of development, clarity and presentation, applicability, and editorial independence. Each question rated on a continuum from strongly agree to strongly disagree with a corresponding score of 1 (*strongly disagree*) to 4 (*strongly agree*). Domain scores can be obtained and standardized by comparing obtained scores to maximum possible scores. Typically, more than one individual uses the instrument to rate the CPG on each question. Results of the assessment of each of the domains are then used to make an overall assessment and recommendation regarding the use of the guideline in practice.

The AGREE instrument has been used by various clinicians and organizations to evaluate CPGs related to diabetes, renal, and other health problems (Qaseem et al., 2007; van Diermen, Aartman, Baart, Hoogstraten, & van der Wall, 2009; Zadvinskis & Grudell, 2010). A group of nurses used it to appraise the National Kidney Foundation's Kidney Disease Outcomes Quality Initiative (KDOQI) CPGs for chronic kidney disease to establish best practice for the screening of renal function before cardiac angiography to prevent contrast-induced nephropathy (Zadvinskis & Grudell). Based on their assessment, the team decided that a practice change was evident, and that a change in their previous order set was needed to reflect a change in standards of care.

To illustrate use of the AGREE instrument, the American Association for Respiratory Care CPG related to endotracheal suctioning of mechanically ventilated patients with artificial airways were reviewed in 2010. Results and overall recommendation are displayed on Table 4.1.

Hopefully, more clinicians will use the AGREE instrument to determine the quality and the applicability of existing CPGs, as well as use the instrument to develop future CPGs.

TABLE 4.1   **Results of the AGREE Instrument**

AGREE Domains	Scores	Comments
Scope and Purpose		
1. The overall objective of the guideline is specifically described.	2	No introductory statement of objective or purpose, although title provides direction. Document includes information on steps to procedure, but no benefits or cost factors are discussed.
2. The clinical question covered by the guideline is specifically described.	4	Title, headings, and specific statements are provided.
3. The patients to whom the guideline is meant to apply are specifically described.	3	Patients with artificial airways who are receiving mechanical ventilation are the focus of the CPG. Adult, pediatric, and neonatal patients are referred to in item 2.2 but no age parameters are provided.
Stakeholder Involvement		
4. The guideline development group includes individuals from all the relevant professional groups.	2	Only MD and RRTs were included. No RNs, PTs, EMT/Paramedics, or unlicensed assistive personnel were included. No family or lay care providers were included.
5. The patients' views and preferences have been sought.	1	No evidence of patient consultation is found. Pain, anxiety, dyspnea, excessive coughing, and bronchspasm are listed as complications, effects that would be of interest to patients and families. Some mention of these effects in the explanations to patients and families would be appropriate to include.
6. The target users of the guideline are clearly defined.	1	Users referred to as "properly trained individuals" and settings listed.
7. The guideline has been piloted among target users.	2	No evidence of any pilot, although prior version was published in 1993
Rigor of Development		
8. Systematic methods were used to search for evidence.	3	Search included last 10 years using Medline, CINAHL, & Cochrane reviews. No search terms provided, no mention of hand searching, or discussion of other guidelines. Search yielded 114 RCTs, six meta-analyses, and 62 review articles.
9. The criteria for selecting the evidence are clearly described.	2	No description was provided for the type of evidence or research methods were included. Use of the GRADE criteria was mentioned.

AGREE Domains	Scores	Comments
10. The methods used for formulating the recommendations are clearly described.	1	No description of article critique or selection methods, number of reviewers, or methods used to resolve reviewer disagreements provided.
11. The health benefits, side effects, and risks have been considered in formulating the recommendations.	3	Adverse events (complications, and contraindications risks) of the procedure were included. No benefits (patient outcomes, survival, QOL, patient symptom control, patient responses) noted although indications for the procedure were included. No discussion comparing one approach to another.
12. There is an explicit link between the recommendations and the supporting evidence.	3	Sources cited for each component although often only one source. GRADE criteria for the overall 10 recommendations.
13. The guideline has been externally reviewed by experts prior to its publication.	1	No mention of external review or review by other provider groups (RN, PT, etc.). No team member with methods expertise noted.
14. A procedure for updating the guideline is provided.	3	Although no timeline for the next review is provided, this update cites the previous document (1993) that is less than 10 years old. Sources cover 1990–2009, all age groups cited, include articles from several disciplines (nursing, respiratory therapy, medicine, physical therapy), and four foreign countries as well as Cochrane reviews and the CDC.

Clarity and Presentation

AGREE Domains	Scores	Comments
15. The recommendations are specific and unambiguous.	3	Recommendations are general and do not provide specific information regarding the applications (e.g., provision of preoxygenation). However, information on those details are found in the other sections of the document.
16. The different options for the management of the condition are clearly presented.	1	Only recommended methods are listed. Only alternatives mentioned are the use of open versus closed suction systems, and deep versus shallow suctioning.
17. Key recommendations are easily identifiable.	3	All recommendations are listed at the end. They should have had a more prominent place in document. No tables, algorithms, and so forth were included.
18. The guideline is s upported with tools for application.	1	None found.

(continued)

TABLE 4.1   **Results of the AGREE Instrument** *(continued)*

AGREE Domains	Scores	Comments
Applicability		
19. The potential organizational barriers in applying the recommendations have been discussed.	1	Not found
20. The potential cost implications of applying the recommendations have been considered.	1	No cost information provided.
21. The guideline presents key review criteria for monitoring and /or audit purposes.	3	Specific information found in the document could be used to measure structure, processes, and patient outcomes if desired. Though not in recommendations per se.
Editorial Independence		
22. The guideline is editorially independent from the funding body.	3	No funding provided thought the organizational sponsor, AARC provided the steering committee. Financial disclosures were included
23. Conflicts of interest of guideline development members have been recorded.	4	Conflicts of interest were included.
Overall Assessment		
Would you recommend these guidelines for use in practice?	Unsure	Because no real discussion of the research is found, it would be difficult to recommend their use.

AARC = American Association for Respiratory Care; CDC = Centers for Disease Control and Prevention; CINAHL = Cumulative Index to Nursing and Allied Health Literature; CPG = clinical practice guidelines; EMT = emergency medical technician; MD = medical doctor; PT = physical therapist; QOL = quality of life; RCTs = randomized clinical trials; RN = registered nurse; RRT = registered respiratory therapist.

■   ASSESSING THE EFFECT ON OUTCOMES IN THE APPLICATION OF CLINICAL PRACTICE GUIDELINES

The work is not done even if the CPG is found to be of high quality and applicable to practice. It is important to carefully implement the CPG in a real practice setting and to subsequently evaluate its effects on the final product, the outcome, through outcomes assessment. Typically, outcome assessment such as development of CPGs or implementation of a practice improvement project, is conducted by a team. Resources and support for the assessment (e.g., personnel, funds, or access to databases, etc.) may come from inside as well as outside the practice site. Researchers or statisticians (e.g., university faculty) within the community can help in planning and in carrying out the assessment process.

When assessing the effect of the application of evidence to practice, outcomes to be assessed should be chosen based on four criteria: salience, objectivity, reality, and common currency (Minnick, 2009). "Salience is the quality of being related to the phenomenon of interest. Objectivity is the ability of the outcome to be measured without bias" (p. 110). Reality is "the extent to which the outcome definition . . . is true to life" (p. 110). Consultation with stakeholders can improve the likelihood that the outcome of interest meets these three criteria. Common currency refers to whether the way the outcome is defined and measured is standardized across settings. Familiarity with literature related to the outcome as well as consultation with others who work with the outcome of interest will help in the identification of any generally accepted definition and method of measurement.

Another quality that may be important is temporality. This is important when the project has a limited implementation period. For example, if a project will be implemented for 3 months, it is important to know whether it is possible to change the outcome over that period, or whether it would be better to use another indicator. To overcome these challenges, one needs to be sure that the definition of outcomes used on the PICO are consistent across the project and aims, and are consistent with the evidence.

The link between the evidence-based improvement intervention (e.g., the application of the CPG) and the outcome to be assessed needs to be clear. Even with clear linkages, at least seven challenges have been identified that interfere in one's ability to trace a direct relationship between the cause (application of an evidence-based intervention) and its effect (effect on the outcome of interest; Minnick, 2009). They include patient adherence to the treatment, inability to control multiple comorbidities; nonclinical (e.g., demographic) differences among participating patients, passage of time between intervention and measurement of the outcome, lack of availability of baseline data, involvement of a many providers in the setting or in the patient's care, and general complexity inherent in today's health care delivery settings. It is important to recognize these challenges and to try to incorporate ways to mitigate these issues in designing the assessment (e.g., use repeated measures methods, collect information on participating patient's demographics and comorbidities from medical records for use as covariates in analysis, compare outcomes that occurred during the same months of the year for both the "before" and "after" groups, etc.). A "broad knowledge of patients, providers, and systems variables" (Minnick, p. 113) as well as substantive support from the practice or institution (time of key stakeholders, financial resources, information technology expertise, staff personnel, etc.) is important to the success of this process.

Data analysis is an important component of outcome assessment (see Chapter 14 on evaluation for more detail). Data linked to the intended outcomes must be collected and analyzed to fully understand the effect of the translated evidence on outcomes. It is likely that any project will require consideration of data related to not only patients, but also data that characterize the context of the care environment (staffing, census, organizational processes, etc.). It is important to enlist expert assistance during the planning phase so that relevant data are included when data are being collected. This is another reason to consider including individuals with knowledge of research and statistical analysis methods on the assessment team. All projects should evaluate, at a minimum, descriptive statistics related to the setting, the project, and its outcomes. Some projects (e.g., those that use the typical quality improvement in pretest and posttest design) might use chi-square or t tests to characterize the differences found between the two times or two groups. And other projects could allow use of correlation techniques to understand results of the project.

■ FUTURE USE OF CLINICAL PRACTICE GUIDELINES TO IMPROVE PATIENT OUTCOMES

Although data supports the effect of guidelines on the processes of care (Cason, Tyner, Saunders, & Broome, 2007; Grimshaw & Russell, 1993; Kornbluth et al., 2006), their effect on outcomes has been scarcely documented (Smith & Hillner, 2001; Worrall, Chaulk, & Freake, 1997). Do they really promote improved outcomes? How can CPGs be best implemented and how can their use be sustained? How can patient outcomes derived from the application of CPGs be assessed, analyzed, and integrated to further improve the CPG and overall care? Additional research is needed, and provider's experiences and insights regarding use of CPGs need to be reported. What is certain is that health care professionals and institutions will continue to be called on to use all available methods to improve the quality and safety of health care delivered so that the most important outcome, patient health, is optimized.

■ REFERENCES

Ackerman, M. H. (1999). What would Vesalius think? *American Journal of Critical Care, 8*(2), 70–71.

Anderson, G. (1993). Implementing practice guidelines. *Canadian Medical Association Journal, 148*(5), 753–755.

Appraisal of Guidelines for Research and Evaluation Collaboration. (2001). *Appraisal of guidelines for research & evaluation (AGREE) instrument.* London, England: Author.

Brooks, B. A., & Barrett, S. (1998). Core competencies for outcomes management in nursing. *Outcomes Management for Nursing Practice, 2*(2), 87–89.

Cabana, M. D., Rand, C. S., Powe, N. R., Wu, A. W., Wilson, M. H., Abboud, P. A., & Rubin, H. R. (1999). Why don't physicians follow clinical practice guidelines? A framework for improvement. *Journal of the American Medical Association, 282*(15), 1458–1465.

Carman, K. L., Maurer, M., Yegian, J. M., Dardess, P., McGee, J., Evers, M., & Marlo, K. O. (2010). Evidence that consumers are skeptical about evidence-based health care. *Health Affairs, 29*(7), 1400–1406. doi: 10.1377/hithaff.2009.0296

Cason, C. L., Tyner, T., Saunders, S., & Broome, L. (2007). Nurses' implementation of guidelines for ventilator-associated pneumonia from the Centers for Disease Control and Prevention. *American Journal of Critical Care, 16*(1), 28–38.

Davis, D. A., & Taylor-Vaisey, A. (1997). Translating guidelines into practice. A systematic review of theoretic concepts, practical experience and research evidence in the adoption of clinical practice guidelines. *Canadian Medical Association Journal, 157*(4), 408–416.

Deaton, C. (2001). Outcomes measurement and evidence-based nursing practice. *Journal of Cardiovascular Nursing, 15*(2), 83–86.

Dennison, C. R., & Hughes, S. (2009). Reforming cardiovascular care: Quality measurement and improvement, and pay-for-performance. *Journal of Cardiovascular Nursing, 24*(5), 341–343.

Donabedian, A. (1985). Explorations in quality assessment and monitoring. Vol. 3. The methods and findings of quality assessment and monitoring: An illustrated analysis. Ann Arbor, MI: Health Administration Press.

Donabedian, A. (2005). Evaluating the quality of medical care. *The Millbank Quarterly, 83*(4), 691–729.

Foster, R. L. (2001). Who is responsible for measuring nursing outcomes? *Journal of the Society of Pediatric Nurses, 6*(3), 107–108.

Grap, M. J. (2009). Not-so-trivial pursuit: Mechanical ventilation risk reduction. *American Journal of Critical Care, 18*(3), 200–309. doi: 10.4037/ajcc2009724

Green, L. W. (2006). Public health asks of systems science: To advance our evidence-based practice, can you help us get more practice-based evidence? *American Journal of Public Health, 96*(3), 406–409.

Grimshaw, J. M. & Russell, I. T. (1993). Effect of clinical guidelines on medical practice: A systematic review of rigorous evaluations. *Lancet, 342*(8883), 1317–1322.

Hammermeister, K., Shroyer, A., Sethi, G. & Grover, F. (1995). Why it is important to demonstrate linkages between outcomes of care and processes and structures of care. *Medical Care, 33*(10 Supplement), OS5–OS16.

Haynes, R. B. (1993). Some problems in applying evidence in clinical practice. *Annals of the New York Academy of Science, 703*, 210–225.

Heater, B. S., Becker, A. M., & Olson, R. K. (1988). Nursing interventions and patient outcomes: A meta-analysis of studies. *Nursing Research, 37*(5), 303–307.

Hughes, R. G. (2008). Chapter 44. Tools and strategies for quality improvement and patient safety. In R. G. Hughes (Ed.), *An Evidence-based handbook for nurses* (pp. 1–39). Washington, DC: Agency for Healthcare Research and Quality. Retrieved from http://www.ahrq.gov/qual/nurseshdbk/docs/HughesR_QMBMP.pdf

Institute of Medicine. (1990). In K. N. Lohr. (Ed.), *Medicare: A strategy for quality assurance.* Washington, DC: National Academy Press.

Institute of Medicine. (2001). *Crossing the quality chasm: A new health care system for the 21st century.* Washington, DC: National Academy Press.

The Joint Commission. (2008). Using evidence-based practice and outcomes management to improve care. *The Joint Commission Benchmark, 10*(3), 9–10.

Joseph, A. M. (2007). The impact of nursing on patient and organizational outcomes. *Nursing Economics, 25*(1), 30–34.

Kingston, M. E., Krumberger, J. M., & Peruzzi, W. T. (2000). Enhancing outcomes: Guidelines, standards, and protocols. *AACN Clinical Issues, 11*(3), 363–374.

Kornbluth, A., Hayes, M., Feldman, S., Hunt, M., Fried-Boxt, E., Lichtiger, S., . . . Young, J. (2006). Do guidelines matter? Implementation of the ACG and AGA osteoporosis screening guidelines in inflammatory bowel disease (IBD) patients who meet the guidelines' criteria. *American Journal of Gastroenterology, 101*(7), 1546–1550.

Kurtzman, E. T., & Corrigan, J. M. (2007). Measuring the contribution of nursing to quality, patient safety and health care outcomes. *Policy, Politics & Nursing Practice. 8*(1), 20–36.

Lohr, K. N. (1988). Outcome measurement: Concepts and questions. *Inquiry, 25*(1), 37–50.

Lohr, K. N., & Field, M. J. (1992). A provisional instrument for assessing clinical practice guidelines. In M. J. Field & K. N. Lohr (Eds.), *Guidelines for clinical practice: From development to use.* Washington DC: Institute of Medicine, National Academy Press.

Marek, K. D. (1997). Measuring the effectiveness of nursing care. *Outcomes Management for Nursing Practice, 1*(1), 8–12.

McGlynn, E. A., Asch, S. M., Adams, J., Keesey, J., Hicks, J., DeCristofaro, A., & Kerr, E. A. (2003). The quality of health care delivered to adults in the United States. *New England Journal of Medicine, 348*(26), 2635–2645.

Minnick, A. F. (2009). General design and implementation challenges in outcomes assessment. In R. M. Kleinpell (Ed.), *Outcome assessment in advanced practice nursing* (pp. 107–118). (2nd ed.). New York, NY: Springer Publishing.

Mitchell, P. H. (2008). Defining patient safety and quality care. In R. G. Hughes (Ed.), *Patient safety and quality: An evidence-based handbook for nurses* (pp. 1–5). Rockville, MD: Agency for Healthcare Research and Quality. Retrieved from http://www.ahrq.gov/qual/nurseshdbk/docs/MitchellP_DPSQ.pdf

Mittman, B. S., & Siu, A. L. (1992). Changing provider behavior: Applying research on outcomes and effectiveness in health care. In S. M. Shortell & U. E. Reinhardt (Eds.), *Improving health policy and management.* Arbor, MI: Health Administration Press.

Mullins, C. D., Baldwin, R., & Perfetto, E. M. (1996). What are outcomes? *Journal of the American Pharmacists Association, NS36*(1), 39–49.

Newhouse, R, & Poe, S. (2005). *Measuring patient safety.* Sudbury, MA: Jones and Bartlett.

Oermann, M. H., & Floyd, J. A. (2002). Outcomes research: An essential component of the advanced practice nurse role. *Clinical Nurse Specialist, 16*(3), 140–144.

Parse, R. R. (2006). Outcomes: Saying what you mean. *Nursing Science Quarterly, 19*(3), 189.

Qaseem, A., Vijan, S., Snow, V., Cross, J. T., Weiss, K. B., Owens, D. K., & Clinical Efficacy Assessment Subcommittee of the American College of Physicians. (2007). Glycemic control and type 2 diabetes mellitus: The optimal hemoglobin A1c targets. A guidance statement from the American College of Physicians. *Annals of Internal Medicine, 147*(6), 417–422.

Rotter, T., Kinsman, L., James, E., Machotta, A., Gothe, H., Willis, J., . . . Kugler, J. (2009) Clinical pathways: Effects on professional practice, patient outcomes, length of stay and hospital costs. *Cochrane Database of Systematic Reviews,* (3), CD006632.

Smith, T. J., & Hillner, B. E. (2001). Ensuring quality cancer care by the use of clinical practice guidelines and critical pathways. *Journal of Clinical Oncology, 19*(11), 2886–2897.

Sox, H. C. (1994). Practice guidelines: 1994. *The American Journal of Medicine, 97*(3), 205–207.

Tablan, O. C., Anderson, L. J., Besser, R., Bridges, C., Hajjeh, R., Centers for Disease Control and Prevention, & Healthcare Infection Control Practices Advisory Committee. (2004). Guidelines for preventing health-care-associated pneumonia, 2003: Recommendations of CDC and Healthcare Infection Control Practices Advisory Committee. *Morbidity and Mortality Weekly Report. Recommendations and Reports/Centers for Disease Control, 53*(RR–3), 1–36.

Tanenbaum, S. J. (2009). Pay for performance in Medicare: Evidentiary irony and the politics of value. *Journal of Health Politics, Policy and Law, 34*(5), 717–746.

van Diermen, D. E., Aartman, I. H., Baart, J. A., Hoogstraten, J., & van der Waal, I. (2009). Dental management of patients using antithrombotic drugs: Critical appraisal of existing guidelines. *Oral Surgery, Oral Medicine, Oral Pathology, Oral Radiology, and Endodontics, 107*(5), 616–624.

Van Driel, M. L., De Sutter, A. I., Christiaens, T. C., & De Maeseneer, J. M. (2005). Quality of care: The need for medical, contextual, and policy evidence in primary care. *Journal of Evaluation in Clinical Practice, 11*(5), 417–429.

Worrall, G., Chaulk, P., & Freake, D. (1997). The effects of clinical practice guidelines on patient outcomes in primary care: A systematic review. *Canadian Medical Association Journal, 156*(12), 1705–1712.

Zadvinskis, I. M., & Grudell, B. A. (2010). Clinical practice guideline appraisal using the AGREE instrument: Renal screening. *Clinical Nurse Specialist, 24*(4), 209–214.

C H A P T E R FIVE

Translation of Evidence for Improving Safety and Quality

Christine A. Goeschel

■ INTRODUCTION

The quality of care in U.S. hospitals is a cause of widespread concern (Murray & Frenk, 2010). This is particularly disquieting because there has been a dramatic increase in quality and patient safety-related activities during the past decade (Leape, 2010). When the Institute of Medicine (IOM) released its seminal reports, *To Err Is Human* in 1999 and *Crossing the Quality Chasm* in 2001, the assertions that between 44,000 and 98,000 preventable deaths occur annually in U.S. hospitals were both startling and riveting. The IOM minimum goal of a 50% reduction in errors over 5 years seemed aggressive but plausible (IOM, 1999, 2001). A Research and Development (RAND) report suggesting that U.S. hospitalized patients receive, on average, half the therapies evidence suggests they should (McGlynn et al., 2003) fueled the urgency for improvement created by the IOM reports. Subsequent national surveys suggested that patient safety was a top priority for hospital leaders, including boards of trustees (Barry, 2005; Callendar, Hastings, Hemsley, Morris, & Peregrine, 2007; Jiang, Lockee, Bass, & Fraser, 2008). High expectations prevailed, yet, just 3 years after the IOM reports were released, health services researchers began voicing concerns over the slow pace of progress (Auerbach, Landefeld, & Shojania, 2007; Leape & Berwick, 2005; Leatherman et al., 2003; Wachter, 2004).

Now, 10 years after *To Err is Human* was released, there is broad agreement that health care is more complex, methods to improve are more challenging, and progress is more elusive than anyone imagined. Health disparities research suggests that there is uneven distribution of improvements in quality of care, and a decline in performance on many measures, when assessed against minority status (Agency for Healthcare Research and Quality [AHRQ], 2009a). Consumer research and front-page news reveal that public frustrations are growing because of the lack of information on quality of care and blatant examples of health care dangers (Consumers Union, 2009; Graham et al., 2004; Weingart et al., 2010). Patient safety and quality of care research suggests that progress is slow, new problems are emerging, and on many national performance measures, either the quality of care stayed the same or got worse during the past decade (Bogdanich, 2010; The Commonwealth Fund Commission, 2008). Health policy research validates that the costs of poor quality of care are rising, regulatory interests are intensifying, and policy approaches to clinical problems are increasing (Leape, 2010; Woodward et al., 2010).

Why has improvement not gone as expected? The authors of *To Err Is Human* recommended four key strategies to improve the quality of care and safety of patients in the United States.

1. Establish a national focus to create leadership, research, tools, and protocols to increase the knowledge base (science) about safety.
2. Develop a nationwide public mandatory reporting system, and encourage health care organizations and practitioners to develop and participate in voluntary reporting systems to identify and learn from errors.
3. Raise performance standards and expectations for improvements in safety through the actions of oversight organizations, professional groups, and group purchasers of health care.
4. Implement safety systems in health care organizations to ensure safe practices at the delivery level.

Unfortunately, a national infrastructure to implement the strategies did not exist. Thus, well-intentioned clinicians, administrators, and policy makers often forged independent, resource-intensive, poorly designed interventions to address the IOM strategies. Moreover, in the absence of empirical guidance and an infrastructure to support improvement, organizations and clinicians often took unwarranted comfort in their patient safety progress by assessing their level of activity rather than measurable improvement. However, without a common patient safety taxonomy, standardized measures, valid data, and rigorous evaluation, it is not surprising that 10 years after the alarm bell sounded, we have few examples of measurable improvement in quality of care or patient safety.

Interest in providing evidence-based, cost-effective, and accountable care has never been higher, and the stakes have never been greater. Infrastructure to support efforts is beginning to emerge, yet, the complexity of where and how to approach this challenge can stifle even the most courageous nursing leader.

If evidence-based practice is "simply the integration of the best possible research evidence with clinical expertise and with patient needs" (Malloch & Porter-O'Grady, 2010, p. 1), what should be the accountability standard when evidence is scant, clinical expertise is diverse, the system of care delivery is evolving, and patients' needs vary widely. Research to answer those questions is flourishing. The study of the diffusion of innovations in health care is increasing exponentially (Greenhalgh, Robert, Macfarlane, Bate, & Kyriakidou, 2004; Rogers, 1995), research on knowledge translation is adding clarity to the phases of moving research evidence into clinical practice, and emerging health services research exploring *knowledge-to-action* (KTA) *translation* is gaining attention by practitioners, policy makers, patients, purchasers, and the public (Graham et al., 2006).

However, although research evolves, patients suffer preventable harm every day, in virtually every health care setting in the country. Nurses have a pivotal role in keeping patients safe and in narrowing the gap between evidence-based practice and common practice. As administrators, educators, researchers, and bedside clinicians, the mandate for nurses to lead patient safety is here and now.

Thus, in full recognition of the nascent nature of the science, this chapter focuses evidence for improving safety and quality within the context of the IOM's four strategic recommendations and offers practical insights and tools for nurse leaders at all levels of practice. This chapter will (a) discuss the importance of viewing health care delivery as a science to discover evidence to improve quality and safety, (b) provide an organizing framework from which to consider patient safety research and translation activities, (c) present an adaptable and proven method to implement patient safety at the unit level (Comprehensive Unit-Based Safety Program [CUSP]), (d) describe a successful patient safety program using CUSP that is being implemented nationally and internationally, and (e) discuss national momentum and ubiquitous barriers as the industry moves from awareness and acknowledgement of quality and patient safety deficits, to accountability for quality of care and patient safety outcomes.

■ HEALTH CARE DELIVERY AS A SCIENCE

Patient safety research and translation are mired in traditional and often archaic systems of health care delivery. Until recently, funding for U.S. health care research focused almost entirely on discovering disease mechanisms and identifying new therapies with minimal investments to identify effective, efficient, and safe delivery of therapies to patients. Thus, errors of omission (failure to provide evidence-based therapies) continue as a significant health care challenge (Hayward, Asch, Hogan, Hofer, & Kerr, 2005; Reason, 2002). Correcting this failure requires viewing health care delivery as a science. This involves conducting rigorous scientific research on methods to improve health care delivery that produces hard data, with clear and measurable results. Only then will it be possible to summarize evidence into clear standards; develop measures; monitor performance with valid, reliable data; hold clinicians and administrators accountable for outcomes; and set explicit national improvement targets. Until now, even when research revealed effective methods to improve patient safety and quality of care, the lack of a national infrastructure to disseminate the knowledge broadly, study its uptake and translation, and evaluate its generalizability through rigorous measurement was an almost insurmountable barrier to progress.

One attempt to address that barrier is a novel program currently underway across the country. The program aims to reduce central line-associated bloodstream infections (CLABSI), a type of infection that is largely preventable, kills thousands of people in the United States each year, and adds well more than a billion dollars of excess cost to the national health care bill (U.S. Department of Health & Human Services [HHS], 2009). However, we know how to dramatically reduce a unit-based method to implement evidence-based care through a method developed by the Johns Hopkins University Quality and Safety Research Group (QSRG). More than 100 ICU teams in Michigan used the model and achieved a 66% reduction in CLABSI and a median CLABSI rate of zero (Pronovost, Berenholtz, Needham, et al., 2006). The teams have, thus far, sustained these improvements for more than 4 years (Pronovost et al., 2010).

The mandate to spread the program that the research demonstrated was effective at Johns Hopkins and in more than 100 intensive care units (ICU) in Michigan, was stimulated by public pressure (Faber, Bosch, Wollersheim, Leatherman, & Grol, 2009), political pressure (Waxman, 2008), and private pressure via philanthropic donations specifically earmarked to replicate the work in other states. Together, those pressures contributed to a national improvement target issued by HHS and an AHRQ-funded national collaborative. The collaborative aims to have all hospitals in every state in the country, the District of Columbia, and Puerto Rico reduce CLABSI to the levels achieved in Michigan; and to have sound data to demonstrate the improvement. The program, "On the CUSP: Stop BSI" (Stop BSI) provides a foundation for the discussions that follow.

■ FRAMEWORK FOR PATIENT SAFETY RESEARCH AND IMPROVEMENT

A precursor to improving patient safety is to understand what activities fall within the rubric. The murky boundaries between health services research, quality improvement, and patient safety often produce duplicative, uncoordinated, and, sometimes, competitive efforts that are resource intensive, counterproductive, and frustrating for participants. Thus, the lack of a simple, yet, meaningful framework for patient safety efforts often impedes the ability of local providers to translate research into practice and assess patient safety progress. The Johns Hopkins University QSRG developed a framework for patient safety research and improvement in response to the growing demand for quality and safety data and for higher quality and safer care (Pronovost et al., 2009). The framework emerged from the IOM strategies for improvement, literature on knowledge transfer and diffusion of innovation, and QSRG experiences implementing collaborative improvement projects (Graham, Harrison, Brouwers, Davies, & Dunn, 2002; Graham & Logan, 2004; Greenhalgh et al., 2004). Although the framework is evolving, preliminary feedback from physicians, nurses, and administrators validates both the need for and utility of this early construct. The framework includes five domains: (a) evaluating patient safety progress, (b) translating evidence into practice, (c) measuring and improving culture, (d) identifying and mitigating hazards, and (e) evaluating the association between organizational characteristics and outcomes. Improving the quality of care and patient safety at a comprehensive level hinges on the need for new knowledge and experience in each of the domains. Stop BSI demonstrates the distinctions, as well as the inter-relatedness of the domains.

Stop BSI: An Exemplar for Patient Safety Research and Improvement

The QSRG/Pronovost model for improvement has three key elements. The first is the CUSP, which provides a five-step framework to address patient safety issues at a local level, and to enhance unit culture (Pronovost et al., 2005). CUSP provides a solid foundation for any unit-based quality and patient safety-improvement activity. CUSP provides education on the science of safety, fosters teamwork and patient-focused relationships, and then builds on caregiver wisdom to identify potential patient harms and create unit-specific solutions. The second element of the program is a model for Translating Evidence into Practice (TRiP; Pronovost, Berenholtz, & Needham, 2008). TRiP seeks to provide behaviorally based guides (often in the form of checklists) to implement evidence-based care. Johns Hopkins QSRG used the TRiP model to produce interventions that can reduce CLABSI. These interventions resulted in dramatic infection reduction at Hopkins and across Michigan. The third critical element is a rigorous system to measure, report, and improve outcomes. The CUSP/TRiP model synthesizes knowledge, technical expertise, and implementation science to achieve a specific, measurable improvement goal. Nursing leadership is integral to success of the program (Goeschel et al., 2006). However, this role places nurses at a crossroad between the way things are and the way things might be.

Adaptive Versus Technical Work

Effective leaders understand the difference between technical and adaptive work (Heifetz, 1994; Heifetz & Linsky, 2002). Technical work addresses problems with known answers and is skill or knowledge based. Adaptive work involves changing attitudes, beliefs, or behaviors and is much more difficult than technical work. Moreover, leaders often issue technical solutions for adaptive problems, which contribute to the failure of many improvement programs. Solving adaptive problems requires time, broad input, and recognition that threats implicit in change are both systemic and personal.

The CUSP/TRiP model to achieve and sustain improvements in patient safety (Pronovost, Berenholtz, et al., 2008) includes both technical work (e.g., create checklists that summarize science) and adaptive work (e.g., efforts to change attitudes, beliefs, and behaviors). Experience at a hospital and state level suggests that it is most effective and efficient when a central group organizes and leads the technical aspects of the project, and local teams lead the adaptive aspects, taking into consideration unit- and hospital-specific resources, cultures, and infrastructures (Pronovost, Berenholtz, Goeschel, et al., 2006). Stop BSI uses this same framework for the national project.

The Comprehensive Unit-Based Safety Program

CUSP is an iterative approach to improve a unit's teamwork and safety culture. Root cause analyses often cite lack of teamwork as a contributing factor, and approximately 65% of all sentinel events are linked to poor communication (The Joint Commission, 2009). CUSP has been associated with teamwork and safety culture improvements (Timmel et al., 2010). CUSP provides structure to improve safety throughout a hospital, yet, is flexible enough to focus on concerns identified by bedside caregivers. The following CUSP steps are both technical and adaptive:

1. Educate on the science of safety.
2. Identify defects in care.
3. Assign executive leader to a unit-level CUSP team.
4. Learn from one defect per month.
5. Implement tools to improve teamwork and safety culture.

Step 1 aims to educate about the science of safety through a short training video and group discussions. Science of safety learning objectives are to (a) accept that safety is part of the work system, (b) appreciate the basic attributes of safe design (standardize work, develop independent checks for important processes, and learn from mistakes), recognize that these attributes apply to technical work and adaptive work, and (c) understand that interdisciplinary teams make wiser decisions because they have diverse and independent input.

Step 2 invites staff to identify "how the next patient will be harmed." It is important to introduce this after most staff has completed science of safety training. Generally, the nurse manager or CUSP team leader facilitates the process, which includes all unit staff, as well as physicians and support staff that frequent the unit (not just nurses). The two-question survey (how is the next patient likely to be harmed on our unit, and what ideas do you have that might reduce this risk?) is distributed at a staff meeting or placed in mailboxes, and a survey drop box is provided for this activity so responses may be candid and anonymous. The team leader compiles the results and shares them at a CUSP/CLABSI team meeting. The team decides which safety hazards pose the greatest threat and develops a plan to work on those hazards first.

Step 3 requires the chief executive officer (CEO) to assign a senior hospital leader as a member of each unit-level CUSP/CLABSI team. The senior leader meets monthly with the team, reviews hazards identified in step 2, participates in the process to select improvement priorities, helps secure the resources and institutional support needed so the team can proceed with their plan, and then holds the team accountable for following through on the plan (Pronovost et al., 2004).

Step 4 teaches teams to learn, not merely recover, from mistakes. Using a simple, structured tool, teams investigate defects in care (Pronovost, Holzmueller, et al., 2006). The tool prompts users to answer what happened, why it happened, what did they do to reduce the risk, and whether their actions actually reduced this risk. The completed one-page written summary of the investigation is shared widely. This helps focus opportunities. For example, some teams discovered that stocking the central line cart was erratic and needed a defined protocol and audit process. Other teams identified that staff did not always follow central line maintenance procedures. These lessons prompted other teams to check their local practice.

Step 5 encourages teams to try tools to improve communication and teamwork. The daily goals checklist is one of the first tools many teams try because it is clearly patient safety focused (Holzmueller, Timmel, Kent, Schulick, & Pronovost, 2009; Pronovost et al., 2003; Schwartz, Nelson, Saliski, Hunt, & Pronovost, 2008). The checklist starts and finishes with a patient focus rather than a nursing or medical focus. It asks: "What patient safety risk does this patient face?", "How can we mitigate them?", and "What do we (the caregiver team) need to do today to move this patient to the next level of care?" Completed during interdisciplinary rounds, the team creates the daily goals form collectively, so that all staff members (e.g., nurses, doctors, therapists) understand the plan and their discipline-specific responsibility to implement the plan.

Use of the CUSP/TRiP model nearly eliminated CLABSI in ICUs at the Johns Hopkins Hospital (Berenholtz et al., 2004), in 103 Michigan ICUs (Pronovost, Berenholtz, et al., 2007), in all Rhode Island ICUs, and in ICUs throughout Spain. It is currently being used in 97% of ICUs in England and in Stop BSI across the United States. However, this is a narrowly focused project, and the national implementation process is not yet tried and true. Moreover, getting to the national project was more happenstance than plan. It is important to understand that path to create the infrastructure needed for future efforts. Many teams involved in Stop BSI are seeing great reductions in CLABSI; they are beginning to grasp the importance of valid data and rigorous measurement, and they want to know "what is next." The answer is a mystery because evidence for how to improve quality of care and patient safety remains limited, and a real path to meaningful national improvement targets and implementation infrastructure has yet to emerge. A quick look at the CUSP/CLABSI path may inform the evolution of a better way.

■ THE PATH TO A NATIONAL CUSP/CLABSI EFFORT TO STOP BSI

In phase 1, QSRG researchers reviewed empiric data, and selected five key procedures that would most likely prevent CLABSI. Primary considerations included numbers needed to treat (NNT) from the empirical literature and barriers to implementation. The aim was to identify interventions with the greatest potential to reduce infections, and fewest barriers to implementation. They compiled these procedures into an easy-to-follow checklist. Nurses and other ICU staff identified potential barriers to using the checklist and developed tactics to overcome those barriers to optimize compliance. The team then pilot tested the intervention in ICUs at Johns Hopkins and measured its performance. They nearly eliminated these infections. TRiP implementation happened in concert with CUSP implementation, as described earlier.

In phase 2, AHRQ awarded the QSRG and Michigan Keystone Center, a patient safety challenge grant to pilot test broad implementation of the program (AHRQ, 2008). Within 3 months of implementing the interventions, the median rate of infection in the 103 participating ICUs plummeted to zero and stayed at zero for 4 years (Pronovost et al., 2010). These infections were reduced by 66%. The work was not easy; it required hospital leaders, doctors, and nurses to implement interventions, improve teamwork, and monitor performance. Nevertheless, the results were well worth the investment. Estimates are that the reduction in infections saved nearly 200 million dollars and 1,500 lives in a single year.

In phase 3, AHRQ and philanthropists are funding a nationwide collaborative project to implement what worked at Hopkins and in Michigan. Most hospitals are trying to reduce these infections, but they need support to be efficient, and to rigorously measure and improve performance. Through this effort, researchers, AHRQ, CDC, state hospital associations, and individual hospitals are collaborating and, through trial and error, are paving the way for future national improvement programs.

Although this approach may be a model not just to eliminate CLABSI but also to address other health care-acquired infections and other types of preventable harm, there are many hurdles to overcome before such efforts can take shape.

Moving From Patient Safety Awareness and Acknowledgment to Accountability

The most recent national health care quality report (AHRQ, 2009b) asserts that we lack the ability to monitor even basic progress in patient safety. Outside of process measures, we have very limited capacity to inform the public or clinicians about the success of our efforts to make patient care safer.

The attributes of quality measures are generally well accepted; they need to be valid, important, useable, and feasible. However, examples of how to successfully apply these attributes and measurably improve care are rare, beyond the CLABSI example previously described. However, federal funders, professional societies, regulators, industry quality leaders, and local providers are beginning to move beyond shining a light on patient safety problems. Just as business and industry leaders understand financial accounting standards and terms and are legally accountable to adhere to standard financial reporting requirements, there is growing recognition that in order for consumers to choose high quality providers, and for health care leaders to be accountable for the patient safety and quality of care, basic standards, common taxonomy, and uniform quality and safety reporting requirements are needed.

Patient safety measures to inform such standards and reporting requirements must evolve. The following challenges require careful consideration. Not all harm is preventable, so it is crucial that patient safety measures focus on measures of preventable harm, use of evidence-based interventions, learning from mistakes or error reports, and culture.

■ VALIDITY

Validity refers to whether a study is able to answer the questions it scientifically intends to answer. There are many types of validity, and they warrant deep understanding and discussion as standards and measures take shape (Berenholtz et al., 2007). For the purposes of evidence for quality and patient safety, it is most important to understand that without a scientific approach to quality and safety improvements, the risk is that erroneous conclusions are drawn from projects, providers may think improvements have occurred when they have not, unintended consequences may occur, and consumers will have no legitimate way to *choose quality* (Pronovost, Miller, & Wachter, 2007; Pronovost, Goeschel, & Wachter, 2008).

■ DATA QUALITY CONTROL

Regardless of the type of performance measure, data quality control has received relatively little attention. The limited literature examining data quality control in quality and patient safety studies raises substantial concern. Policy makers, hospital leaders, and clinicians make important decisions based on the assumption that quality improvement project results are accurate.

Quality-control methods are critical to help ensure the accuracy of any effort to collect, analyze, and report data (Needham et al., 2009).

■ PRIORITIZING QUALITY IMPROVEMENT TARGETS

Problems are immense and resources are limited. It is crucial to prioritize what we measure and what resources we commit to measuring both clinical performance and patient outcomes. The number of *measures for mandated reporting is growing exponentially with seemingly little consideration of what is important*. Although there are attempts to prioritize quality improvement targets (the National Quality Forum's [NQF] Quality Partners is one strategy), much more needs to be done in this regard. Systematic ways to prioritize national quality measurement incorporating both prediction models of disease burden and risk mitigation models need to be developed. Tools and methods that are successful in other industries such as aviation may be applicable.

■ USEABLE MEASURES

The current method of providing national measures of performance that are high-level surrogates for actual performance is viewed critically by many clinicians, who favor quality metrics that are collected locally and have faced validity. National surrogate measures do not allow the public to evaluate local quality, and unique local measures do not allow consumers to make an informed choice about their provider and to *comparison shop*. Ideally, measures should be scalable, and the ultimate unit of measure should be the patient, clinician, or patient care area. Once these measures are developed and implemented, they may be aggregated to provide hospital, health system, state, and national information. The elimination of CLABSI in ICUs is an example of how this might be done.

■ FEASIBLE

Once measures are developed, there are undeniable challenges to the feasibility of collecting data to monitor progress. There are strong trade-offs between manual-based data collection and the opposite extreme of using discharge data collection that, although feasible, suffers from lack of validity. New data mining strategies using advanced information technologies offer huge potential to close this gap. Quality and patient safety scientists will need to consider how to achieve standardized definitions of preventable harms and ways to incorporate the data elements into electronic medical records, easing the burden of manual data collection without forfeiting the validity of the measures used to monitor progress. Such solutions will present both operational and policy challenges. For example, this will likely require joint documentation between nurses and physicians; one of many changes in historical practice patterns that nurse and physician leaders will need to embrace to enhance patient safety. In addition, organizations will need to pay for the investment of clinical time into development of information technologies. Without that investment, there is a potential that hospitals may "automate" ineffective paper and delivery system processes.

Regulatory, Market, and Professional Society Influences to Improve Safety

Analogous to the "perfect storm," it seems as although conditions are finally right for patient safety to actually improve, although the storm is long brewing and not yet here. Many anticipatory gestures of the past decade have been well intentioned but wasteful, and some clinicians, administrators, and agencies that are in the storms' path have "hunkered down," seemingly to wait it out, hoping the storm would blow over and nothing would change. However, a critical mass of industry leaders are clearly committed to improving patient safety, are willing to learn from their own mistakes, and, in unprecedented fashion, are willing to work together to support patient safety research, implementation research, and dissemination research, all with an unwavering focus on improved health care delivery. Hope is on the horizon.

The Patient Safety and Quality Improvement Act of 2005 (S. 544; AHRQ, 2010) was passed after years of debate and revision. The goal was a national law to make it easier for providers to report and learn from medical errors. It took 3 years for AHRQ to issue the first proposed rules to implement that legislation (February 2008), and the law took effect in 2009. More than 80 patient safety organizations are AHRQ certified as of June 1, 2010 and efforts are underway to develop systematic and industry-wide methods to learn from the patient safety data collected by PSOs to improve care.

Public reporting of hospital quality and safety data is increasing in both the United States and abroad. As data is reported, there are new challenges regarding what to report and how to use reported data. Scientific and policy discussions focus on the strength of the evidence for what is reported, whether reported data is sound and equally important, whether the reported data is useful to stimulate improvement activity (Battles & Stevens, 2009; Benn et al., 2009; Jha, Orav, & Epstein, 2009; Pham et al., 2010; Rosenthal & Riley, 2001; Rothberg, Morsi, Benjamin, Pekow, & Lindenauer, 2008).

Accrediting bodies developed standards highlighting the importance and delineating accountability for quality and safety within hospitals (Joint Commission on Accreditation of Healthcare Organizations, 2003; NQF, 2005). The Joint Commission reports that whereas compliance with its safety goals and standards is high, there has been limited change in the safety outcomes that it monitors (www.jointcommissionreport.org). However, it continues to refine standards and safety goals, align them with emerging evidence, and enlist the support of scientific partners and professional societies in a model of collaborative effort that is novel and promising (Farrell, 2009; The Joint Commission, 2008).

The NQF (www.qualityforum.org) continues to add to its list of consensus standards (which are now more than 600), has a list of safe practices that are updated every 2 years, and for the third time since its 2003 inception, NQF is revisiting and refining its widely embraced list of serious reportable events.

The Centers for Medicare and Medicaid services (www.cms.gov) is paying for performance (P4P), although the list of measures adopted by CMS has generated some controversy over the existence and strength of the evidence for the measures selected (Centers for Medicare & Medicaid Services, 2010) and the sheer number of measures (anticipated to top 50 by 2011, and 75 by 2012, with an expectation that there will be a capacity for direct electronic data capture for some measures). However, the mere existence of a P4P process from the largest payer in the country has expedited efforts to develop valid measures for quality and safety outcomes.

Industry quality leaders such as the Institute for Healthcare Improvement (IHI) continue to shine a light on pressing quality and safety issues (Batalden & Davidoff, 2007; Berwick, 2009; Conway, 2008), encourage providers to become more efficient and effective (Berwick, 2003), and provide a forum for quality improvement, patient safety education, and training at all levels within health care, from board members to frontline staff.

Business groups such as Leapfrog (www.leapfroggroup.org) are aligning their standards for hospital performance with industry efforts such as reducing CLABSI.

Funders such as AHRQ are not only testing the waters with novel approaches to implement evidence for quality and safety on a national level; they are exploring diverse ways to "push" evidence for research that they funded into the field (www.innovations.ahrq.gov, www.psnet.ahrq.gov).

Perhaps, most importantly, health policy leaders are also on board, and the recent health policy reform legislation has specific language and provisions to expedite improvement. The Patient Centered Outcomes Research Act of 2009 sets the stage for the consideration of health delivery as science.

The efforts are aligned, the momentum is building, and the potential is real. Nurses, however, must help lead the transformation, or it is doomed to falter. No other discipline is closer to the core work, regardless of the setting, regardless of the patient population, regardless of the delivery model.

■ CONCLUSIONS

Patient safety is a nascent science and valid evidence for how to improve is scant. However, on a daily basis, nurses are part of the provider team that is charged with making it happen. At this early stage of scientific development, it is critical that above all else, nurses understand the importance of their voice, keep patients as their North Star, remember that the science is new to everyone, and commit to be part of leading the evolutionary process. There are few answers for ways to improve patient safety, or how to translate emerging evidence into practice most effectively. We must learn together: nurses, doctors, patients, administrators, and regulators. Every paradigm we have in health care came from an age when scientific discovery was slow, all data was patient-specific, and we considered many of the most distressing outcomes inevitable. All of that has changed. Now we must change as well. The future is ours, and although it may seem murky, chaotic, and uncertain, it is rich with the potential for breathtaking progress.

■ REFERENCES

Agency for Healthcare Research and Quality. (2008). *Press release: AHRQ awards $3 million to help reduce central line-associated bloodstream infections in hospitals ICUs.* Retrieved from http://www.ahrq.gov/news/press/pr2008/clabipr.htm

Agency for Healthcare Research and Quality. (2009a). *National healthcare disparities report.* Rockville, MD: Author.

Agency for Healthcare Research and Quality. (2009b). *National healthcare quality report.* Rockville, MD: Author.

Agency for Healthcare Research and Quality. (2010). *Patient safety organizations.* Retrieved from http://www.pso.ahrq.gov/index.html

Auerbach, A. D., Landefeld, C. S., & Shojania, K. G. (2007). The tension between needing to improve care and knowing how to do it. *The New England Journal of Medicine, 357*(6), 608–613.

Barry, D. R. (2005). Governance: Critical issues for hospital CEO and boards. *Frontiers of Health Services Management, 21*(3), 25–29.

Batalden, P. B., & Davidoff, F. (2007). What is "quality improvement" and how can it transform healthcare? *Quality & Safety in Health Care, 16*(1), 2–3.

Battles, J. B., & Stevens, D. P. (2009). Adverse event reporting systems and safer healthcare. *Quality & Safety in Health Care, 18*(1), 2.

Benn, J., Koutantji, M., Wallace, L., Spurgeon, P., Rejman, M., Healey, A., & Vincent, C. (2009). Feedback from incident reporting: Information and action to improve patient safety. *Quality & Safety in Health Care, 18*(1), 11–21.

Berenholtz, S. M., Pronovost, P. J., Lipsett, P. A., Hobson, D., Earsing, K., Farley, J. E., . . . Perl, T. M. (2004). Eliminating catheter-related bloodstream infections in the intensive care unit. *Critical Care Medicine, 32*(10), 2014–2020.

Berenholtz, S. M., Pronovost, P. J., Ngo, K., Barie, P. S., Hitt, J., Kuti, J. L., . . . Dorman, T. (2007). Developing quality measures for sepsis care in the ICU. *Joint Commission Journal on Quality and Patient Safety, 33*(9), 559–568.

Berwick, D. M. (2003). Disseminating innovations in health care. *The Journal of the American Medical Association, 289*(15), 1969–1975.

Berwick, D. M. (2009). What 'patient-centered' should mean: Confessions of an extremist. *Health Affairs, 28*(4), w555–w565.

Bogdanich, W. (2010, Jan. 23). Radiation offers new cures, and ways to do harm. *The New York Times,* Retrieved from www.nytimes.com/2010/01/24/health/24radiation.html

Callendar, A. N., Hastings, D. A., Hemsley, M. C., Morris, L., & Peregrine, M. W. (2007). Corporate responsibility and health care quality: A resource for health care boards of directors. Washington, DC: U.S. Department of Health and Human Services, American Health Lawyers Association.

Centers for Medicare & Medicaid Services. (2010). *Hospital-acquired conditions.* Retrieved from http://www.cms.hhs.gov/HospitalAcqCond/06_Hospital-Acquired_Conditions.asp

The Commonwealth Fund Commission on a High Performance Health System. (2008). *Why not the best? Results from the national scorecard on U.S. health system performance, 2008.* New York, NY: Author.

Conway, J. (2008). Getting boards on board: Engaging governing boards in quality and safety. *Joint Commission Journal on Quality and Patient Safety, 34*(4), 214–220.

Faber, M., Bosch, M., Wollersheim, H., Leatherman, S., & Grol, R. (2009). Public reporting in health care: How do consumers use quality-of-care information? A systematic review. *Medical Care, 47*(1), 1–8.

Farrell, R. P. (2009). *National patient safety goals for 2009—universal protocol.* Oakbrook Terrace, IL: Joint Commission Resources. Retrieved from http://www.jcrinc.com/NPSG-Universal-Protocol

Goeschel, C. A., Bourgault, A., Palleschi, M., Posa, P., Harrison, D., Tacia, L. L., . . . Bosen, D. M. (2006). Nursing lessons from the MHA keystone ICU project: Developing and implementing an innovative approach to patient safety. *Critical Care Nursing Clinics of North America, 18*(4), 481–492.

Graham, I. D., Harrison, M. B., Brouwers, M., Davies, B. L., & Dunn, S. (2002). Facilitating the use of evidence in practice: Evaluating and adapting clinical practice guidelines for local use by health care organizations. *Journal of Obstetric, Gynecologic, and Neonatal Nursing, 31*(5), 599–611.

Graham, I. D., & Logan, J. (2004). Innovations in knowledge transfer and continuity of care. *The Canadian Journal of Nursing Research, 36*(2), 89–103.

Graham, I. D., Logan, J., Harrison, M. B., Straus, S. E., Tetroe, J., Caswell, W., & Robinson, N. (2006). Lost in knowledge translation: Time for a map? *The Journal of Continuing Education in the Health Professions, 26*(1), 13–24.

Graham, M. J., Kubose, T. K., Jordan, D., Zhang, J., Johnson, T. R., & Patel, V. L. (2004). Heuristic evaluation of infusion pumps: Implications for patient safety in intensive care units. *International Journal of Medical Informatics, 73*(11–12), 771–779.

Greenhalgh, T., Robert, G., Macfarlane, F., Bate, P., & Kyriakidou, O. (2004). Diffusion of innovations in service organizations: Systematic review and recommendations. *The Milbank Quarterly, 82*(4), 581–629.

Hayward, R. A., Asch, S. M., Hogan, M. M., Hofer, T. P., & Kerr, E. A. (2005). Sins of omission: Getting too little medical care may be the greatest threat to patient safety. *Journal of General Internal Medicine, 20*(8), 686–691.

Heifetz, R. A. (1994). *Leadership without easy answers.* Cambridge, MA: Belknap Press of Harvard University Press.

Heifetz, R. A., & Linsky, M. (2002). *Leadership on the line: Staying alive through the dangers of leading.* Boston, MA: Harvard Business School Press.

Holzmueller, C. G., Timmel, J., Kent, P. S., Schulick, R. D., & Pronovost, P. J. (2009). Implementing a team-based daily goals sheet in a non-ICU setting. *Joint Commission Journal on Quality and Patient Safety, 35*(7), 384–388.

Institute of Medicine. (1999). In L. T. Kohn, J. M. Corrigan, and M. S. Donaldson (Eds.), *To err is human: Building a safer health system.* Washington, DC: National Academy Press.

Institute of Medicine. (2001). *Crossing the quality chasm: A new health system for the 21st century.* Washington, DC: National Academy Press.

Jewell, K., & McGiffert, L. (2009). *To err is human—to delay is deadly.* Yonkers, NY: Consumers Union.

Jha, A. K., Orav, E. J., & Epstein, A. M. (2009). Public reporting of discharge planning and rates of readmissions. *The New England Journal of Medicine, 361*(27), 2637–2645.

Jiang, H. J., Lockee, C., Bass, K., & Fraser, I. (2008). Board engagement in quality: Findings of a survey of hospital and system leaders. *Journal of Healthcare Management, 53*(2), 121–134.

The Joint Commission. (2008). *NPSG 02.05.01 standardized approach to hand-offs.* Retrieved from http://www.jointcommission.org/sentinel_event_statistics_quarterly

The Joint Commission. (2010). *Sentinel event statistics.* Retrieved from http://www.jointcommission .org/sentinel_event_statistics_quarterly

The Joint Commission on Accreditation of Healthcare Organizations. (2003). 2004 national patient safety goals. Retrieved from http://www.jointcommission.org

Leape, L. L. (2010). *Transparency and public reporting are essential for a safe health care system.* The Commonwealth Fund. Retrieved from http://www.commonwealthfund.org/Content/Publications/Perspectives-on-Health-Reform-Briefs/2010/Mar/Transparency-and-Public-Reporting-Are-Essential-for-a-Safe-Health-Care-System.aspx

Leape, L. L., & Berwick, D. M. (2005). Five years after To Err Is Human: What have we learned? *The Journal of the American Medical Association, 293*(19), 2384–2390.

Leatherman, S., Berwick, D., Iles, D., Lewin, L. S., Davidoff, F., Nolan, T., & Bisognano, M. (2003). The business case for quality: Case studies and an analysis. *Health Affairs, 22*(2), 17–30.

Malloch, K., & Porter-O'Grady, T. (2010). *Introduction to evidence-based practice in nursing and health care* (2nd ed.). Sudbury, MA: Jones and Bartlett Publishers LLC.

McGlynn, E. A., Asch, S. M., Adams, J., Keesey, J., Hicks, J., DeCristofaro, A., & Kerr, E. A. (2003). The quality of health care delivered to adults in the United States. *The New England Journal of Medicine, 348*(26), 2635–2645.

Murray, C. J., & Frenk, J. (2010). Ranking 37th—measuring the performance of the U.S. health care system. *The New England Journal of Medicine, 362*(2), 98–99.

National Quality Forum. (2005). Hospital governing board and quality of care: A call to responsibility. *Trustee: The Journal for Hospital Governing Boards, 58*(3), 15–18.

Needham, D. M., Sinopoli, D. J., Dinglas, V. D., Berenholtz, S. M., Korupolu, R., Watson, S. R., . . . Pronovost, P. J. (2009). Improving data quality control in quality improvement projects. *International Journal for Quality in Health Care, 21*(2), 145–150.

Patient Centered Outcomes Research Act of 2009. Retrieved June 17, 2011 from http://www.chsr .org/The%20Patient-Centered%20Outcomes%20Research%20Act%20of%202009.pdf

Pham, J. C., Colantuoni, E., Dominici, F., Shore, A., Macrae, C., Scobie, S., . . . Pronovost, P. J. (2010). The harm susceptibility model: A method to prioritise risks identified in patient safety reporting systems. *Quality and Safety in Health Care, 19*(5), 440–445.

Pronovost, P., Berenholtz, S., Dorman, T., Lipsett, P. A., Simmonds, T., & Haraden, C. (2003). Improving communication in the ICU using daily goals. *Journal of Critical Care, 18*(2), 71–75.

Pronovost, P., Needham, D., Berenholtz, S., Sinopoli, D., Chu, H., Cosgrove, S., . . . Goeschel, C. (2006). An intervention to decrease catheter-related bloodstream infections in the ICU. *The New England Journal of Medicine, 355*(26), 2725–2732.

Pronovost, P., Weast, B., Rosenstein, B., Sexton, J. B., Holzmueller, C. G., Paine, L., . . . Rubin, H. R. (2005). Implementing and validating a comprehensive unit-based safety program. *Journal of Patient Safety, 1*(1), 33–40.

Pronovost, P. J., Berenholtz, S. M., Goeschel, C. A., Needham, D. M., Sexton, J. B., Thompson, D. A., . . . Hunt, E. (2006). Creating high reliability in healthcare organizations. *Health Services Research, 41*(4 Pt. 2), 1599–1617.

Pronovost, P. J., Berenholtz, S. M., Goeschel, C. A., Thom, I., Watson, S. R., Holzmueller, C. G., . . . Sexton, J. B. (2007). Improving patient safety in Michigan intensive care units. *Journal of Critical Care, 22*, 1–5.

Pronovost, P. J., Berenholtz, S. M., & Needham, D. M. (2008). Translating evidence into practice: A model for large scale knowledge translation. *British Medical Journal, 337*, a1714.

Pronovost, P. J., Goeschel, C. A., Colantuoni, E., Watson, S., Lubomski, L. H., Berenholtz, S. M., . . . Needham, D. (2010). Sustaining reductions in catheter related bloodstream infections in Michigan intensive care units: Observational study. *British Medical Journal, 340*, c309.

Pronovost, P. J., Goeschel, C. A., Marsteller, J. A., Sexton, J. B., Pham, J. C., & Berenholtz, S. M. (2009). Framework for patient safety research and improvement. *Circulation, 119*(2), 330–337.

Pronovost, P. J., Goeschel, C. A., & Wachter, R. M. (2008). The wisdom and justice of not paying for "preventable complications". *The Journal of the American Medical Association, 299*(18), 2197–2199.

Pronovost, P. J., Holzmueller, C. G., Martinez, E., Cafeo, C. L., Hunt, D., Dickson, C., . . . Makary, M. A. (2006). A practical tool to learn from defects in patient care. *Joint Commission Journal on Quality and Safety, 32*(2), 102–108.

Pronovost, P. J., Miller, M., & Wachter, R. M. (2007). The GAAP in quality measurement and reporting. *The Journal of the American Medical Association, 298*(15), 1800–1802.

Pronovost, P. J., Weast, B., Bishop, K., Paine, L., Griffith, R., Rosenstein, B. J., . . . Davis, R. (2004). Senior executive adopt-a-work unit: A model for safety improvement. *Joint Commission Journal on Quality and Safety, 30*(2), 59–68.

Reason, J. (2002). Combating omission errors through task analysis and good reminders. *Quality and Safety in Health Care, 11*(1), 40–44.

Rogers, E. (Ed.). (1995). *Diffusion of innovations* (4th ed.). New York, NY: Free Press.

Rosenthal, J., & Riley, T. (2001). *Patient safety and medical errors: A roadmap for state action*. Portland, ME: National Academy for State Health Policy.

Rothberg, M. B., Morsi, E., Benjamin, E. M., Pekow, P. S., & Lindenauer, P. K. (2008). Choosing the best hospital: The limitations of public quality reporting. *Health Affairs, 27*(6), 1680–1687.

Schwartz, J. M., Nelson, K. L., Saliski, M., Hunt, E. A., & Pronovost, P. J. (2008). The daily goals communication sheet: A simple and novel tool for improved communication and care. *Joint Commission Journal on Quality and Patient Safety, 34*(10), 608–613, 561.

Timmel, J., Kent, P. S., Holzmueller, C. G., Paine, L. A., Schulick, R. D., & Pronovost, P. J. (2010). Impact of the Comprehensive Unit-based Safety Program (CUSP) on safety culture in a surgical inpatient unit. *Joint Commission Journal on Quality and Patient Safety, 36*(6), 252–260.

U.S. Department of Health & Human Services. (2009). *HHS action plan to prevent healthcare-associated infections.* Retrieved from http://www.hhs.gov/ophs/initiatives/hai/infection.html

Wachter, R. M. (2004). The end of the beginning: Patient safety five years after 'to err is human'. *Health Affairs,* Supp Web Exclusives: W4-534–545.

Waxman (2008). Retrieved June 17, 2011 from http://oversight-archive.waxman.house.gov/story.asp?id=2187

Weingart, S. N., Toro, J., Spencer, J., Duncombe, D., Gross, A., Bartel, S., . . . Connor, M. (2010). Medication errors involving oral chemotherapy. *Cancer, 116*(10), 2455–2464.

Woodward, H. I., Mytton, O. T., Lemer, C., Yardley, I. E., Ellis, B. M., Rutter, P. D., . . . Wu, A. W. (2010). What have we learned about interventions to reduce medical errors? *Annual Review of Public Health, 31,* 479–497.

CHAPTER SIX

Translation of Evidence for Leadership

Mary Terhaar

Leaders whose organizations thrive in the demanding environment of industry today have an aptitude and a discipline for connecting people with purpose (Fullen, 2009). These effective leaders know their people, know their strengths and passions, and put them to work in service of a well-focused vision articulated as compelling strategic intent (Kotter, 1990). Leadership in nursing is no different: The success of the organization depends on connecting people with purpose.

The work of translating evidence into practice provides a perfect vehicle through which to accomplish such connections and improve outcomes for patients, organizations, and communities. The challenge is to create environments and cultures that systematically support the work of translation, reward initiative, and accelerate the success of engaged individuals and the projects they undertake. Because health care systems are complex, they are likely to change in less linear, less predictable ways, as contrasted with systems in simpler industries (Rorbach et al., 2006). As a result, nurse leaders need to develop structures, processes, and resources for translation that simultaneously promote fidelity with the target innovation and suitable adaptation to assure success in the target environment (Leape & Berwick, 2005). Although fidelity and adaptability may appear in opposition, both play a critical role in a type of creative tension that produces results.

Improving public health and financial accountability will not be achieved without effective leadership. Accountable leaders will rise to the challenges set by the Institute for Medicine to reduce error (2000), achieve true quality (2001), and transform the workplace (2004) to achieve outcomes. The report To Err is Human (2000) directs health care as an industry to reduce error in meaningful ways that will translate to significantly improved public health. The report Crossing the Quality Chasm (2001) calls clinicians, leaders and managers to deliver on the investment in research by developing ways to translate its application and improve outcomes. The report Keeping Patients Safe: Transforming the Work Environment of Nurses (2004) calls for resolution of the root causes of error and poor quality. Evidence has bearing for the targets set, strategies selected, implementation of operations and innovations, and evaluation of performance. Leaders need evidence for their practice and need to act on evidence for clinical practice as well.

The purpose of this chapter is to present a body of knowledge about leadership that applies to the work of translation. Culture and environment are addressed in other chapters, and so the focus here will be on the strategies and practices of leaders, whose nursing staff surf the wave of translation and evidence-based practice to attain professional success and practice excellence.

■ LEADERS

Leaders help organizations cope with change. They motivate and inspire people to achieve a compelling vision (Kotter, 1990). Leaders can be recognized by their active stance toward goals, high level of personal engagement, clear orientation to opportunity, and inspiring energy (Zaleznik, 1977). They create environments that invite people to connect to the mission by improving their own work products, as well as the work of the team (Laschinger et al., 2004).

An Informed and Engaged Executive

Key to consistent, successful penetration of evidence-based practice throughout a nursing organization is an informed executive that establishes translation as a critical component of the strategic plan, with strong links to the business performance targets. Knowledge of the mechanics of translation, as well as workforce responses to the work, positions the executive to lead effectively (Sredl, 2008). Specifically, practiced ability to search the literature, evaluate the evidence, and draw trustworthy conclusions will help secure the greatest gain from translation activities. Just as translation has yet to penetrate clinical practice, so too knowledge of translation and expertise, with respect to its application, remain underdeveloped among the nurse executives who set performance targets and allocate resources for practice (Sredl, 2008). Educating leadership, resourcing it effectively, grounding all strategy deeply in evidence, and highlighting accomplishments that derive from translation will help to develop the knowledge and expertise organizations will need for consistent, effective performance improvement based on application of evidence.

Today's nursing workforce is diverse in age, experience, and educational preparation. Forty-five percent (45.4%), the largest subset of practicing nurses, have earned associates degrees, 34.2% have earned baccalaureate degrees, and the remaining 20.4% have earned diplomas. Between 2004 and 2008, the education of RNs changed. Those whose initial education was a diploma decreased from 25.6% to 20.4%, whereas those prepared with associate degrees rose from 42.9% to 45.4%, and those entering practice with bachelor of science in nursing (BSN) degrees rose from 31.0% to 33.7% (Health Resources and Services Administration [HRSA], 2010).

The result of this shift is that the significant majority of the workforce has not developed the foundation for evaluation of evidence or translation of research as a component of their curriculum. Effective engagement of this segment of the workforce in translation and evidence-based practice requires leadership by example (Ferguson, Milner, & Snelgrove-Clarke, 2004). Leadership is required to consistently and clearly articulate the rationale for decisions based on evidence and to build systems that support practicing nurses as they develop the skills and critical thinking strategies required to discipline practice with sound evidence. Yet, nurses have a clear preference for social learning above more traditional pedagogies (Ferguson et al.). This asserts a claim on nursing leaders to model and teach the basics for translation even as it requires them to make available resources and tools to facilitate the work. Partnerships with academics are likely to prove constructive in these endeavors (Springer, Corbett, & Davis, 2006) but will not substitute for nursing leadership with experience and understanding of the mechanics and the benefits of translation.

Promote Evidence-Based Management Practices

A growing body of literature makes strong connections between staffing and outcomes (Lacey et al., 2007; Needleman, Beurhaus, Mattke, Stewart, & Zelevinsky, 2002). Patient outcomes improved when registered nurses provided a higher proportion of the care, and when patients had access to more hours of care by registered nurses (Aiken, Clarke, Sloane, Sochalski, & Silber, 2010).

In one systematic review including six studies of acute care hospitals, an overall incidence of adverse events was reported to be 9.2% of which 43.5% could have been prevented (Cho, Hwang, & Kim, 2008; de Vries, Ramrattan, Smorenburg, Gouma, & Boermeester, 2008). Nursing care in the form of monitoring and intervention would have been central to reducing the risk of such adverse events (Lucero, Lake, & Aiken, 2009). And yet, social pressures to contain cost conspire to reduce the numbers of nurses available to conduct such protective surveillance. The result is diminished quality of care (Aiken, Clarke, Sloane, Sochalski, & Silber, 2002; Hanrahan, Kumar, & Aiken, 2010) that is reported in the literature as error, incomplete nursing action, missed opportunity, undetected risk, and failure to rescue.

Failure to Rescue

Higher numbers of nursing hours provided by registered nurses were associated with lower incidence of failure to rescue ($P = .05$), in the event of shock, pneumonia, cardiac arrest, upper gastrointestinal bleeding, sepsis, and deep vein thrombosis (Needleman et al., 2002). These findings were reported from a study in which 799 hospitals from 11 states participated. The review included 5,075,969 medical patients and 1,104,659 surgical discharges.

Among surgical patients with comorbid mental illness, staffing and education of nurses influenced outcomes (Kutney-Lee & Aiken, 2008). Among 228,433 surgical patients, 4.7% had a serious mental health condition complicating their diagnosis (5.8%; $n = 188$), as compared with patients without complications (7.4%; $n = 4,265$). Patients with mental health conditions experienced more postoperative complications (30.6%; $n = 3,259$) and, yet, failure to rescue was significantly lower. For patients with mental health complications, length of stay (LOS) was found to be 17.4% longer. However, when LOS was contrasted for these patients admitted to hospitals where more than 40% of the nursing staff were prepared at the baccalaureate level, patients in hospitals where less than 20% of the staff had similar education had an LOS 14.8% longer. Educational preparation influenced failure to rescue and LOS. The same is true for staffing. Both relationships were identified for a particularly challenging and risk-prone population.

These findings are consistent with earlier studies of staff-to-patient ratios (Aiken, Clarke, Sloane, et al., 2008) and educational preparation (Aiken, Clarke, Cheung, Sloane, & Silber, 2003). Society asks hospitals and providers to more carefully husband health care dollars, even as it demands better outcomes. Quality nursing care lies at the center of the fulcrum because nursing provides the surveillance system that can identify when resource allocation efforts interfere with outcomes attainment. Nursing can change the resource equation to assure targets are obtained. Among the most trusted of the professions, nursing can advocate for providers from many disciplines to engage and intervene for effective problem solving. Nursing can mobilize colleagues as appropriate to complete the team, reduce delay, avoid omission, and increase the quality of care. This is only possible if nurses are available, present, educated, and empowered to take this role.

Maximize the Workforce Capabilities of RNs

Deploying nurses in appropriate numbers with necessary complements of skill is required to assure that required nursing actions are executed, and this is associated with quality and safety (Aiken et al., 2003, 2005, & 2008). In one study of 8,670 practicing nurses, 40% reported leaving at least three tasks incomplete at the end of a shift. These incomplete nursing actions were found to explain the largest portion of variance (B = -0.21, $SE + 0.004$; $P < .001$) in quality when factored with workload and patient safety issues (Sochalski, 2004).

Nurses do not consistently meet all needs of patients and have described in detail the nature of the activities and interventions they cannot complete (Lucero et al., 2009). Nurses from 168 hospitals across Pennsylvania self-report failure to update plans of care (42%), provide comfort for and talk with patients (40.3%), provide skin care and back rubs (31.7%), educate patients and families (28.5%), document interventions and responses (21.4%), attend to oral hygiene (20.8%), and complete discharge preparation (12.9%).

Because unmet needs for nursing care have been related to decrease in overall quality, strategies that increase the ability of nurses to complete their work hold potential to increase the quality and improve outcomes. Increasing staffing by one full-time RN per patient day produces increased quality as measured by decreased hospital-associated mortality in critical care (odds ratio, 0.91; 95% confidence interval; 0.86–0.96), surgical care (odds ratio, 0.84; 95% confidence interval; 0.80–0.89), and medical care (odds ratio, 0.94: 95% confidence interval; 0.94–0.95). Ninety-six studies from a total of 2,858 were included in a meta-analysis of outcomes associated with staffing. A dose response for nurse staffing was consistent across studies. Reducing patient load in critical care from 3.3 to 2 was associated a 6% reduction in death. Reducing patient load on medical units from 5 to 2 decreased death rate by 38%, and in surgical units reducing assignments from 5 to 2.8 was associated with a 35% reduction. Nursing staffing was consistently effective as a means to reduce mortality (Kane, Shamliyan, Mueller, Duval, & Wilt, 2007). Identifying the dose of nursing required for quality outcomes is a complex challenge and so proscribing the correct dose for an individual unit or population is as well. Manojlovich et al. (2011) reviewed findings from 100 studies and found RN: patient ratio and RN hours per patient day predicted MRSA infection rates and falls. The team concluded nursing dose is a critical concern for patients, nurses, leadership, and society.

■ ACTIVE STANCE TOWARD GOALS

Effective leaders work in ways that distribute both responsibility and credit: decentralization is the key (Kotter, 1990). In industry, decentralization is commonly accomplished by deploying teams and task forces. These are groups of workers, close to the customer or the service, and deployed to meet a particular challenge or respond to a specific customer need. Teams and taskforces used in nursing usually focus on well-defined assignments that are limited in time and scope, and frequently consultative in nature. These teams may make recommendations to an executive that often retains authority for the decisions, or they may themselves have authority by charge, charter, structure, or policy.

In successful organizations, inclusive strategies drive decisions close to the point of service (Fullen, 2008). In nursing, participative management, implemented as shared governance, has been demonstrated effective as a means to improve quality, customer satisfaction, staff retention, cost management, and to satisfy market demands (Porter-O'Grady, 2004). So persuasive are the results that Practice Standard 1 of the Pathway to Excellence requires *Nurses Control the Practice of Nursing* for a nursing organization to earn Magnet recognition (American Nurses Credentialing Center [ANCC], 2008). Nurses may accomplish the work of translation in teams on patient care units or in inclusive structures that by design cut across all patient care areas, specialties, roles, levels of education, and experience. Regardless, effective nurse leaders distribute responsibility and accomplishment across the nurses responsible for care and outcomes (American Association of Colleges of Nursing [AACN], 2010).

If the work of nursing were effectively managed by traditional, centralized, top-down structures, then practice would be error-free, because command and control has historically been the dominant design. This, however, is not the case (Crow, 2006). The original Magnet hospital studies and the impressive body of work to follow has established that linear, hierarchical structures do not produce the best results with respect to health care because people and health are nonlinear in nature.

Effective nurse leaders hardwire application of evidence in the day-to-day work of nursing. In a high-performing nursing institution, translation is the norm; not a special project (Stetler et al., 1999, 2003, 2007). Data and responsibility are woven into the work of translation, quality, safety, and performance improvement (Institute of Medicine [IOM], 2004). These processes harness industry of nursing to improve service, outcomes, and capacity. They are approaches that create an active stance toward goals and an orientation toward opportunities.

■ ORIENTATION TO OPPORTUNITY

Nurses Improve Practice

Magnet organizations are poised to be the innovators of future best practices to improve nursing practice, including development of patient partnerships, implementation and translation of evidence-based practice, and dissemination and translation of new technologies (Wolf, Triolo, & Ponte, 2008). In 2008, the ANCC announced a new model for the Magnet recognition program that translates the original 14 forces of magnetism into five model components: (a) transformational leadership; (b) structural empowerment; (c) exemplary professional practice; (d) new knowledge, innovations, and improvements; and (e) empirical outcomes. The five components are interrelated. For example, meeting the transformational leadership component requires that the leader acquires, evaluates, and translates evidence into organizational decision making, and continuous improvement to foster structural empowerment, exemplary professional practice, and implementation of new knowledge into

practice. This new model includes sources of evidence and empiric outcomes that, by definition, accentuate transformational nursing leadership (Meredith, Cohen, & Raia, 2010).

Magnet hospitals report improved patient outcomes, including lower morbidity and
mortality rates and increased satisfaction. These improvements are accompanied by improved
outcomes for nurses as well, including decreased needle sticks, burnout, and turnover (Clarke,
2007; Friese, Lake, Aiken, Silber, & Sochalski, 2008). Cumulatively, the result is higher
nurse satisfaction and improved financial performance across the organization (Armstrong &
Laschinger, 2006; Armstrong, Laschinger, & Wong, 2009; Brady-Schwartz, 2005).

The impressive outcomes reported by Magnet hospitals result from the infrastructure
and culture they share. Nurses in these facilities are empowered to solve problems, educated
to do so effectively, and supported with staffing patterns that reflect a value for the their contribution as knowledge workers, critical thinkers, and problem solvers (Kane-Urabazzo, 2006;
Aiken et al., 2001, 2008, 2009). This translates to improved safety and quality outcomes
(Laschinger et al., 2001, 2006, 2008; Armstrong, et al., 2009). Physician staffing patterns have
the same effect. Staffing to the population, volume and acuity improves outcomes (Pronovost
et al., 2002). New nurses, brought to the bedside in ways that communicate respect and value
are less likely to experience burnout and less likely to experience burnout and other negative
outcomes that can compromise care (De Wolf et al., 2010; Laschinger et al., 2010).

The evidence on reducing variability in practice and assuring consistent application
of evidence to improve outcomes also makes clear that engaged nurses improve practice.
Pronovost (Pronovost et al., 2010; Goeschel et al., 2011; Sexton et al., 2011) worked with
teams of physicians, nurses, therapists, and others in the ICU to develop checklists that
helped to reduce variability in practice, and resulted in decreased rate of infection, length of
stay, cost per case and sequelae. Gawande (2009), in his bestseller about checklists, professionals, and practice outcomes, emphasizes the critical importance of providing nurses with
tools and gravitas to address practice issues. A modest tool such as a checklist, although
dismissed by some, holds potential to improve performance not as a substitute for critical
thinking, but, rather, as a trigger for details that can be lost among the competing demands
of complex clinical cases, practice environments, and health care systems. Simple strategies
such as the checklist are well suited to practice environments where variability is found within
nursing, medicine, and other disciplines as well.

Although the engagement of nurses in translation contributes significantly to its success, the pace of change is not without negative impact (Crow, 2006). This knowledge makes
clear that nurses' participation in planning and evaluation is key. Such involvement can di-
minish unintended negative consequences and, as a result, mitigate the negative effects of
constant change in the practice environment (Clarke, 2007; Cheney, 2008).

■ THE WORK ENVIRONMENT OF NURSES

Climate

Work climate refers to the perceptions of the work environment including perceptions of
decision making, justice, leadership and other norms held by those who practice in it (Stone
et al., 2005). In a meta analysis of 6 studies funded by the Agency for Health Care Quality, in
which 80,000 health care workers participated, perceptions of climate including leadership,

organizational structure, supervision, behaviors of the group, emphasis on quality, and work design accounted for 24–65% of the variance in satisfaction. These findings make clear the importance of the work environment with respect to satisfaction and ultimately performance of staff. Managing the climate for practice is essential to providing safe care (Stone et al., 2007a), promoting safety for staff (Stone et al., 2006a & 2006b) and retaining qualified nurses (Stone et al., 2007b) and each outcome supports the other.

If climate has to do with perceptions of the practice environment, then primary nursing, education, supervision and violence prevention interventions have been supported as effective practices in that climate (Schalk, Bijl et al., 2010). The managers themselves and their ability to express authentic caring about staff constibute positively to perceptions of the work environment. This translates to a favorable climate for practice (Wade et al., 2008) as does a perception of fairness in dealings with reports (Williams et al., 2006). The same would hold true for Shared Governance which enjoys well documented success. (Porter-O'Grady, 2000 & 2001). This approach to inclusive leadership and decision making translates to a climate where practicing nurses are involved and have a sense of potency in decisions that affect their work and work environment).

Infrastructure and perceptions of a supportive work environment are central to the body of work related to Magnet hospitals. Magnet hospitals are those able to present evidence of the presence of the Forces of Magnetism. They share a climate, culture, and environment in which nursing thrives and produces significant constructive outcomes for patients, the institution, for practicing nurses, other professionals and the community (Smith et al., 2006). As a result of significant investment in practice, these hospitals report perceptions among the nurses who practice in them that the culture and the climate support excellence. (Schmalenberg & Kramer, 2008).

Health care lags behind other high-stakes industries with respect to reducing error. Health care has been slow to heighten awareness of risk, recognize potential for failure, focus on adaptability, create readiness for the unexpected, emphasize knowledge and expertise above title and credential, encourage a big-picture perspective, and develop flexibility to flatten any structure as needed. These process improvements are widely recognized as effective in other industries (Weick & Sutcliffe, 2001). Like other industries beginning the work of consistently producing error-free outcomes, health care has relied more heavily on technology than knowledge workers or well-engineered systems despite a growing body of knowledge about effective leadership practices capable of reducing error and risk (Frankel, Leonard, & Denham, 2006).

A solid base of evidence supports involvement of nurses in decisions that impact practice, including work design, work flow, and work process. Such involvement improves clinical, quality, operational, and financial outcomes (Porter-O'Grady, 2004, 2009). It contributes to satisfaction and retention of nurses (Lacey et al., 2007; Laschinger, Finegan, Shamian, & Wilk, 2004; Moore & Hutchison, 2007).

The IOM report *Keeping Patients Safe: Transforming the Work Environment of Nurses* (2004) summarized the evidence, and made five recommendations for nurses and nurse leaders to improve the quality and safety of the nursing work environment:

1. Nurses should participate in *decision making* at all levels—work design and work flow issues.
2. Promote *evidence-based management practices*.

3. Maximize the *workforce capabilities of RNs* and identify the need of RN staffing for each patient care unit per shift.
    a. Recommended that nursing homes have at least one RN on duty at all times.
    b. Recommended that staffing levels increase as the number of patient increases.
4. *Work and workspace design* to prevent and mitigate errors.
    a. Recommended that nursing shifts be limited to 12 hours in any 24-hour period, and no more than 60 hours in a 7-day stretch.
5. Create and sustain a *culture of safety* (IOM, 2004).

Fair and Just Culture

Change in any organization has the potential to stimulate resistance, which ranks high among the reasons that innovations fail. People whose work is impacted by any innovation need to trust that the new approach is safe and valid, need confidence in the leadership driving change, and need to believe that outcomes will be maintained or improved. A practice environment characterized by justice in expectations and treatment across members (distributive) and as a base for policy (procedural) is referred to as a fair and just culture. Such a culture is associated with improved retention, satisfaction, performance, and quality (St-Pierre & Holmes, 2010).

Cameron and Masterson (2000) identified this significant aspect of the change process as the *leader–member exchange* (LMX). *LMX* has been noted to affect perceived fairness in interpersonal interaction and policy (Piccolo, Bardes, Mayer, & Judge, 2008). Although evidence suggests that leaders create this sense of fairness and justice in the workplace, achieving financial performance and productivity targets conspire to decrease the number of managers and leaders available to accomplish this important work. The increased requirements placed on managers, as they take on relatively more responsibility, have been characterized as distributive injustice on the managers themselves (Thorpe & Loo, 2003). It extends to the entire staff inasmuch as it threatens to keep leaders from the important work of creating a fair and just culture for all (St-Pierre & Holmes, 2010).

> Nurse leaders can create an environment in which every member of the team feels a responsibility and is accountable for ensuring that the value of keeping patients safe is upheld. Moving toward a just culture requires that nurse leaders hold themselves and staff accountable as errors are disclosed. This accountability includes understanding why errors occur and identifying what systems, processes, and conditions are at fault. Nurse leaders are also accountable to manage staff so that at-risk behaviors are identified and managed to reduce the risk of error.

The following is the three-behavior model by David Marx (2001):

- Honest human errors made in the context of error-prone systems
- At-risk behavior (should be aware, failure to recognize)
- Reckless behavior (conscious disregard), including intentional rule violations

Evidence-based leadership will discriminate between these three classes and respond in a way that is effective to manage the behavior. The effective leader will recognize human error and focus on solutions rather than blame, will monitor for and mitigate risky behaviors, and will manage and eliminate recklessness.

Executive Rounds

Collaborative walk rounds by leaders and providers have been demonstrated to provide a counterbalance to the pressures of the market for financial outcomes above quality. Such rounds can increase engagement and accountability and improve outcomes (Frankel et al., 2003, 2006). They help to establish a strategic and tactical focus on safety, service, and operations (Pronovost, 2004; Gawande, 2009). In one study, 48 sets of rounds were conducted monthly on 47 different patient care units. Executive leaders, nurses, and others engaged in direct patient care addressed near misses and operational failures with the goal of identifying and mitigating the cause. Data were entered into a log-enabling metalevel analysis of the sources of errors across the organization. (Frankel et al., 2003). From a quality improvement perspective, the data from the journal indicated all parties participating in the rounds found them to be productive. From a leadership perspective, executives engaged in discussions about direct patient care are better informed because they approach decisions that affect that care and the individuals who provide it.

Including executives in clinical rounds assures high-level decisions about resources and environment are informed by real challenges both clinicians and patients face. Such rounds enable leadership to put a practical and personal face on the data shared in dashboards and reports (Denham et al., 2005, 2006). Potentially uncomfortable for the executive, exposure to the point of service translates to informed decisions and improved outcomes. Successful industries have long been aware of the risk of failure which is useful in planning to avoid it. Leaders who participate in work rounds can have a move vivid understanding of both the risk and the implications of failure, and this can translate into an environment more conducive to practice (Frankel et al., 2006).

Interprofessional Collaboration

In a recent Cochrane Review, five randomized controlled trials were found to focus on strategies to enhance interprofessional collaboration. All five were found to have design flaws or methodological weaknesses: sample sizes were small and interventions were varied (walking rounds, video-conferencing, audio-conferencing, case studies, and team meetings). Some measured length of stay and others measured charge per case. Improvement was not consistently reported (Zwarenstein, Goldman, & Reeves, 2009). As a result, further study with larger samples and consistent methods and interventions are needed to support evidence-based collaborative practice.

Rounds are a means to strengthen collaboration. Executive rounds, referred earlier, achieve context and impact for decisions made in board rooms. But daily work rounds, made by physicians, nurses, all disciplines engaged in care and leadership, facilitate clear and direct communication and problem solving along with education and decision support. These rounds decrease mortality, sequelae, and error (Pronovost et al., 1999, 2001). Interprofessional communication is at the anecdote to frustration and root causes of medication error (Manojlovich & DeCicco, 2007).

Team Training

Training for teams to enhance functioning and communication has been proven effective in multiple studies (Cooper & Gaba, 2002; Helmreich & Musson, 2000; Leonard, Graham, &

Bonacum, 2004). The IOM (2004) built on this work in its third report titled *Keeping Patients Safe: Transforming the Work Environment of Nurses*. The document provides a roadmap for nurse leaders with detailed recommendations for staffing, skill sets, work, workspace, shifts, culture, and structure.

Developing the ability of physicians, nurses, and others engaged in patient care to work effectively as teams is one strategy with potential to improve collaboration, quality of care, and the work environment. In one elective, medical students were introduced to non-physician caregivers with the goals of developing understanding, improving communication, introducing the possibilities for collaboration, demonstrating how services offered by other professionals complement the work of the physicians, and improving the students' skill in communicating with nonphysicians. At the close of the 2-week long precepted rotation with a nonphysician professional, students reported a sense of empowerment as a result of their new skills and understanding (Pathak, Hotzmueller, Haller, Pronovost, 2010).

Training for teams is not effective without a culture that values and supports the behaviors on a day-to-day basis. So the "team" must be situated within culture and permeate all work. It is also true that teamwork is learned. Accommodation is needed in the education for caregiving professionals. Traditionally proved in the silos of nursing schools apart from medical schools, social work schools, and other professional schools, effective education for health care professionals needs to incorporate scenarios and team activities where the realities of practice and the interdependence of work comes into clear focus and, in so doing, becomes more effective (Frankel et al., 2006).

Performance Envelope

For any strategy to take root, leadership is required. The work of quality needs to be visible, compelling, and pervasive across the organization and needs a champion with the visibility, authority, tenacity, data, and credibility to take the team through many waves of change (Denham, 2005, 2006). The notion of the performance envelopment proposes to reverse a late adopter position of executive and financial officers by engaging this level of leadership in systems design that promotes safety and eliminates conditions that limit initiative and capability of people from all disciplines engaged in service delivery on the frontline and in support positions (Denham, 2010). The performance envelopment is the safe zone of performance within systems design limits, and includes recognizing the capabilities of people. Success begins and ends with leadership (Denham, 2010).

Sustained Improvement Based on Evidence

Pronovost et al. (2011) determined that bloodstream infections per 1,000 catheter days could be reduced, and improved performance sustained, in critical care units across the state of Michigan. The team implemented five recommendations from the Centers for Disease Control and Prevention including: (a) washing hands before insertion, (b) using full-barrier precautions, (c) preparing the skin with chlorhexidine before insertion, (d) using the femoral site only when use of another site is impossible, and (e) removing catheters as soon as the patient's condition permits. Eighty-seven percent (87%) of the 103 intensive care units originally participating in the project reported a total of 1,532 intensive care unit months of data, comprising 300–310 catheter days as part of a second study focused on sustainability.

Catheter-related bloodstream infection rates reported as mean scores decreased from 7.7 at baseline to 1.3 at 16–18 months and 1.1 at 34–36 months following implementation. During the same period, bloodstream infection rates were unchanged. The intervention designed to reduce catheter-related infections was considered to be specific and effective, and produced sustained improvement in the target measure (Hyzy et al., 2010).

Operations

Operations of the work environment are significant for practice. In a systematic review of the literature including 9000 titles and abstracts, focused on practice environment, Schalk et al. (2010) identified strategies documented as effective to improve the environment. These included very basic items: primary nursing, education tools, individualized care, supervision, and violence prevention. Each of these strategies was supported as effective in only 1 or 2 quality studies. So, while they have face value and empirical evidence to support application, they lack a strong and deep empirical base.

■ ROLE OF ORGANIZATION IN TRANSLATION

Leaders strategically develop capacities that drive innovation, critical to successful translation of evidence, into meaningful performance improvement. These include will, ideas, and execution. Will takes the form of clearly developed aims communicated and embraced across the enterprise. Ideas come from a workforce and leadership constantly engaged in achieving excellence (Reinertsen, Bisognano, & Pugh, 2008). Execution is the discipline to manage performance to targets, to use data to evaluate progress, and to refine plans of action to achieve aims.

Transforming Care at the Bedside

The Transforming the Care at the Bedside (TCAB) initiative, a national program of the Robert Wood Johnson Foundation (RWJF) and Institute for Healthcare Improvement (IHI) began in July 2003 and concluded in August 2008. With so much care being delivered in hospital medical/surgical units, and with an estimated 35%–40% of unexpected hospital deaths occurring on such units, the RWJF and the IHI created an initiative called *Transforming Care at the Bedside* to improve care on medical/surgical units and to increase the amount of time nurses spend caring for patients at the bedside. The initiative was built around improvements in four main categories (Figure 6.1): (a) safe and reliable care, (b) vitality and teamwork, (c) patient-centered care, and (d) value-added care processes (IHI, 2008). TCAB started with 10 hospitals, but has been so successful that more than 5 hospitals have joined the TCAB Learning and Innovation Community, and 68 hospitals are participating in the American Organization of Nurse Executives TCAB Collaborative. The key to this success is leadership support for and implementation of evidence-based management practices such as communication models that support consistent and clear communication among caregivers; professional support programs such as preceptorships and educational opportunities; and redesigned workspaces that enhance efficiency and reduce waste (Rutherford, Lee, & Greiner, 2008; Viney, Batcheller, Houston, & Belcik, 2006).

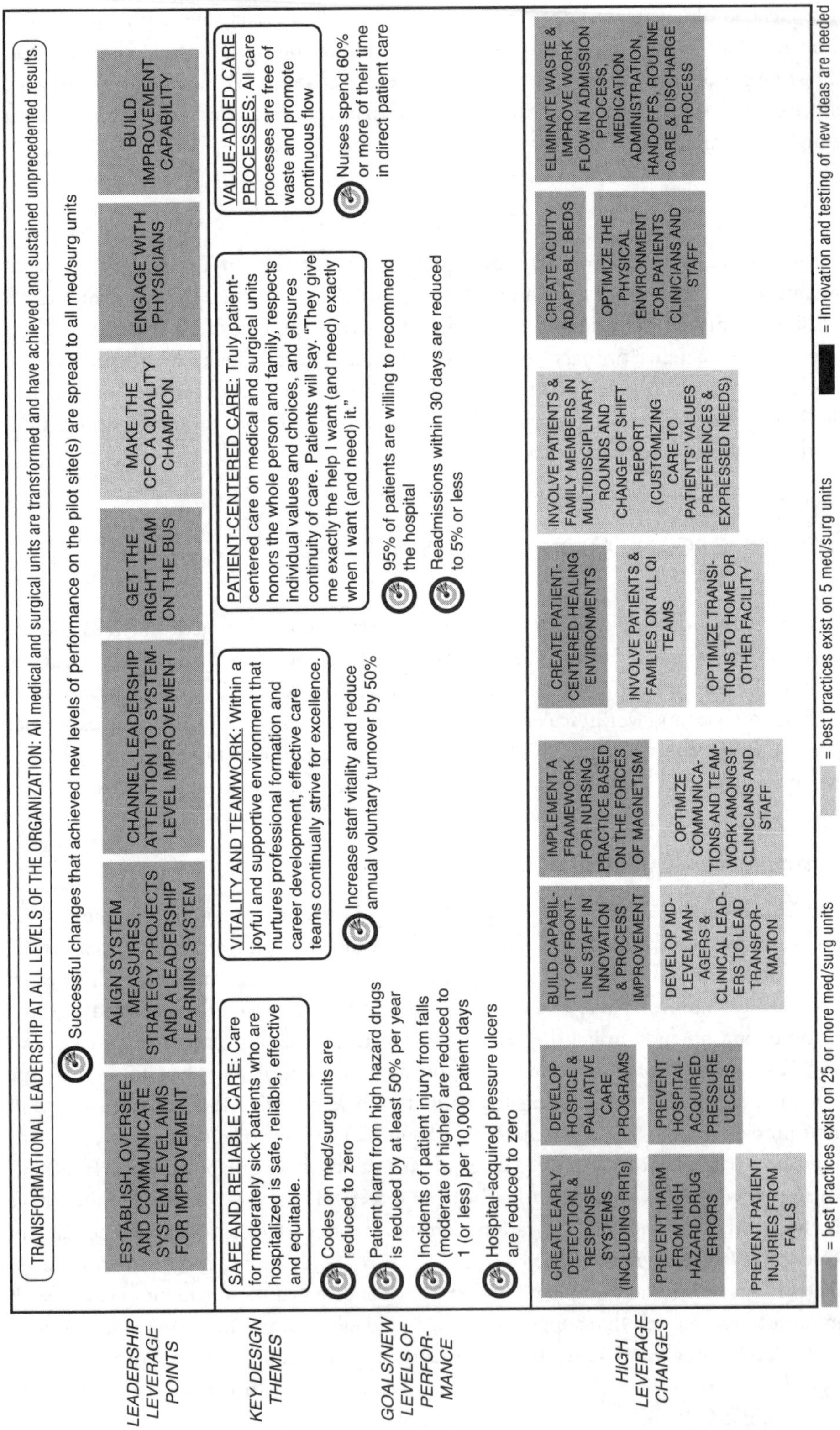

TRANSFORMATIONAL LEADERSHIP AT ALL LEVELS OF THE ORGANIZATION: All medical and surgical units are transformed and have achieved and sustained unprecedented results.

⊘ Successful changes that achieved new levels of performance on the pilot site(s) are spread to all med/surg units

LEADERSHIP LEVERAGE POINTS

| ESTABLISH, OVERSEE AND COMMUNICATE SYSTEM LEVEL AIMS FOR IMPROVEMENT | ALIGN SYSTEM MEASURES, STRATEGY PROJECTS AND A LEADERSHIP LEARNING SYSTEM | CHANNEL LEADERSHIP ATTENTION TO SYSTEM-LEVEL IMPROVEMENT | GET THE RIGHT TEAM ON THE BUS | MAKE THE CFO A QUALITY CHAMPION | ENGAGE WITH PHYSICIANS | BUILD IMPROVEMENT CAPABILITY |

KEY DESIGN THEMES

__SAFE AND RELIABLE CARE:__ Care for moderately sick patients who are hospitalized is safe, reliable, effective and equitable.

__VITALITY AND TEAMWORK:__ Within a joyful and supportive environment that nurtures professional formation and career development, effective care teams continually strive for excellence.

__PATIENT-CENTERED CARE:__ Truly patient-centered care on medical and surgical units honors the whole person and family, respects individual values and choices, and ensures continuity of care. Patients will say. "They give me exactly the help I want (and need) exactly when I want (and need) it."

__VALUE-ADDED CARE PROCESSES:__ All care processes are free of waste and promote continuous flow

GOALS/NEW LEVELS OF PERFOR-MANCE

⊘ Codes on med/surg units are reduced to zero

⊘ Patient harm from high hazard drugs is reduced by at least 50% per year

⊘ Incidents of patient injury from falls (moderate or higher) are reduced to 1 (or less) per 10,000 patient days

⊘ Hospital-acquired pressure ulcers are reduced to zero

⊘ Increase staff vitality and reduce annual voluntary turnover by 50%

⊘ 95% of patients are willing to recommend the hospital

⊘ Readmissions within 30 days are reduced to 5% or less

⊘ Nurses spend 60% or more of their time in direct patient care

HIGH LEVERAGE CHANGES

CREATE EARLY DETECTION & RESPONSE SYSTEMS (INCLUDING RRTs)	DEVELOP HOSPICE & PALLIATIVE CARE PROGRAMS	BUILD CAPABILITY OF FRONT-LINE STAFF IN INNOVATION & PROCESS IMPROVEMENT	IMPLEMENT A FRAMEWORK FOR NURSING PRACTICE BASED ON THE FORCES OF MAGNETISM	CREATE PATIENT-CENTERED HEALING ENVIRONMENTS	INVOLVE PATIENTS & FAMILY MEMBERS IN MULTIDISCIPLINARY ROUNDS AND CHANGE OF SHIFT REPORT (CUSTOMIZING CARE TO PATIENTS' VALUES PREFERENCES & EXPRESSED NEEDS)	CREATE ACUITY ADAPTABLE BEDS	ELIMINATE WASTE & IMPROVE WORK FLOW IN ADMISSION PROCESS, MEDICATION ADMINISTRATION, HANDOFFS, ROUTINE CARE & DISCHARGE PROCESS
PREVENT HARM FROM HIGH HAZARD DRUG ERRORS	PREVENT HOSPITAL-ACQUIRED PRESSURE ULCERS	DEVELOP MID-LEVEL MANAGERS & CLINICAL LEADERS TO LEAD TRANSFORMATION	OPTIMIZE COMMUNICATIONS AND TEAMWORK AMONGST CLINICIANS AND STAFF	INVOLVE PATIENTS & FAMILIES ON ALL QI TEAMS		OPTIMIZE THE PHYSICAL ENVIRONMENT FOR PATIENTS CLINICIANS AND STAFF	
PREVENT PATIENT INJURIES FROM FALLS				OPTIMIZE TRANSITIONS TO HOME OR OTHER FACILITY			

▮ = best practices exist on 25 or more med/surg units   ▮ = best practices exist on 5 med/surg units   ▮ = Innovation and testing of new ideas are needed

FIGURE 6.1   The TCAB model. From Robert Wood Johnson Foundation and Institute for Healthcare Improvement (IHI).

Microsystems

Recent work in clinical microsystems promises to provide a framework for leaders and teams intending to improve systems and outcomes (Reis, Scott, & Rempel, 2009). Leadership, at the level of the microsystem, focuses on day-to-day challenges of infrastructure and operations.

> Clinical microsystems are the small, functional, front-line units that provide most health care to most people. They are the essential building blocks of larger organizations and of the health system. They are the place where patients and providers meet. The quality and value of care produced by a large health system can be no better than the services generated by the small systems of which it is composed. (Nelson et al., 2002, p. 473)

The microsystems approach is inclusive and democratic, with results informed by processes in the hands of those who execute the work (Batalden, Nelson, Edwards, Godfrey, & Mohr, 2003). In nursing and health care, clinical microsystems engage clinicians who provide direct services in ongoing work to improve quality. As a result, larger numbers of caregivers are informed in detail about the work. They grow competent and confident to identify potential practice issues. In so doing, they improve quality and performance. They develop skills and confidence to address problems in real time and decrease their tolerance of recalcitrant practice problems (Williams, Dickinson, Robinson, & Allen, 2009).

A microsystems approach is based on the body of evidence that draws a clear connection between the nurses' work environment and the quality of care (Ulrich, Woods, et. al, 2007). Investment in the practice environment and the work of nursing yields improved outcomes. This is the basis for microsystems, the platform for nurse leaders to achieve meaningful, sustained process, and quality improvements, and the process to be used to connect people with purpose.

■ CONCLUSIONS

In my graduate education, I had a wise faculty member who liked to quote A. A. Milne (1928):

> Here is <u>Edward Bear</u>, coming downstairs now, bump, bump, bump on the back of his head . . . sometimes he thinks there really is another way if only he could stop bumping a minute and think about it.

Translation offers a means to stop bumping on the back of our heads: to terminate the cycle of habitual practice, to substitute evidence for opinion. Leading by example would necessitate that managers, administrators, and executives evaluate evidence and apply strong and valid findings in innovation focused on carefully selected, well-crafted quality aims. Nurse leaders must establish culture through modeling a spirit of inquiry and speaking the evidence-based practice and translation language, and develop the organization's capacity through knowledge and skill building and using performance to drive improvement. To do so would enable these leaders to connect people with purpose, to facilitate organizational learning, and position their enterprise for the challenges in health care to come.

■ REFERENCES

Aiken, L. H., Clarke, S. P., Cheung, R. B., Sloane, D. M., & Silber, J. H. (2003). Educational levels of hospital nurses and surgical patient mortality. *Journal of American Medical Association, 290*(12), 1607–1623.

Aiken, L. H., Clarke, S. P., Sloane, D. M., Lake, E. T. & Cheney, T. (2008). Effects of hospital care environment on patient mortality and nurse outcomes. *Journal of Nursing Administration, 38*(5), 223–229.

Aiken, L. H., Clarke, S. P., Sloane, D. M., Lake, E. T., & Cheney, T. (2009). Effects of hospital care environment on patient mortality and nurse outcomes. *Journal of Nursing Administration, 39*(7–8 Suppl.), S45–S51.

Aiken, L. H., Clarke, S. P., Sloane, D. M., Sochalski, J. A., & Silber, J. H. (2002). Hospital staffing and patient mortality, nurse burnout, and job dissatisfaction. *Journal of American Medical Association, 288*(16), 1987–1993.

Aiken, L. H., Clarke, S. P., Sloane, D. M., Sochalski, J. A., & Silber, J. H. (2010). Hospital nurse staffing and patient mortality, nurse burnout, and job dissatisfaction. *Journal of the American Medical Association 288*(16), 1987–1993.

Aiken, L. H., Clarke, S. P., Sloane, D. M., Sochalski, J. A., Busse, R., Silber J. H., Clarke, H., . . . & Shamian, J. (2001). Nurses' reports on hospital care in five countries. *Health Affairs, 20*(3), 43–53.

Aiken, L. H., Havens, D. S., Sloane, D. M. (2009). The magnet nursing services recognition program. *American Journal of Nursing, 100*(3), 2635.

American Association of Colleges of Nursing (2010). Retrieved from http://www.nursecredentialing .org/Pathway.aspx

American Nurses Credentialing Center. (2008). *A new model for ANCC's Magnet Recognition Program.* ANCC Website. Retrieved from http://www.nursecredentialing.org/Pathway.aspx

Armstrong, K. J., & Laschinger, H. (2006). Structural empowerment, magnet hospital characteristics, and patient safety culture: Making the link. *Journal of Nursing Care Quality, 21*(2):124–132.

Armstrong, K. J., Laschinger, H., & Wong, C. (2009). Workplace empowerment and magnet hospital characteristics as predictors of patient safety climate. *Journal of Nursing Care Quality, 24*(1), 55–62.

Batalden, P. B., Nelson, E. C., Edwards, W. H., Godfrey, M. M., & Mohr, J. J. (2003). Microsystems in health care: Part 9. Developing small clinical units to attain peak performance. *Joint Commission Journal on Quality and Patient Safety, 29*(11), 575–585.

Brady-Schwartz, D. C. (2005). Further evidence on the Magnet recognition program: Implications for nursing leaders. *Journal of Nursing Administration, 35*(9), 397–403.

Cameron, A., & Masterson, A. (2000). Managing the unmanageable? Nurse Executive Directors and new role developments in nursing. *Journal of Advanced Nursing, 31*(5), 1081–1088.

Cheney, T. (2008). Effects of hospital care environment on patient mortality and nurse outcomes. *Journal of Nursing Administration, 38*(5), 223–229.

Cho, S. H., Hwang, J. H., & Kim, J. (2008). Nursing staffing and patient mortality in intensive care units. *Nursing Research, 57*(5), 322–330.

Clarke, S. P. (2007). Hospital work environments, nurse characteristics, and sharps injuries. *American Journal of Infection Control, 35*(5), 302–309.

Cooper, J. B.,& Gaba, D. (2002). No myth: Anesthesia is a model for addressing patient safety. *Anesthesiology, 97*(6), 1335–1337.

Crow, G. (2006). Diffusion of innovation: The leaders' role in creating the organizational context for evidence-based practice. *Nursing Administration Quarterly, 30*(3), 236–242.

Denham, C. R. (2005). Patient safety practices: Leaders can turn barriers into accelerators. *Journal of Patient Safety, 1*(1), 41–55.

Denham, C. R. (2010). Greenlight issues for the CFO: Investing in patient safety. *Journal of Patient Safety, 6*(1), 52–56.

Denham C. R. (2006). Leaders need dashboards, dashboards need leaders. *Journal of Patient Safety, 2*(2), 45–53.

Denham, C. R., Bagian, J., Daley, J., Edgman-Levitan, S., Gelinas, L., O'Leary, D., . . . Wachter, R. (2005). No excuses: The reality that demands action. *Journal of Patient Safety, 1*(3),170–175.

de Vries, E. N., Ramrattan, M. A., Smorenburg, S. M., Gouma, D. J., & Boermeester, M. A. (2008). The incidence and nature of in-hospital adverse events: A systematic review. *Quality & Safety in Healthcare, 17*(3), 216–223.

De Wolfe, J. A., Perkin, C. A., Harrison, M. B., Laschinger, S., Oakley, P., Peterson, J., & Seaton, F. (2010). Strategies to prepare and support preceptors and students for preceptorships: A systematic review. *Nurse Educator, 35*(3), 98–100.

Ferguson, L., Milner, M., & Snelgrove-Clarke, E. (2004). The role of intermediaries: Getting evidence into practice. *Journal of Wound Ostomy Continence Nursing, 31*(6), 325–327.

Frankel, A., Graydon-Baker, E., Neppl, C., Simmonds, T., Gustafson, M., & Gandhi, T. K. (2003). Patient safety leadership WalkRounds. *Joint Commission Journal of Quality & Safety, 29*(1), 16–26.

Frankel, A. S., Leonard, M. W., & Denham, C. R. (2006). Fair and just culture, team behavior, and leadership engagement: The tools to achieve high reliability. *Health Services Research, 41*(4 Pt. 2), 1690–1709.

Friese, C. R., Lake, E. T., Aiken, L. H., Silber, J. H., & Sochalski, J. (2008). Hospital nurse practice environments and outcomes for surgical oncology patients. *Health Services Research, 43*(4), 1145–1163.

Friese, C. R., Earle, C. C., Silber, J. H., & Aiken, L. H. (2010). Hospital characteristics, clinical severity, and outcomes for surgical oncology patients. *Surgery, 147*(5), 602–609.

Fullen, M. (2009). *Six secrets of change.* San Francisco, CA: Jossey Bass.

Gawande, A. (2009). *The checklist manifesto: How to get things right.* New York, NY: Metropolitan Books.

Goeschel, C. A., Berenholtz, S. M., Culbertson, R. A., Jin, L., & Pronovost, P. J. (2011). Board quality scorecards: Measuring improvement. *American Journal of Medical Quality,* 1–17.

Hanrahan, N. P., Kumar, A., & Aiken, L. H. (2010). Adverse events associated with organizational factors of general hospital inpatient psychiatric care environments. *Psychiatric Services, 61*(6), 569–574.

Health Resources and Services Administration (2010). *The registered nurse population: Initial findings from the 2008 National Sample Survey of Registered Nurses.* Washington, DC: U.S. Department of Health and Human Services. Health Resources and Services Administration.

Helmreich, R. L., & Musson, D. M. (2000). Surgery as team endeavor. *Canadian Journal of Anesthesia, 47*(5), 391–392.

Hyzy, R. C., Flanders, S. A., Pronovost, P. J., Berenholtz, S. M., Watson, S., George, C., . . . Auerbach, A. D. (2010). Characteristics of intensive care units in Michigan: Not an open and closed case. *Journal of Hospital Medicine, 5*(1), 4–9.

Institute for Healthcare Improvement (2008). *Transforming care at the bedside.* Retrieved from http://www.ihi.org/IHI/Programs/StrategicInitiatives/TransformingCareAtTheBedside.htm

Institute for Medicine. (2000). *To err is human: building a safer health system*. Washington, DC: National Academies Press.

Institute for Medicine. (2001). *Crossing the quality chasm*. Washington, DC: National Academies Press.

Institute for Medicine (2004). *Keeping patients safe: Transforming the work environment of nurses*. Washington, DC: National Academies Press.

Kane, R. L., Shamliyan, T. A., Mueller, C., Duval, S., & Wilt, T. J. (2007). The association of registered nurse staffing levels and patient outcomes: Systematic review and meta-analysis. *Medical Care, 45*(12), 1195–1204.

Kotter, J. P. (1990). What leaders really do. *Harvard Business Review, 68*(3), 103–111.

Kramer, M., & Schmalenberg, C. (2008). The practice of clinical autonomy in hospitals: 20,000 nurses tell their story. *Critical Care Nurse, 28*(6), 58–71.

Kramer, M., Schmalenberg, C., & Maguire, P. (2010). Nine structures and leadership practices essential for a magnetic (healthy) work environment. *Nursing Administration Quarterly, 34*(1), 4–17.

Kutney-Lee, A., & Aiken, L. H. (2008). Effect of nurse staffing and education on the outcomes of surgical patients with comorbid serious mental illness. *Psychiatric Services, 59*(12), 1466–1469.

Lacey, S. R., Cox, K. S., Lorfing, K. C., Teasley, S. L., Carroll, C. A., & Sexton, K. (2007). Nursing support, workload, and intent to stay in magnet, magnet-aspiring, and non-magnet hospitals. *Journal of Nursing Administration, 37*(4), 199–205.

Laschinger, H. K. S. (2008). Effect of empowerment on professional practice environments, work satisfaction, and patient care quality: Further testing the Nursing Worklife Model. *Journal of Nursing Care Quality, 23*(4), 322–330.

Laschinger, H. K. S., Finegan, J. E., Shamian, J., & Wilk, P. (2004). A longitudinal analysis of the impact of workplace empowerment on work satisfaction. *Journal of Organizational Behavior, 25*(4), 527–545.

Laschinger, H. K. S., & Leiter, M.P. (2006). The impact of nursing work environments on patient safety outcomes: The mediating role of burnout/engagement. *Journal of Nursing Administration, 36*(5), 259–267.

Laschinger, H. K. S., Shamian J, Thomson D. (2001). Impact of magnet hospital characteristics on nurses' perceptions of trust, burnout, quality of care, and work satisfaction. *Nursing Economics, 19*(5), 209–219.

Leape, L. L., & Berwick, D. M. (2005). Five years after To Err Is Human: What have we learned? *Journal of the American Medical Association, 293*(19), 2384–2390.

Leonard, M., Graham, S., & Bonacum, D. (2004). The human factor: The critical importance of effective teamwork and communication providing safe care. *Quality & Safety in Healthcare, 13*(Suppl 1), i85–i90.

Lucero, R. J., Lake, E. T., & Aiken, L. H. (2009). Variations in nursing care quality across hospitals. *Journal of Advanced Nursing, 65*(11), 2299–2310.

Manojlovich, M., Sidani, S., Covell, C., & Antonakos, C. (2011). Nursing dose: Linking staffing variables to adverse patient outcomes. *Nursing Research, 60*(4):214–220.

Manojlovich, M., & DeCicco B. (2007). Healthy work environments, nurse–physician communication, and patients' outcomes. *American Journal of Critical Care, 16*(6), 536–543.

Marx, D. (2001). *Patient safety and the "just culture": A primer for health care executives*. New York, NY: Columbia University. Available at the Agency for Healthcare Research and Quality website (http://psnet.ahrq.gov/resource.aspx?resourceID=1582) or directly at http://www.mers-tm.org/support/Marx_Primer.pdf

Masterson, S. S., Lewis, K., Goldman, B. M., & Taylor, M. S. (2000). Integrating justice and social exchange: The differing effects of fair procedures and treatment of work relationships. *The Academy of Management Journal, 43*(4), 738–748.

Meredith, E. K., Cohen, E., & Raia, L. V. (2010). Transformational leadership: Application of magnet's new empiric outcomes. *Nursing Clinics of North America, 45*(1), 49–64.

Milne, A. A. (1928). *The house at Pooh corner.* New York, NY: Dutton Children's Books.

Moore, S. C., & Hutchison, S. A. (2007). Developing leaders at every level: Accountability and empowerment actualized through shared governance. *The Journal of Nursing Administration, 37*(12), 564–568.

Needleman, J., Buerhaus, P., Mattke, S., Stewart, M., & Zelevinsky, K. (2002). Nurse-staffing levels and the quality of care in hospitals. *New England Journal of Medicine, 346*(22), 1715–1722.

Nelson, E. C., Batalden, P. B., Huber, T. P., Mohr, J. J., Godfrey, M. M., Headrick, L. A., & Wasson, J. H. (2002). Microsystems in health care: Part 1. Learning from high performing front-line clinical units. *Joint Commission Journal of Quality Improvement, 28*(9), 472–493.

Pathak, S., Holzmueller, C. G., Haller, K. B., & Pronovost, P. J. (2010). A mile in their shoes: Interdisciplinary education at the Johns Hopkins University School of Medicine. *American Journal of Medical Quality, 25,* 462–467.

Piccolo, R. F., Bardes, M., Mayer, D. & Judge T. (2008) Does high quality leader–member exchange accentuate the effects of organizational justice? *European Journal of Work and Organizational Psychology, 17*(2), 273–298.

Porter-O'Grady, T. (2000). Governance at the crossroads. Post-millenium trustees face difficult decisions in a new age of health care. *Health Progress, 81*(6), 38–41, 55.

Porter-O'Grady, T. (2001). Is shared governance still relevant? *Journal of Nursing Administration, 31*(10), 468–473.

Porter-O'Grady, T. (2004). Shared governance: Is it a model for nurses to gain control over their practice? *Online Journal of Issues in Nursing, 9*(1), 1. Retrieved from www.nursingworld. org/MainMenuCategories/ANAMarketplace/ANAPeriodicals/OJIN/TableofContents/Volume92004/No1Jan04/Overview.aspx

Porter-O'Grady, T. (2009). Creating a context for excellence and innovation: Comparing chief nurse executive leadership practices in magnet and non-magnet hospitals. *Nursing Administration Quaterly, 33*(3), 198–204.

Pronovost, P. J., Angus, D. C., Dorman, T., Robinson, K. A., Dremsizov, T. T., & Young, T. L. (2002). Physician staffing patterns and clinical outcomes in critically ill patients: A systematic review. *Journal of the American Medical Association, 288*(17), 2151–2162.

Pronovost, P. J., Goeschel, C. A., Colantuoni, E., Watson, S., Lubomski, L. H., Berenholtz, S. M., . . . Needham, D. (2010). Sustaining reductions in catheter related bloodstream infections in Michigan intensive care units: Observational study. *British Medical Journal, 340,* c309. doi: 10. 1136/bmj.c309

Pronovost, P. J., Jenckes, M. W., Dorman, T., Garrett, E., Breslow, M. J., Rosenfeld, B. A. . . . Bass, E. (1999). Organizational characteristics of intensive care units related to outcomes of abdominal aortic surgery. *Journal of the American Medical Association, 281*(14), 1310–1317.

Reinertsen, J. L., Bisognano, M., & Pugh, M. D. (2008). *Seven leadership leverage points for organization-level improvement in health care* (2nd ed.). Cambridge, MA: Institute for Healthcare Improvement.

Reis, M. D., Scott, S. D., & Rempel, G. R. (2009). Including parents in the evaluation of clinical microsystems in the neonatal intensive care unit. *Advances in Neonatal Care. 9*(4), 174–179.

Rorbach, L. A., Grana, R., Sussman, S., & Valente, T. W. (2006). Type II translation: Transporting prevention interventions from research to real-world settings. *Evaluation and the Health Professions, 29*(3), 302–333.

Rutherford, P., Lee, B., & Greiner, A. (2004). *Transforming care at the bedside.* IHI Innovation Series white paper. Boston, MA: Institute for Healthcare Improvement. Retrieved from www.IHI.org

St-Pierre, I., & Holmes, D. (2010). The relationship between organizational justice and workplace aggression. *Journal of Advanced Nursing, 66*(5), 1169–1182.

Schalk, D. M., Biji, M. L., Halfens, R. J., Hollands, L., & Cummings, G. G. (2010). Interventions aimed at improving the nursing work environment: A systematic review. *Implementation Science, 5,* 34. doi:10.1186/1748-5908-5-34

Schmalenberg, C., & Kramer, M. (2008). Essentials of a productive nurse work environment. *Nursing Research, 57*(1), 2–13.

Sexton, B., Berenholtz, S. M., Goeschel, C. A., Watson, S. R., Holzmueller, C. G., Thompson, D. A., Hyzy, R. C., Marsteller, J. A., Schumacher, K., & Pronovost, P. J. (2011) Assessing and improving safety climate in a large cohort of intensive care units. *Critical Care Medicine, 39*(5), 934–939.

Smith, H., Tallman, R., & Kelly, K. (2006). Magnet hospital characteristics and northern Canadian nurses' job satisfaction. *Nursing Leadership (Toronto, Ontario), 19*(3), 73–86.

Springer, P. J., Corbett, C., & Davis, N. (2006). Enhancing evidence-based practice through collaboration. *The Journal of Nursing Administration, 36*(11), 534–537.

Sochalski, J. (2004). Is more better? The relationship between nurse staffing and the quality of nursing care in hospitals. *Medical Care, 42*(2 Suppl.), II67–II73.

Sredl, D. (2008). Evidence-based nursing practice: What US nurse executives really think. *Nurse Researcher, 15*(4), 51–67.

Stetler, C. B., & Caramanica, L. (2007). Evaluation of an evidence-based practice initiative: Outcomes, strengths and limitations of a retrospective, conceptually-based approach. *Worldviews on Evidence-Based Nursing, 4*(4), 187–199.

Stone, P. W., Harrison, M. I., Feldman, P., Linzer, M., Peng, T., Roblin, D., Scott-Cawiezell, J., Warren, N., & Williams, E. (2005). Organizational climate of staff working conditions and safety: An integrative model. In K. Henriksen, J. B. Battles, E. S. Marks, et al. (Eds.). *Advances in Patient Safety: From Research to Implementation.* Rockville, MD: Agency for Health Care Research and Quality.

Stone, P. W., & Gershon, R. R. (2006). Nurse work environments and occupational safety in intensive care units. *Policy, Politics, and Nursing Practice, 7*(4), 240–247.

Stone, P. W., Larson, E. L., Mooney-Kane, C., Smolowitz, J., Lin, S. X., & Dick, A. W. (2006). Organizational climate and intensive care unit nurses' intention to leave. *Critical Care Medicine, 34*(7), 1907–1912.

Stone, P. W., Mooney-Kane, C., Larson, E. L., Horan, T., Glance, L. G., Zwanziger, J., & Dick, A. W. (2007). Nurse working conditions and patient safety outcomes. *Medical Care, 45*(6), 571–578.

Stone, P. W., Mooney-Kane, C., Larson, E. L., Pastor, D. K., Zwanziger, J., & Dick, A. W. (2007). Nurse working conditions, organizational climate, and intent to leave in ICUs: An instrumental variable approach. *Health Services Research, 42*(3 Pt 1), 1085–1104.

Thorpe, K., & Loo, R. (2003). Balancing professional and personal satisfaction of nurse managers: Current and future perspectives in a changing health care system. *Journal of Nursing Management, 11*(5), 321–330.

Ulrich, B. T., Buerhaus, P. I., Donelan, K., Norman, L., & Dittus, R. (2007). Magnet status and registered nurse views of the work environment and nursing as a career. *Journal of Nursing Administration, 37*(5), 212–220.

Ulrich, B. T., Woods, D., Hart, K. A., Lavandero, R., Leggett, J., & Taylor, D. (2007). Critical care nurses' work environments: Value of excellence in beacon units and magnet organizations. *Critical Care Nurse, 27*(3), 68–77.

Viney, M., Batcheller, J., Houston, S., & Belcik, K. (2006). Transforming care at the bedside: Designing new care systems in an age of complexity. *Journal of Nursing Care Quality, 21*(2), 143–150.

Wade, G. H., Osgood, B., Avino, K., Bucher, G., Bucher, L., Foraker, T., . . . Sirkowski, C. (2008). Influence of organizational characteristics and caring attributes of managers on nurses' job enjoyment. *Journal of Advanced Nursing, 64*(4), 344–353.

Weick, K. E., & Sutcliffe, K. M. (2001). *Managing the unexpected: Assuring high performance in an age of complexity.* San Francisco, CA: Jossey Bass.

Williams, L. L. (2006). The fair factor in matters of trust. *Nursing Administration Quarterly 30*(1), 30–37.

Williams, I., Dickinson, H., Robinson, S., & Allen, C. (2009). Clinical microsystems and the NHS: A sustainable method for improvement? *Healthcare Organization & Management, 23*(11), 119–132.

Wolf, G., Triolo, P., & Ponte, P. R. (2008). Magnet recognition program: The next generation. *Journal of Nursing Administration, 38*(4), 200–204.

Zaleznik, A. (2004). Managers and leaders: Are they different. *Clinical Leadership Management Review, 18*(3), 171–177.

Zwarenstein, M., Goldman, J., & Reeves, S. (2009). Interprofessional collaboration: Effects of practice-based interventions on professional practice and healthcare outcomes. *Cochrane Database of Systematic Reviews,* 3, CD000072. doi: 10.1002/14651858.CD000072.pub2

C H A P T E R   SEVEN

Translation of Evidence for Education

Anne E. Belcher

■ INTRODUCTION

According to Emerson and Records (2008), "the ultimate imperative facing nursing today is the creation of a culture that values the practice of nursing education and expands evidence-based education through the design, testing, and refinement of education strategies from nursing and other disciplines" (p. 359). These authors define evidence-based nursing education practice as "the validation, generation, application, and perpetuation of those methods that facilitate the preparation of skilled and thoughtful nurses who function in a constantly evolving, global health environment" (p. 361). The scholarly process of evidence-based education includes the following:

1. Asking the question
2. Searching for the best evidence using critical appraisal
3. Considering the characteristics, preferences, and values of the students when designing learning activities
4. Implementing and evaluating educational change

Nurse educators, whether in an academic or practice setting, need to generate the scholarship of teaching and learning (SoTL), as well as translate existing SoTL into their educational planning, implementation, and evaluation.

■ RECOMMENDATIONS FROM REPORTS ON NURSING EDUCATION

The Institute of Medicine (IOM, 2003) report, *Health Professions Education: A Bridge to Quality*, has its overarching vision for the reform of health professions education to enhance the quality and safety of patient care: "All health professionals should be educated to deliver patient-centered care as members of an interdisciplinary team, emphasizing evidence-based practice, quality improvement approaches, and informatics" (p. 121).

The report indicates that, in the case of evidence-based practice, there is no standardized definition of evidence.

The existing definitions include evidence that can be quantified, such as randomized controlled trials; evidence based on qualitative research; evidence that exists in institutional databases; and evidence derived from the knowledge and experi-ence of experts and peers, including inductive reasons. (p. 122)

Misunderstandings and misconceptions regarding the definition continue to present challenges, especially with regard to the implementation of evidence-based practice across the professions. Recommendation 8 includes the focus on "the link between the (core) compe-tencies and evidence-based education" (p. 134).

The Carnegie Foundation report, *Educating Nurses: A Call for Radical Transformation* (Benner, Sutphen, Leonard, & Day, 2010), addresses the issue of development for nursing faculty. The questions raised with regard to studying the goals and outcomes of teaching, as well as evalu-ating their choice of teaching strategies, are applicable to all nurses who teach and include:

- What kinds of responses are expected from students during a classroom session?
- What kinds of imaginative access to the practice does the class provide?
- What is the level of information presented and represented in the exchange of questions and answers between students and teachers?
- What is the extent of integration between classroom and clinical education? (p. 223).

One can readily see the applicability of these questions to the teaching of students, staff, patients, and families, with a realization that the "classroom" may be a patient room or home and that the "clinical education" may focus on self-care.

■ EVALUATING THE EDUCATION EVIDENCE FOR NURSING—WHAT DO WE KNOW?

When considering the evaluation of education evidence for nursing, the answer to the ques-tion "what do we know?" is "not very much." Many years ago, when nursing research was in its infancy, the focus of the studies conducted was on the students, the teachers, and the curricula. As the profession evolved, the focus shifted to clinical problems and away from educational issues. It is impressive that Tanner, Holzemer, and others persevered with their Society for Research in Nursing Education and the Journal of Nursing Education during those years when clinical research was being funded and publicized and rewarded. Because the profession has become aware of the nursing faculty shortage, there has been increasing attention given to educational research, although funding for this focus continues to lag significantly behind that allocated to clinical research. Consequently, the evidence for educa-tion is limited; although fortunately, organizations such as the National League for Nursing promote the importance of nursing education research. The challenge facing today's nurse educators is the implementation of teaching strategies that promote professional role devel-opment, clinical competency, and critical-thinking skills.

Even with the increasing emphasis on nursing education research, the numbers of studies that have been replicated is small, so that translation is still a significant challenge. There is a need for doctoral students and faculty to identify educational questions that have been studied and to seek verification of the results of those studies. In addition, we need to appreciate the research conducted by our colleagues in education and in other health profes-sions because their work provides us with meaningful findings that are applicable to nursing education.

Within that context, there are factors that affect the translation of existing research that should guide future research. These factors include the nature of the learners; the nature of the faculty/teachers; the characteristics of the content to be presented; educational theories, such as the theory of multiple intelligence learning; learning styles; and information processing. Each of these factors will be discussed in the following sections.

The Nature of the Learners

Health professions programs are attracting larger numbers of older, nontraditional students and career changers, as well as increasing numbers of students from ethnic minorities. Today's nursing education programs have a mix of students from the baby boom generation, generation X, and millennial generation Y/Net who demonstrate unique differences in various ways, including their use of the Internet. Likewise, nurses in the practice setting represent all of these generations, and staff development educators are challenged to teach using various technologies and to teach the nurses how to use the technologies in their practice. As Weiner (2008) observed, mobile devices and pervasive wireless networks are redefining the ways in which we live, work, plan, and learn. Therefore, faculty and students need to acknowledge this redefinition and integrate these technologies into teaching and learning. Weiner's observation can also be applied to patients and their families, as can the description of these individuals as being of various generations and ethnic minorities. Nurses who conduct patient/family education are increasingly challenged to be culturally competent in the delivery of content and supervision of skill development in the practice setting.

The Nature of the Faculty/Teachers

Almost a third of current nursing faculty are older than the age of 55 and, as these faculty members retire, nursing schools are losing some of their most experienced teachers. These teachers not only provide students with proven instructional strategies, but they also mentor new faculty. The recruitment and retention of novice teachers is complicated by salary differentials and the lack of comprehensive orientation and support as they develop their educator role. The same issues apply in the practice site where experienced staff development and patient educators are likewise retiring in large numbers and are not being succeeded by advanced practice nurses who value the educator role. Many current nurse educators are baby boomers who are challenged to learn how to use new technologies. It is critically important that nurses who function in a faculty/teacher role acquire the skills needed to meet the needs of various generations and that they value the positive effect of evidence-based strategies. This becomes the challenge for current faculty who need to use not only cognitive but also affective teaching strategies to instill this value into future faculty and teachers.

Characteristics of the Content to Be Presented

The complex practice of nursing is often addressed in schools of nursing by adding more content to the curriculum/courses without consideration of the changing nature of our practice and the need to be able to access resources, rather than memorizing facts and figures that may already be outdated. Many of these same issues apply in staff development and patient education; the emphasis should realistically be on access to resources rather than learning specific information. Romiszowski (1999) offers the helpful suggestion, via levels of analysis of instructional design, that teachers focus on the selection of content on materials worth learning and not known. These screens could be used to determine what is essential content not previously provided to or experienced by the learners.

■ EDUCATIONAL THEORIES—FRAMEWORKS FOR EVIDENCE TRANSLATION

Although there are numerous educational theories from which to choose from, the focus of this chapter is on pedagogy, andragogy, learning styles, information processing, and Gardner's theory of multiple intelligence learning (see Exhibit 7.1 for a listing of each of these theories, the evidence base, and suggested uses of each in face-to-face and online teaching).

Pedagogy is the theory, methods, and activities for maximizing teaching and learning. However, the term pedagogy has also been used to describe teaching in a broader sense. With regard to adult learners, there are several interpretative pedagogies that focus on exploring, deconstructing, and critiquing experiences. These pedagogies empower the student, decenter the authority, encourage social action, and develop new knowledge. They include critical pedagogy, feminist pedagogy, postmodern discourse, and phenomenology (Billings & Halstead, 2009).

Andragogy (Knowles, 1970) refers to principles of adult learning, which are relevant to the increasing number of more mature students entering into and practicing nursing. These adults are typically highly motivated and committed to learning. They bring a wealth of knowledge and experience from their prior education, work, and family. They benefit from educational experiences in which the teacher is sensitive to the individual and is actively engaged with them in their learning. As noted by Bankert & Kozel (2005) with regard to empowering the adult learner, diminishing learning boundaries and allowing for autonomy and responsibility enable the adult learner to reflect on past experiences and interactions; he or she will in turn become self-directed in discovering information and new meanings relevant to practice. These researchers go on to say that "support for adult learners can be achieved by creating a caring learning environment that is founded on partnerships and collaboration, mutual respect and commitment, self-direction, and creativity" (p. 229). Other aspects of adult learning that are important are (a) delineating the usefulness/practical value of the information being taught; (b) building on the learner's past experiences; (c) matching the goals of instruction with those of the learner to the greatest extent possible; and (d) creating a learning environment where the learner does not have fear of failure.

Learning Styles

There is evidence in learning style research that students can master any information when the material is presented in a format that matches their learning preference (Denig, 2004). *Learning styles* refers to the ways in which, and the conditions under which, learners most efficiently and effectively perceive, process, store, and recall what they are trying to learn (James & Gardner, 1995) and how they prefer to approach learning (Cassidy, 2004). For example, O'Hare (2002) found that when nurses were taught new and difficult

---

EXHIBIT 7.1

Educational Theories: Frameworks for Evidence Translation

Pedagogy

Critical pedagogy

Evidence base: Marginalization proposed as guiding concept for valuing diversity in nursing knowledge; relinquish faculty authority and empower students to identify injustices and imbalances in power, and guide analysis of issues and support action for change; assignments can include deconstruction of the issue

Use in face-to-face teaching: Written assignments, field trips, experience with professional lobbyist organizations

Use in online teaching: Written assignments

Feminist pedagogy

Evidence base: Commitment to the emancipation of women; concepts and principles can be used when emphasizing group dynamics, interpersonal relationships, power, and authority; personal lived experience as the content for analysis

Use in face-to-face teaching: Cooperative learning

Use in online teaching: Journal writing

Postmodern discourse

Evidence base: Truth is constantly being constructed and is in process; application appropriate in climates in which ambiguity is possible; faculty work with students to develop appreciation of multiple ways of understanding socially constructed systems

Use in face-to-face teaching and in online teaching: Exercises can be used to encourage pluralistic appreciation

Phenomenology

Evidence base: Goal is to understand human experience; restructures relationship between knowledge and skill because of the holistic view of the phenomena of interest in the human being

Use in face-to-face teaching: Faculty selects phenomena that are relevant to course content and explore them in classroom; there are an unlimited number of anecdotal phenomena from which faculty and students can draw

Use in online teaching: Expanded database formats, case studies, anecdotal recordings, to name a few

(continued)

EXHIBIT 7.1

Educational Theories: Frameworks for Evidence Translation *(Continued)*

Andragogy

Evidence base: Adults are self-directed and problem-centered; need and want to learn useful information that can be readily adapted

Use in face-to-face teaching: Collaborative relationship and use of democratic process; course materials sequenced according to learner readiness; use of internships and a "practica"

Use in online teaching: Independent study and inquiry projects; reflective journal writing, portfolios

Learning styles

Evidence base: Indicates the preferred educational conditions that will help the student to learn as much as possible; instruments used to identify include Knowles's principles of adult learning (see text about andragogy) and Kolb's learning styles inventory

Use in face-to-face teaching: Useful when tutoring or counseling students; need for faculty to use varied styles so as to create active learners in classroom

Use in online learning: Provide students with options for meeting course and module objectives so that they can choose based on their preferred learning style

Information-processing theories

Evidence base: Focus is on ways in which individuals perceive, organize, and remember large amounts of information; memory viewed as complex organized system

Use in face-to-face and online teaching: Need to not reward memorization in didactic portion of curriculum; need to emphasize the need to apply expected knowledge in the practice setting

Gardner's theory of multiple intelligences

Evidence base: Qualities identified in all categories can contribute to an optimal patient encounter in nursing; faculty can focus on each student's unique profile and use their strengths to enhance contributions to practice; there is a need to develop teaching strategies to complement all multiple intelligence categories

Use in face-to-face teaching and in online teaching: Student helped to use the multiple intelligence theory for self-evaluation and for the evaluation of others materials through teaching methods that matched their learning style preferences, they scored higher on standardized achievement examinations. Her work focused on comparing traditional versus learning-style presentations of course content in adult health nursing with baccalaureate students. Accepting the diversity of learning styles helps the teacher to make informed decisions about program development, instructional design, and learning experiences.

Friedman and Alley (1984) developed six principles of learning style:

- Both the style by which the teacher prefers to teach and the style by which the learner prefers to learn can be identified.
- Teachers need to guard against relying on teaching strategies and tools that match their own preferred learning styles.
- Teachers are most helpful when they assist learners in identifying and in learning using their own preferred style.
- Learners should have the opportunity to learn using their own preferred style.
- Learners should be encouraged to diversify their style preferences.
- Teachers can develop specific learning activities that reinforce each style.

Information processing is a cognitive perspective that emphasizes the thinking process: thought, reasoning, the way information is encountered and stored, and memory functioning (Sternberg, 2006). Tracking learning through the various stages helps the teacher and the learner to assess what happens to information as it is perceived, interpreted, and remembered by each learner. This may, in turn, suggest ways of improving the structure of the learning situation, as well as how to correct distortions, misconceptions, and errors in learning. Strategies of value to the teacher and the learner include:

- Having the learner describe how they believe they learn
- Asking the learner to describe what they are thinking as they learn
- Evaluating learner mistakes
- Giving close attention to the learner's inability to remember or demonstrate information

Gardner's theory of *multiple intelligence* (MI) *learning* provides a conceptual framework for designing classroom activities that promote an interactive learning environment. In his 1983 publication, *Frames of Mind*, Gardner identified the components of MI learning, noting that it is possible to determine one's intellectual profile and to use this profile to enhance educational experiences. In a 1999 publication, he defined *intelligence* as a "biopsychological potential to process information that can be activated in a cultural setting to solve problems or create products that are of value in a culture" (Gardner, 1999, pp. 33–34).

When MI-inspired learning was implemented with adult learners, it was observed to reduce teacher directedness, to increase student initiative and control, to increase the authenticity of the learning experience, and to make learning more relevant (Kallenbach & Viens, 2004).

Amerson (2006) noted that nursing education can use the concepts of MI to "create learning environments that will encourage active participation by building on the student's natural intelligence profile" (p. 194). Nicholson-Nelson (1998) supports the principle that teaching methods need to be designed by faculty to match learners' intelligence.

Reis (2008a) provides examples of the application of Gardner's (2003) eight categories of multiple intelligence to instructional strategies as follows:

- Linguistic—reading, discussion
- Logic–mathematical—charts, thinking games
- Kinesthetic—doing, demonstrations
- Spatial—handouts, overheads
- Musical—using/creating songs
- Interpersonal—small group activities
- Intrapersonal—journal writing, reflecting
- Naturalistic—outdoor activity, treasure hunts

The use of various strategies accommodates highly diverse groups of learners who reflect the populations of nursing students, nurses, and patients/families with whom we interact.

■ EVIDENCE FOR ACADEMIC EDUCATION

The strategies described in this section are "tried and true" or relatively new on the education scene. Evidence for the use of each is primarily anecdotal; therefore, educational research is needed to validate the observed benefit of each to the learner.

Face-to-face education is the traditional approach in which the teacher is the "sage on the stage," using primarily lecture as the instructional modality. This type of education is described as a "one-size-fits-all" approach that is scheduled for set times in set places (O'Neil, Fisher, & Newbold, 2009). On the positive side, Caruso and Kvavik (2005) found that students, although wanting to be linked into the Internet, do want lots of face-to-face time as well.

The rapid expansion of *online/distance education* has provided "the professional development and accountability for nurses, promoting lifelong, self-directed learning and the ability to reach a very diverse student population" (Cantrell, O'Leary, & Ward, 2008, p. 548). Other benefits of online education include the ability of students and practicing nurses to attend class on their own schedule while eliminating travel time, parking problems, and child care expenses. Characteristics of a strong online program are flexibility, provision of a personal touch, computer guidance, well-constructed courses, and ongoing evaluation by learners and teachers. Learning activities are organized around learning outcomes that address both content mastery and learning skill development. The media chosen to deliver courses should be pedagogically effective, receptive to different learning styles, and sensitive to the time and place limitations of the students. There needs to be more independent and interactive learning as well as more individualized learning experiences that appeal to the learners' individual learning styles. According to a report by Eduventures (2005), nursing programs continue to be the leading adopters of online learning, particularly for delivery of continuing education. In addition, many nurses use online learning to earn advanced degrees while remaining active in their practice. "The nursing education market is one of the best examples of the success of online learning in the health disciplines" (p. 48).

Hybrid education/blended learning is a thoughtful fusion of face-to-face and online course delivery, with both synchronous and asynchronous elements. It offers students and faculty an approach that avoids either/or choices and the "downsides" of online and face-to-face experiences. It provides a way to extend and enhance the educational experience in an effective and efficient manner. According to Reis (2008b), blended learning is the "organic integration of thoughtfully selected and complementary face-to-face and online approaches and technologies" (p. 3). Students are asked to assume increased responsibility for their learning but must be given control of the learning experience; faculty are encouraged to adopt new approaches, to incorporate collaborative activities, and to develop technological skills.

Self-directed learning (SDL) incorporates such skills as definition of personal objectives, appreciation of the dynamics of behavioral change, information acquisition/assimilation, and self-evaluation that are acquired within the context of a respectful and facilitative learner–teacher relationship. SDL, as perceived by students and faculty, includes the following essential characteristics: (a) students and faculty must understand the value of empowering learners to take increasing responsibility for decisions related to learning; (b) students engaged in SDL undergo a transformation that begins with negative feelings (i.e., frustration, confusion, and dissatisfaction) and ends with confidence and skills for lifelong learning; and (c) faculty development is needed to ensure high levels of teacher competency in facilitating SDL (Lunyk-Child et al., 2001).

Problem-based learning (PBL) is that "which results from the process of working toward the understanding or resolution of a problem" (Barrows & Tamblyn, 1980, p. 12). Students are presented with a clinical situation or professional issue. The goals of PBL are to "(1) construct an extensive and flexible knowledge base, (2) develop effective problem-solving skills, (3) develop self-directed, lifelong learning skills, (4) help students to become effective collaborators, and (5) assist students in becoming intrinsically motivated to learn" (Hmelo-Silver, 2004, p. 240). This strategy is best used with small groups, especially when active learning is an objective of the teacher. Whereas there is mixed evidence about the level of knowledge acquisition, anecdotal evidence indicates that students benefit from the applicability of the learning to the clinical situation.

Collaborative learning is described as classroom strategies that require students to work in small groups and to receive recognition based on group performance on the assignment. Cabrera, Nora, Bernal, Terenzini, and Pascarella (1998) indicated that "collaborative learning restructures the classroom away from the traditional lecture to small group work requiring intensive interactions between students and their faculty member while working through complex projects" (p. 2). There is evidence that use of this strategy has a positive effect on students' cognitive development and long-term retention of knowledge. It has been found that women and minorities prefer this learning style (Adams, 1992). Because this strategy is designed to foster group membership skills, promote positive interpersonal relationships, and make the learning situation more comfortable (McKeachie & Svinicki, 2006), individual students' achievement may be more difficult to measure but the benefits for learning to cooperate/collaborate are important, especially for a practice discipline.

Executive style education provides learners with the opportunity to come together as a cohort for intensive immersion in one or more courses. This format may be for a week, a weekend, or some other variation; it challenges the teacher to maintain learner interest and attention for often long periods, but the use of active learning strategies will keep the learners engaged. When students must travel long distances for course delivery, this style can meet their need for concentrated time and attention to learning. Many students now have full-time positions from which they do not wish to take a leave of absence. Executive style education enables them to take planned vacation time or personal leave time for coursework (K. White, personal communication, September 15, 2010).

■ EVIDENCE FOR PATIENT AND FAMILY EDUCATION

Readiness Assessment

Readiness to learn is defined as the time when the learner shows an interest in learning the knowledge and/or skills necessary to maintain or regain optimal health. When a patient or family member asks a question, the time is often prime for learning. Assessing readiness requires that the teacher understand what needs to be taught, collect and validate that information, and then apply such methods as observation, interviewing, and reviewing data in the chart. Lichtenthal (1990) defined PEEK as being the four types of readiness to learn:

- Physical readiness—includes measures of ability, the complexity of the task, environmental effects, health status, and gender
- Emotional readiness—includes anxiety level, support system, motivation, risk-taking behavior, frame of mind, and developmental stage
- Experiential readiness—level of aspiration, past coping mechanisms, cultural background, locus of control, and orientation
- Knowledge readiness—present knowledge base, cognitive ability, learning disabilities, and learning styles

The value of determining the physical readiness of the learner lies in the teacher's ability to plan the level of the content, the number of steps into which the learning task should be divided, the arrangement of the learning environment, the length of the learning session, and the value placed on learning based on gender.

The value of determining emotional readiness of the learner lies in the teacher's need to provide a comfortable emotional climate, both intrinsic and extrinsic motivation, focus on the "here and now" versus the future, and attention to the developmental status and needs of the learner.

The value of determining experiential readiness of the learner lies in the teacher's need to appeal to the learner's level of aspiration, to build on past effective coping strategies, to incorporate cultural variables, and to address the locus of control with the selection of instructional strategies.

The value of determining the knowledge readiness of the learner lies in the teacher's need to determine the learner's present knowledge base; to identify and direct learning based on the learner's cognitive ability, as well as learning and reading disabilities; and to address the learner's learning style in the presentation of material and experiences.

The teacher must determine not only if an interpersonal relationship has developed with the learner, but also if prerequisite knowledge and skills have been mastered, if the learner displays motivation, and if the plan for teaching matches the developmental level of the learner.

Motivation

Motivation has been defined as a psychological force that moves one toward some type of action (Haggard, 1989). It has also been described as a willingness of the learner to embrace learning (Redman, 2007). Motivation is the result of both internal and external factors: personal attributes, environmental influences, and relationship systems. Rules that set the stage for motivation include: (a) the state of optimum anxiety, (b) learner readiness, (c) realistic goal setting, (d) learner satisfaction/success, and (e) uncertainty-reducing or uncertainty-maintaining dialogue.

■ TECHNOLOGY IN EDUCATION

Bastable (2008) noted that educators in the information age are developing into facilitators of learning rather than providers of content; their goal is to help learners learn how "to refine a problem, to find the information they need, and to critically evaluate the information they find" (p. 521). With this goal in mind, educators need to reconceptualize their role as a facilitator of learning, a consumer of technology, and an evaluator of the use and effect of technology. This section has as its focus technologies for use in the laboratory (simulation), in the classroom, and in the practice setting, as well as academic uses of emerging technologies.

Academic Uses of Emerging Technologies

Skiba (2008) observed that "digital natives tend to communicate in the moment using instant messaging (IM), text messaging, blogging, expressing themselves on social networking sites, and now sending tweets" (p. 499; for a comprehensive list of academic technology uses, examples and support suggestions, see the article by Weiner, 2008).

In a recent report from eSchoolNews (2009), U.S. Education Secretary Arne Duncan stated that schools and colleges should deliver course content to students' cell phones. His advocacy comes as smart phones—iPhones, Blackberrys, and other devices that access the Internet—become more evident in lecture halls and in practice sites. As an example of their use, nursing students of Ball State University download course materials—such as electronic nursing manuals, lab books, medical dictionaries, diagnosis literature, to name a few—onto their mobile devices.

Instant messaging (IM) enables two individuals to exchange real-time text messages that allow for quick questions and clarifications. Each individual must register and provide a unique user name. Many instructors use this format for virtual office hours.

Text messaging, also known as "texting," refers to "the exchange of brief written messages between mobile phones over cellular networks" (Wikipedia, 2010, para. 1). The most frequent application of the service is person-to-person messaging, but text messages are also used to interact with automated systems, such as a school, college, or university's use of the system to alert students, faculty, and staff about emergent situations on the campus.

Peer-to-peer networks (P2P) connect two locations over the Internet and allow the addition of two-way audio and video if web cameras and headsets are provided. Products such as Skype can be used to connect instructors to the school or practice site with either preceptors or students at a distance for virtual site visits or advising. *Web conferencing* provides for a class of a more traditional nature, wherein a teacher presents material and engages the learners in a live verbal discussion. Examples of the products used include WebEx, Adobe Connect, Elluminate Live!, and Microsoft Live Meeting. Each of these products has two components: the first allows the users to share whatever is on their desktop, such as PowerPoint slides, web pages, and personal computer (PC)-based applications; the second is the ability to share audio where the students can hear the teacher and can talk to each other (Trangenstein, 2008).

Discussion boards for substantive posting, as seen in such platforms as Blackboard (www .blackboard.com), provide the teacher with the opportunity to assign topics for discussion for the students and can include the requirement that students respond to/critique one another's comments. This strategy keeps the learners engaged in the learning, provides them with the opportunity to comment on topics, and gives the teacher data with which to assess "classroom participation" in a substantive way.

Blogs/Web logs are writing tools that are easy to use and can enhance nurses' writing, communication, collaboration, reading, and information-gathering skills (Maag, 2005). The individual writer provides his or her opinion on a particular subject and allows others to leave their comments. A nursing school blog might motivate students to post their responses to case studies, artwork, and creative thoughts.

Twitter is an online application that is defined by Wikipedia (2010c) as

> A social networking service that enables its users to send and read messages known as tweets. Tweets are text-based posts of up to 140 characters displayed on the author's profile page and delivered to the author's subscribers who are known as followers. (para. 1)

Skiba (2008) suggested several ways to use Twitter with students: (a) to communicate about what we learn at conferences; (b) to notify students of an important change in plans (i.e., class is cancelled); (c) to reach a large group of colleagues like preceptors, who may not have easy access to e-mail; (d) to teach collaborative writing skills; and (e) to provide quick answers to questions from students about assignments, readings, and so forth.

Wikis are a collaboration tool through which multiple participants can contribute to the authorship of a document or project. Each participant can manage, edit, and organize content on a website using a standard Web browser. Changes are tracked and become a part of the site's record.

Virtual reality has been described as a revolution that has the potential for bridging the gap between knowledge and application of knowledge to practice. Skiba (2008) identified three trends that she believes support this "revolution": (a) touch screens; (b) rise in social networking phenomenon; and (c) gaming. Nongaming virtual worlds such as Second Life, in which avatars can be created to serve as guides to learning, are becoming increasingly popular in nursing education. An *avatar* is a computer user's representation of one's self or an alter ego, usually in the form of a three-dimensional model or a two-dimensional icon (picture). The term can also refer to the personality connected with the screen name or "handle" of the Internet user (Wikipedia, 2010a).

YouTube, according to Wikipedia (2010d), is a "video-sharing website on which users can upload and share videos" (para. 1). It is operated as a subsidiary of Google, which uses Adobe Flash video technology "to display a wide variety of user-generated content, including movie clips, TV clips, and music videos, as well as amateur content such as video blogging and short original videos" (para. 2).

Faculty and students often use clips from YouTube to illustrate communication, skills, and professional issues (http://www.youtube.com).

Technology in the Laboratory

Historically, the technology in the laboratory setting has consisted of inert models, equipment, and supplies that were used by faculty and students to "simulate" various skills, including medication administration, insertion of catheters, and intravenous therapy, to name a few.

In recent years, the development of low-definition and high-definition manikins and complex equipment has dramatically changed the laboratory environment.

Simulation offers a unique mode for experiential learning and evaluation. It also provides a risk-free environment in which learners can practice skills without fear of harming a patient. As defined by the National Council of State Boards of Nursing (2005), a simulated learning experience imitates the work environment and requires the learner to demonstrate procedural techniques, decision making, and critical thinking. Simulated learning experiences that integrate feedback, debriefing, or guided reflection have demonstrated the learners' ability to link theory and practice, to synthesize knowledge, and to promote insight (Bruce, Bridges, & Holcomb, 2003). The topology of simulation includes task trainers, computer-based programs, virtual reality, high-fidelity human patient simulators, and standardized patients. Each of these categories has a specific purpose in teaching and validating clinical skills (Decker, Sportsman, Puetz, & Billings, 2008).

The use of simulation requires strategic planning. Nurse educators must acquire the knowledge and skills needed to use this strategy, to develop realistic evidence-based case scenarios, and to design and validate standardized and reliable testing methods (Decker et al., 2008). In addition, Dillon, Boulet, Hawkins, and Swanson (2004) described the challenges of cost and time commitments, development of scoring methods, appropriate selection of simulated experiences, the issue of simulation not being completely realistic, and the need to validate whether the skills demonstrated in the simulated environment are transferred by the learner to the patient care setting.

Schiavenato (2009) noted that there is a dearth of data to support the effectiveness of simulation in nursing education. She raises such questions as:

- What is the effect of simulation replacing clinical experience versus simulation augmenting clinical experience?
- Which simulation is best in a given setting?
- What is the cost benefit of the human patient simulator?

Tackling the basic question of the *why* of simulation in nursing should "encourage the empirical execution of simulation, clarification of goals and outcomes, and facilitation of research, such as the evaluation of competing technologies and the investigation of evidence-based pedagogical and clinical practices" (p. 393).

Technology in the Classroom

In addition to active learning strategies in the classroom, faculty are now incorporating other technologies to enhance their delivery of content. For many years, faculty have used audio and video enhancements to their lectures, including audiotapes of breath and heart sounds, interviews, and music (also on CDs and the radio); movies on DVDs; videotapes and links to videocasts (i.e., YouTube); overhead transparencies; and PowerPoint presentations. There are general principles that have been identified as guides to the selection of technology for the classroom:

- The teacher must be familiar with the content of the medium.
- Print and nonprint materials have been shown to change learner behavior.
- There is no tool that is inherently better than another.

- Tools should complement the instructional methods and behavioral objectives.
- The materials should reinforce and supplement (not replace) the teacher's role.
- Tools should be appropriate for the learning environment, such as the size of and seating in the classroom, acoustics, lights, and audio-visual (AV) resources.
- Media should complement the developmental stages, educational level, and sensory abilities of the learners.
- The message must be "accurate, valid, authoritative, up to date, state of the art, appropriate, unbiased, and free of any unintended messages" (Bastable, 2008, p. 475).

Some of the newer technologies that have been found to promote learning in the classroom include:

Student response systems (clicker technology), which involves the teacher's use of a computer with an attached receiver; the computer projects a presentation for students to view. Questions can be displayed with possible answers; students have wireless keypads and select the answer they believe is correct by pushing the corresponding number or letter. Answers are sent to the receiver, the software collects the results, and the aggregate data are graphically displayed within the presentation for all participants to see. The system also stores individual student answers on all questions so that the teacher can use the data for grading purposes if desired. There is evidence that students are more engaged in the classroom when clickers are used (Bruff, 2009). Students have been found to review readings and other assigned materials prior to class in preparation for the clicker quiz, and their interactions during the clicker question presentation revealed engaged thinking processes (Berry, 2009).

Streaming video is a sequence of "moving images" that are sent in compressed form over the Internet and displayed by the viewer as they arrive. Features of streaming video are that the files remain on the server and must be viewed on a computer with an Internet connection. Some students prefer streaming video over podcasting, which indicates that each method meets different types of learner needs.

Podcasting (iPOD broadCAST) is an audio broadcast that has been converted to an MP3 file or other audio file format for playback in a digital music player. Features include the student's ability to download the recording to his or her computer or portable audio device. The podcast offers the student anywhere/anytime learning. Students report the value of podcasts as a study method that they use at home or while commuting or exercising. Podcasts are viewed as an adjunct to, not a replacement for, classroom experiences.

■ TECHNOLOGY IN THE PRACTICE SETTING

Personal Digital Assistants

McLeod and Mays (2008) noted that "the challenge for nursing education is to harness the power of (such technologies as) PDAs to empower students to navigate, evaluate, select, and synthesize information to support real-time evidence-based practice at the point of care" (p. 584). The true "tipping point" in the evolution of personal digital assistants (PDAs) was the "provision of ubiquitous wireless Internet connectivity and the consequent development of mobile browsers that enabled users to access online databases of clinical logs, health records, evidence-based guidelines, and peer-reviewed journals" (McLeod & Mays, p. 584). The typical suite for the student and faculty to purchase includes a drug reference, a drug interaction guide, a laboratory reference, a disease reference, a medical dictionary, and a drug calculation program. Other software can be added on an "as-needed" basis: for example, health assessment and procedures manuals, population-specific software, and other specialized applications that can be used to enhance and prolong the value of the PDA.

Electronic Clinical Log

Typhon's student tracking systems (http://www.typhongroup.com) are an example of electronic clinical logs that offer an alternative for documenting the types of clinical experiences in which learners are involved. Desirable features include ease of use, web entry of data, standardized data entry, flagging of selected records for review or comment, and creation of student portfolios.

■ CONCLUSION

There is an ever-evolving need to translate evidence for education into educational programming, whether it be in the academic or practice setting. The IOM and the Carnegie Foundation are two of the numerous organizations whose recommendations for nursing education include the need for translation of evidence-based educational strategies. What we know about the nature of the learners, the nature of the faculty/teachers, and the content to be presented should guide us in our work.

Although there are numerous educational theories that can serve as frameworks for evidence translation, the ones which seem most useful in nursing education are pedagogy, andragogy, learning styles, information processing, and the theory of multiple intelligence. Nurse educators should test one or more of these in the learning environment and perhaps use the best of each for their particular learners and content.

Evidence for academic education is described in this chapter with regard to methods for delivering content to learners: face-to-face, online education, hybrid education/blended learning, self-directed learning, and executive style. These methods were selected for review because of their applicability to the learners and anecdotal evidence of their increasing popularity with both nursing students and nursing staff. It can be expected that patients and families will in the future likewise request these methods for initial learning or review of information. We have been slow to test these methods in the clinical setting, especially with patients and families whose need for education is growing exponentially. Although the evidence for patient and family education to date focuses on readiness assessment and motivation, these concepts are also applicable to nursing education in both the academic and practice settings.

Technology is becoming an indispensable part of education, whoever the learners. The examples of technology described in this chapter—simulation, student response systems, streaming video, PDAs/electronic clinical log, instant messaging, text messaging, P2P networks, blogs, twitter, wikis, podcasting, virtual reality, YouTube, and Web conferencing—are not inclusive but reflect the growing number of options for teachers and learners. Each of these technologies is being tested in educational settings and, as the results are published, translation of findings will grow exponentially. Likewise, these technologies will be used to share translation of evidence for education in the years to come.

■ REFERENCES

Adams, M. (1992). Cultural inclusion in the American college classroom. *New Directions for Teaching and Learning, 49*, 5–17.

Amerson, R. (2006). Energizing the nursing lecture: Application of the theory of multiple intelligence learning. *Nursing Education Perspectives, 27*(4), 194–196.

Bankert, E. G., & Kozel, V. V. (2005). Transforming pedagogy in nursing education: A caring learning environment for adult students. *Nursing Education Perspectives, 26*(4), 227–229.

Barrows, H., & Tamblyn, R. (1980). *Problem-based learning: An approach to medical education.* New York, NY: Springer Publishing.

Bastable, S. B. (2008). *Nurse as educator: Principles of teaching and learning for nursing practice* (3rd ed.). Sudbury, MA: Jones and Bartlett.

Benner, P., Sutphen, M., Leonard, V., & Day, L. (2010). *Educating nurses: A call for radical transformation.* San Francisco, CA: Jossey-Bass.

Berry, J. (2009). Technology support in nursing education: Clickers in the classroom. *Nursing Education Perspectives, 30*(5), 295–298.

Billings, D. M., & Halstead, J. A. (2009). *Teaching in nursing: A guide for faculty* (3rd ed.). St. Louis, MO: Saunders Elsevier.

Bruce, S., Bridges, E. J., & Holcomb, J. B. (2003). Preparing to respond: Joint Trauma Training Center and USAF Nursing Warskills Simulation Laboratory. *Critical Care Nursing Clinics of North America, 15*(2), 149–162.

Bruff, D. (2009). *Teaching with classroom response systems: Creating active learning environments.* San Francisco, CA: Jossey-Bass.

Cabrera, A. F., Nora, A., Bernal, E. M., Terenzini, P. T., & Pascarella, E. T. (1998, November). *Collaborative learning: Preferences, gains in cognitive and affective outcomes, and openness to diversity among college students* (ERIC Document Reproduction Service No. ED427589). Paper presented at the Annual Meeting of the Association for the Study of Higher Education, Miami, FL.

Cantrell, S. W., O'Leary, P., & Ward, K. S. (2008). Strategies for success in online learning. *Nursing Clinics of North America, 43*(4), 547–555.

Caruso, J. B., & Kvavik, R. B. (2005). *ECAR study of students and information technology, 2005: Convenience, connection, control, and learning.* Boulder, CO: EDUCAUSE Center for Applied Research.

Cassidy, S. (2004). Learning styles: An overview of theories, models, and measures. *Educational Psychology, 24*(4), 419–444.

Decker, S., Sportsman, S., Puetz, L., & Billings, L. (2008). The evolution of simulation and its contribution to competency. *The Journal of Continuing Education in Nursing, 39*(2), 74–80.

Denig, S. J. (2004). Multiple intelligences and learning styles: Two complementary dimensions. *Teachers College Record, 106*(1), 96–111.

Dillon, G. F., Boulet, J. R., Hawkins, R. E., & Swanson, D. B. (2004). Simulations in the United States Medical Licensing Examination (USMLE). *Quality & Safety in Health Care, 13*(Suppl. 1), i41–i45.

Eduventures. (2005). *Health education: Consumer demand drives new opportunities for institutions.* Boston, MA: Author.

Emerson, R. J., & Records, K. (2008). Today's challenge, tomorrow's excellence: The practice of evidence-based education. *Journal of Nursing Education, 47*(8), 359–370.

eSchoolNews. (2009). *Cell phones used to deliver course content.* Retrieved from http://www.eschoolnews.com

Friedman, P., & Alley, R. (1984). Learning/teaching styles: Applying the principles. *Theory into Practice, 23*(1), 77–81.

Gardner, H. (1983). *Frames of mind.* New York, NY: Basic Books.

Gardner, H. (1999). *Intelligence reframed: Multiple intelligence for the 21st century.* New York, NY: Basic Books.

Gardner, H. (2003, April). *Multiple intelligences after 20 years.* Invited address presented at the annual meeting of the American Educational Research Association, Chicago.

Haggard, A. (1989). *Handbook of patient education.* Rockville, MD: Aspen.

Hmelo-Silver, C. E. (2004). Problem-based learning: What and how do students learn? *Educational Psychology Review, 16*(3), 235–266.

Institute of Medicine of the National Academies. (2003). *Health professions education: A bridge to quality.* Washington, DC: The National Academies Press.

James, W. B., & Gardner, D. L. (1995). Learning styles: Implications for distance learning. *New Directions for Adult and Continuing Education, 67*(1), 19–31.

Kallenbach, S., & Viens, J. (2004). Open to interpretation: Multiple intelligences theory in adult literacy education. *Teachers College Record, 106*(1), 58–66.

Knowles, M. (1970). *The modern practice of adult education: Andragogy versus pedagogy.* New York, NY: The Association Press.

Lichtenthal, C. (1990). *A self-study model on readiness to learn.* Unpublished manuscript.

Lunyk-Child, O. L., Crooks, D., Ellis, P. J., Ofosu, C., O'Mara, L., & Rideout, E. (2001). Self-directed learning: Faculty and student perceptions. *Journal of Nursing Education, 40*(3), 116–123.

Maag, M. (2005). The potential use of "blogs" in nursing education. *Computers, Informatics, Nursing, 23*(1), 16–24.

McKeachie, W. J., & Svinicki, M. (2006). *McKeachie's teaching tips: Strategies, research, and theory for college and university teachers.* Boston, MA: Houghton Mifflin.

McLeod, R. P., & Mays, M. Z. (2008). Back to the future: Personal digital assistants in nursing education. *Nursing Clinics of North America, 43*(4), 583–592.

National Council of State Boards of Nursing. (2005). *Clinical instruction in prelicensure nursing programs.* Retrieved from https://www.ncsbn.org/Final_Clinical_Instr_Pre_Nsg_programs.pdf

Nicholson-Nelson, K. (1998). *Developing students' multiple intelligence.* New York, NY: Scholastic Professional Books.

O'Hare, L. (2002). *Effects of traditional versus learning-style presentations of course content in adult health nursing on the achievement and attitudes of baccalaureate nursing students.* Unpublished doctoral dissertation, St. John's University, Queens, NY.

O'Neil, C. A., Fisher, C. A., & Newbold, S. K. (2009). *Developing online learning environments in nursing education* (2nd ed.). New York, NY: Springer Publishing.

Redman, B. K. (2007). *The practice of patient education: A case study approach.* St. Louis, MO: Mosby Elsevier.

Reis, R. (2008a). But, we didn't mean to teach porn: The power of play in teaching and learning. *Tomorrow's Professor.* Retrieved from http://ctl.stanford.edu

Reis, R. (2008b). The future—The era of engagement. *Tomorrow's Professor.* Retrieved from http://ctl.stanford.edu

Romiszowski, A. J. (1999). *Designing instructional systems: Decision making in course planning and curriculum design.* London, England/New York, NY: Routledge Falmer.

Schiavenato, M. (2009). Reevaluating simulation in nursing education: Beyond the human patient simulator. *Journal of Nursing Education, 48*(7), 388–394.

Skiba, D. J. (2008). Nursing education 2.0: Twitter & tweets. Can you post a nugget of knowledge in 140 characters or less? *Nursing Education Perspectives, 29*(2), 110–112.

Sternberg, R. J. (2006) *Cognitive psychology* (4th ed.). Belmont, CA: Thomson/Wadsworth.

Trangenstein, P. A. (2008). Electronic toolkit for nursing education. *Nursing Clinics of North America, 43*(4), 535–546.

Weiner, E. E. (2008). Supporting the integration of technology into contemporary nursing education. *Nursing Clinics of North America, 43*(4), 497–506.

Wikipedia (2010a). *Avatar.* Retrieved from http://en.wikipedia.org/wiki/Avatar

Wikipedia (2010b). *Text messaging.* Retrieved from http://en.wikipedia.org/wiki/Text_messaging

Wikipedia (2010c). *Twitter.* Retrieved from http://en.wikipedia.org/wiki/Twitter

Wikipedia (2010d). *YouTube.* Retrieved from http://en.wikipedia.org/wiki/YouTube

CHAPTER EIGHT

Translation of Evidence for Health Policy

Kathleen M. White

In order to advocate effectively for lifesaving legislation, advocates must have clear and compelling scientific evidence to provide a basis for policy change.
—Millie Webb, *Mothers Against Drunk Driving*

Understanding the policy process is critical to incorporation of newly generated research evidence into health care practice and policy. However, there is a large gap between the research and policy worlds. Lavis and colleagues (2002) paraphrased a title of a journal article to describe the gap between research and policy as "the paradox of health services research: if it is not used, why do we produce so much of it?" Why don't we see consistent translation of new scientific evidence into public policy? How might the interactions between researchers and policymakers become more relevant to real world problems? What strategies will improve knowledge translation into health care policy? Brownson, Royer, Ewing, and McBride (2006) suggested that researchers and policymakers are "travelers in parallel universes"; yet, linking scientific advances to public policy has tremendous promise to advance the health and well-being of the population (Brownson et al., 2006). Brownson, Chriqui, and Stamatakis (2009) discussed the importance of implementing evidence-based policy, citing that the 10 great public health achievements of the 20th century, such as seat belt laws, tobacco control, and injury prevention, were model achievements because of a policy change. However, they found that only 6.5% of the sponsors of these achievements provided details that showed that the policies or laws were based on scientific information. There are two ways how research findings are communicated; first by establishing relevance to current issues and second by using a local example to frame the effects of a policy impact, which are critical to knowing when and how quickly the research will be considered for use. Effective methods of dissemination and implementation are needed to put evidence in real world settings, including the policy environment (Brownson & Jones, 2009).

■ POLICY AND THE POLICY PROCESS

Policy is defined as the choices a society, an organization, or a group makes regarding its goals and priorities and how it will allocate its resources to those priorities. The design of policy involves specifying ends or goals to be pursued, the means for achieving those goals, and reflects the values, beliefs, and attitudes of those designing the policy (Mason, Chaffee, & Leavitt, 2011).

Public policy is defined as any action by local, state, or national government that is in response to demands of society to achieve desired goals, values, and practices. Public policy includes laws, regulations, organization/agency guidelines, private sector initiatives, and national or international specialty initiatives.

Health policy specifically addresses how and by whom health care is delivered and financed, environmental influences on health, and has direct and indirect impact on people's health. The World Health Organization (WHO) defines health policy as an agreement or consensus on the health issues, goals, and objectives to be addressed, the priorities among those objectives, and the main directions for achieving them.

The policy process, whether for any public policy or heath care policy in particular, is generally the same and goes through five steps: (a) getting on the public agenda, (b) policy formulation, (c) policy adoption, (d) policy implementation, and (e) policy evaluation (Anderson, 2011). There are several approaches to policymaking, and the decision making that ensues as policies are developed. The first is the *rational* or *linear approach* to policy decision making. Derived from classic economic theory, this approach is considered to be rational, not only because it has a logical and linear sequence, but also because it assumes full information, comparing all possible alternatives to solve the problem. The limitations to this approach are evident, primarily because an exhaustive analysis of benefits and costs to every possible alternative for dealing with a problem is not practical; it is time consuming and expensive. The *incremental approach*, also referred to as incrementalism, involves small steps to policy change. Many who are involved in the policy process argue against making radical changes and are reluctant to change things too quickly; consequently, policies get tweaked over time rather than dramatically changed all at once. Using this more practical approach, only few of the many possible alternatives are considered and tend to be the ones that involves only small changes in existing policy rather than radical innovations. Changes are made only "at the margin." Another approach to the policy decision making is known as the *garbage can approach*. This approach considers that at any particular time there is a mix of problems and possible solutions, and that this mix of problems and solutions determines the policy outcome.

Kingdon's *multiple streams approach* (2003) to policy decision making explains three streams (problem, policy, and politics) to implement evidence-based policy and to communicate and package the policy. This approach attempts to explain why some problems and alternatives are recognized and considered for the policy agenda, whereas others are not. The first stream is the *problem*. It is in this stream that problems come to the attention of policymakers, and the decision is made that something must be done about it or it goes away. Problems come to attention through triggering events, feedback, or new knowledge. The *policy* stream is when alternatives or solutions are generated by the policy community. During this time in the policy process, new knowledge or ideas must be considered feasible and practical to implement to reach the policy agenda. The *politics* stream includes the current context in which the problem and policy streams are operating within, including national mood, organized interests, and current events. When these three streams converge at a given point in time, a problem is recognized, a viable solution is identified, and a change occurs in the political stream. Kingdon (2003) says that a "window of opportunity" opens, and a policy change can be enacted.

■ WHY IS TRANSLATION OF RESEARCH TO POLICY DIFFICULT?

An often cited and important systematic review of evidence from 24 interview studies on facilitators and barriers to the use of research evidence by policymakers yielded weak results (Innvaer, Vist, Trommald, & Oxman, 2002). The use of the evidence was largely descriptive and qualitative and provided limited support for commonly held beliefs. They found that the degree to which evidence is used directly or selectively varies in relation to different types of decision makers and different types of policy questions. In the review of 24 articles, common barriers (and their frequency in parentheses) to the use of research evidence in policymaking were identified:

- Absence of personal contact between researchers and policymakers (11/24)
- Lack of timeliness or relevance of research (9/24)
- Mutual mistrust, including perceived political naivety of scientists and scientific naivety of policymakers (8/24)
- Power and budget struggles (7/24)
- Poor quality of research (6/24)
- Political instability or high turnover of policy-making staff (5/24)

They also identified the most common facilitators (and their frequency) of use of research in policymaking from the review:

- Personal contact between researchers and policymakers (13/24)
- Timeliness and relevance of the research (13/24)
- Research that included a summary with clear recommendations (11/24)
- Good quality research (6/24)
- Research that confirms current policy or endorsed self-interest (6/24)
- Community pressure or client's demand for research (4/24)
- Research that included effectiveness data (3/24)

Finally, the review also identified five strategies to increase policymakers' use of research for policymaking, focusing on what the researcher should do. The researcher should (a) have a personal and close two-way communication with the policymaker; (b) ensure that research is perceived as timely, relevant, and of high quality; (c) include effectiveness data; (d) argue that research is relevant to the demands of policymakers and the community; and (e) provide policy recommendation reports, along with the technical research reports.

Lavis, Lomas, Hamid, and Sewankambo (2006) identified four challenges to translating new research evidence to practice and policy: (a) research evidence competes with other ideas in the decision making process, (b) decision makers may not value research evidence, (c) the new research evidence may not be relevant, and (d) research evidence is often not easy to use or understand.

Brownson et al. (2006) identified eight major challenges to the translation of research to policy. Their research found that most important challenge to the translation of research to policy is the clash of cultures between the researcher and the policymaker, citing that even with sound scientific data, some policies do not get implemented because of lack of public support or competing policy issues. This clash of cultures or "two communities" view will be discussed later in the chapter. The second challenge is poor timing. The generation of new knowledge is not predictable and does not coincide with issues being on the public agenda. Third, ambiguous findings, is the frustration that policymakers have with research results. Brownson et al. (2006) suggest that policymakers want precise estimates, and researchers often provide confidence intervals that are difficult to sell or project. Fourth, balancing objectivity and advocacy is a debate in the research community and is another challenge to translation of research to policy. The debate questions whether a scientist might lose research objectivity if they take an active role in the policy process versus their obligation to report research findings in a timely and understandable manner and advocate for those results to become policy. Another challenge identified in this research is that of personal demands and the scientist's lack of time to be involved in advocacy and policymaking. Information overload and, conversely, the lack of relevant data are both challenges to translating research to policy. Policymakers are limited by the amount of information they can process. The effective communication of research findings in a relevant, timely, and compelling manner is necessary to inform the process. Finally, the mismatch of randomized thinking with nonrandom problems has always plagued the use of research data for policymaking. Brownson et al. (2006) suggest that the use of case studies or anecdotes to increase relevance and impact analysis to understand the value is an important consideration for researchers.

Later, Brownson et al. (2009) identified eight specific barriers to implementing effective evidence-based health policy: (a) a lack of value placed on prevention, (b) an insufficient evidence base, (c) mismatched time horizons, (d) the power of vested interests, (e) researchers isolated from the policy process, (f) complex and messy policy-making process, (g) individuals in one discipline not understanding the policy-making process, and, finally, (h) practitioners lacking the skills to influence evidence-based policy.

■ THEORY AND ORGANIZING FRAMEWORKS FOR TRANSLATION OF EVIDENCE TO POLICY

Research processes include a question, specifically designed methods to answer the question, data collection, analysis, and interpretation (Lavis, 2006). The public policy-making process is less linear, more unpredictable, and the vicissitudes of debate and politics can cause the issue to languish with uncertain outcome.

The classic literature on technology transfer raised the question about who is responsible for ensuring the application of new technology (Kamien & Schwartz, 1975; Lynch & Gregor, 2003). This responsibility debate, referred to as the technology-push or the need- or demand-pull, refers to the source and motivation for the innovation. The source is either the scientist who develops the innovation (technology-push), or the demand for the innovation based on perceived need (demand-pull). According to this *push–pull* theory, an innovation is likely to occur and be applied when a means to develop the innovation and the need for it are simultaneously recognized. This debate has been applied to other disciplines, and more recent discussions in the translation literature have focused on a science-push versus a user-pull debate. The science-push is the development of new knowledge driven by science. The user-pull is making evidence available when there is demand from policymakers for evidence to drive policy.

Nathan Caplan's two communities theory (1979) attempted to explain the use or non-use of research for policymaking as a symptom of the cultural or behavioral gap between researchers and policymakers. The theory posits that there are cultural differences between the research and policy-making communities, that they have different views of the world explained as a gap in values, language, reward systems, and professional affiliations. For example, the researcher is mainly concerned with pure science and esoteric issues, whereas the policymaker is more interested in immediate relevance and has an action orientation. This simple dichotomy of use versus nonuse between the two communities must be acknowledged and understood, but researchers and policymakers cannot be complacent or assume that this is the way it has to be. Caplan, Morrison, & Stambaugh (1975) also found that these two groups—the researchers and the policymakers—see themselves and each other differently. The social scientists in the research saw themselves as rational, objective, and open to new ideas, and they saw the policymakers as action and interest oriented and indifferent to evidence and new ideas. The policymakers saw themselves as responsive, action-oriented, and pragmatic, and saw the scientists as naïve, jargon-ridden, and lacking in practicality. To have an impact on developing and implementing evidence-based policy, the two groups must develop a mutual understanding of the important policy questions and the evidence that is needed to answer them.

Carol Weiss (1979) discusses the three meanings of research as (a) data, (b) ideas, or (c) argumentation, and research is only one of many sources of information used by policymakers. She views that the goal of research is to clarify and accelerate opinion to contribute to the policy process. Her work adds another dimension to the use/nonuse discussion and suggests that it is not a simple dichotomy of use and non-use, but that translation of new knowledge is built on a gradual shift in conceptual thinking over time. She posits that the real decision making is "consideration for use," and she argues that there is an "enlightenment function" of research. She identifies seven models or meanings of research use:

- Knowledge-driven—application of basic research
- Problem-solving—communication of research on agreed upon problem to the policymaker
- Enlightenment—education of the policymaker
- Political—rationalization for previously agreed upon decision
- Tactical—requesting additional information to delay action
- Interactive—competing information sources that implies a search for policy-relevant information
- Intellectual enterprise—policy research as one of many intellectual pursuits

The challenge for the research community is to improve the use of research findings in policymaking. There are numerous frameworks found in the literature that attempt to explain decision making (or lack of decision making) and translation (or lack of translation) of new knowledge into the policy process.

Lavis, Robertson, Woodside, McLeod, and Abelson (2003) developed an organizing framework for knowledge transfer into policy and posits that the push–pull tug of knowledge transfer can be loosened by attention to the message and the target audience. The framework has five key elements: (a) the *message* or how an actionable message should be developed and transferred to decision makers, (b) the *target audience* or *to whom* should the research knowledge be transferred, (c) the *messenger* or *by whom* should the research knowledge be transferred, (d) the *knowledge transfer process* or how should the research knowledge be transferred, and (e) the *evaluation* or use of objective performance measures to evaluate the effect of the transfer of the research knowledge. Lavis et al. (2003) suggests that there are four key target audiences to consider: general public, service providers, managerial decision makers, and policy decision makers, and that the message should be crafted individually to each target audience. He also stresses the importance of stakeholder involvement in the development of health care policy.

There are other models or frameworks for translation of research into policymaking worth mentioning. Dobbins, Ciliska, Cockerill, Barnsley, and DiCenso's (2002) *framework for dissemination and utilization of research for health-care policy and practice* describes a process for the adoption of research evidence into health care decision making. The framework includes the complex interrelationships between the individual, the organization, the environment, and the innovation. This framework uses Everett Rogers's five stages for the diffusion of innovation to describe the journey of the innovation into practice policy: knowledge, persuasion, decision, implementation, and confirmation. Schmid, Pratt, and Witmer (2006) developed a framework for public policy relevant to physical activity, and Rütten et al. (2003) apply the concept of *logic of events* in a model that is determined by wants, abilities, duties, and opportunities to develop and carry out health policy and evaluate impact.

Gold (2009) developed a framework from the literature, showing 10 pathways through which research may be used in policymaking and the factors that mediate the translation of research into messages that are communicated to and used buy policymakers. The 10 pathways are divided into:

1. Traditional pathways where meritorious findings drive use (big bang, gradual accumulation and diffusion, and formal synthesis);
2. Intermediaries help to communicate the research messages (researchers as communicator and experts, formal intermediary-brokered translation, and the mass media); and
3. Users seek to enhance the value of research (commissioned synthesis around policy problems, user-commissioned studies, users provide input into new research, and researcher as user).

Of course, a single pathway is rarely seen, and a composite of these pathways is more realistic and should be the focus of translation efforts to incorporate new knowledge into policy. The additional value that this analysis adds is the emphasis on the linkages of the pathways and building bridges between the research and user communities. Gold (2009) emphasizes the importance of a publicly available repository of research findings and synthesis of those findings not only around important public policy agenda issues, but also in emerging health care problems and issues to raise awareness and to stimulate further research on important topics.

Weinick and Shin (2003), as part of work for the Agency for Healthcare Research and Quality, developed a framework for developing data-driven capabilities to support policy decision making. The framework has four stages and focuses on the importance of stakeholders in making policy decisions. The first stage is *definition and priorities* that includes articulating a common definition of the policy problem among the stakeholders, clarifying stakeholder concerns and priorities, and understanding what questions need to be answered with evidence. The second stage is *generating data* or determining what data are available to support a policy decision. This stage involves assembling a matrix of all available data sources, including an evaluation of what the data represent and confidence in the data, determining the available measures, identifying the need for new or additional data, and developing an inventory of current and past initiatives. The third stage is *assessment* or explaining what the data say about the current state of the problem, undertaking activities that include analyzing data, clarifying the limitations of current knowledge, and disseminating the findings. The fourth and final stage is *action*. The main activity of the action stage is selecting a policy option that is supported by the data. This includes evaluating the impact of past and current initiatives and any unintended consequences, estimating the short- and long-term effects of the options, and making the policy recommendation. This stage should also include an evaluation of values at issue, anticipation of the outcomes of policy options, and development of a plan for communication of the policy choice.

In 2007, the WHO did a review of the capacity issues underlying different aspects of the relationship between researchers and policymakers (Green & Bennett, 2007). Green and Bennett (2007) used a framework to guide the process, to show that there is not a linear relationship between the generation of evidence and policymaking, and that there are many factors involved in the relationship of how new knowledge gets translated into policy. The framework first describes four functional processes: (a) priority setting for research, (b) knowledge generation and dissemination, (c) evidence filtering and amplification, and (d) the policy process. As evidence-informed (this framework does not use evidence-based policy) policymaking occurs, it is recognized that there are many direct and indirect influences on the policymaking, including ideology and values, ability to use the evidence, personal experience and intuition, special interests, and external influences. There are many examples of this filtering and amplification of evidence in the policy arena. Special interests often use this as a way to pick out or *filter* their particular research outputs, translate them into policy messages, and attempt to influence policymakers. The next level of concern for the framework is the various organizations that are carrying out the functions described previously and their interrelationships. They identified their organizations as funding bodies, research institutions, advocacy organizations, the media, think tanks, and government bodies. Finally, the framework includes certain organizational capacities that the organizations must have to carry out the functions, such as leadership and governance, adequate and sustainable resources, and communication and networks. These all operate with a broader national context and wider environment that includes external funders, external research organizations, and external advocacy groups. The added value of this framework to the discussion of translation of research to policymaking is the previously recognized important role of the organization in the policymaking process and to help researchers and policymakers understand what works for whom, and in what circumstances.

■ STAKEHOLDERS OR THE RESEARCH USER GROUP

Knowledge translation for evidence-based policy has been described as a unidirectional flow of information that resulted in a specific policy. If the flow of information was from the researcher to the policymaker, it was called the science-push or knowledge-driven model (Jacobson, Butterill, & Goering, 2003). Conversely, if the policymaker commissioned the information to address a policy problem, it was referred to as a demand-pull or problem-solving model.

Jacobson et al. (2003) developed a framework for knowledge translation: understanding user context from a review of literature and their own experience. The framework contains five domains: (a) the user group, (b) the issue, (c) the research, (d) the researcher–user relationship, and (e) the dissemination strategies. Within each domain, the authors pose questions to the researcher that can serve as a way of organizing the translation to the user group.

The first domain is the *user group*. There are many questions posed under this domain organizing the questions, and they focus on the context in which the user group operates; the morphology, politics, and decision-making practices of the user group; how the user group uses information; and experience with translation.

User Group Questions (Jacobson et al., 2003)

In what formal or informal structures is the user group embedded?

What is the political climate surrounding the user group?

To whom is the user group accountable?

Are changes expected in any of these?

How big is the user group?

How centralized is the user group?

How institutionalized is the user group?

What are the politics within the user group?

What kinds of decisions does the user group make?

What is the user group's attitude toward decision making?

What criteria does the user group use to make decisions?

What actions are available to the user group?

What are the stages or phases of the user group's decision-making work?

What is the user group's pace of work?

What sources of information does the user group access and use?

How does the user group process information (i.e., how does it access, disseminate, and apply information internally)?

For what purposes does the user group use information?

Has the user group demonstrated an ability to learn?

What incentives exist for the user group to use research? Is the user group cynical about research and researchers?

How sophisticated is the user group's knowledge of research methods and terminology?

Does the user group have a history of being involved in knowledge translation?

What knowledge translation structures and processes already exist?

What resources does the user group devote to knowledge translation?

What are the user group's expectations of the researcher? Of the knowledge translation process?

How many user group members will be involved in the knowledge translation process? Who are they?

The second domain is the *issue* and includes questions about the effect of the issue on the user group, how the user group currently deals with the issue and whether this is changing or not, whether there is uncertainty or conflict surrounding the issue, and what are the risks associated with the issue (Jacobson et al., 2003).

The *research* itself is the third domain and encourages the researcher to think about the source, focus, and methodology of the research; the quality, consistency, and ambiguity of the research; the relevance of the research to the user group, such as whether the research has an immediate application, whether it is action oriented, and whether it is compatible with the user group's expectations or priorities; and, finally, what the implications of the research are for the user group and how politically charged they are (Jacobson et al., 2003).

The fourth domain is the *research–user relationship* and focuses the researcher on the linkage between the researcher and the user group, how much trust and rapport exist, do they have a history of working together, how frequently they have contact with one another, and whether the researcher and the user group have agreed on the outcomes of the translation and about the responsibilities and interactions each will have during knowledge translation (Jacobson et al., 2003).

The final domain deals with how the translation will be organized and the *dissemination strategies* that will be used during the translation, such as how to communicate, format, detail needed, use of feedback and reminders, and to what extent and in what ways should the researcher continue to be available to the user group after the conclusion of translating the knowledge (Jacobson et al., 2003).

Attention to these domains by the researcher will improve translation planning and implementation and raise awareness of the information needed by users that can increase the uptake of the research results. The early involvement of multiple stakeholders with specific vested interests is more likely to develop consensus and yield a user-friendly policy that can be successfully implemented and sustained (Irvin et al., 2007; Nieva et al., 2005).

■ SELECTED TRANSLATION OF EVIDENCE TO POLICY

Sorian and Baugh recognized the importance of state participation in setting health policy based on evidence. They raised the following questions: (a) How useful is policy research in making policy decisions? (b) Is research information getting to policymakers in a timely and useful manner? and (c) How can the needs of researchers and policymakers be better aligned? In an attempt to answer these questions, researchers from Georgetown University's Institute for Health Care Research and Policy and the T. Baugh and Company marketing firm conducted a telephone survey of state-based health policymakers. They interviewed 97 legislators, 97 legislative staff members, and 87 executive managers of health-related state agencies (Sorian & Baugh, 2002) to identify pathways and factors that could assist communicating health policy research findings to state policymakers. Results of the survey showed that 53% of the respondents only skim materials and that they never get to 35% of the material. They reported that 49% of the information they receive is not relevant, and when probed about what would make it relevant, 67% said they needed the information to be focused on current debate or 25% on real people. They also identified what made information least useful to them: 36% said when the information is not relevant or focused on real problems; 22% said when it is too long or dense; 20% reported information not to be relevant when it was too theoretical, technical, or used jargon; and 19% were concerned about bias.

Pollack, Samuels, Frattaroli, and Gielen (2010) discussed numerous examples of proven-effective injury prevention measures, such as passenger restraint devices, smoke alarms, residential sprinklers, and motorcycle and bicycle helmets. Their experience has shown that personal contact between researchers and policymakers and timely conveyance of easy-to-understand information that is relevant to the policy context facilitates the acceleration of translation of knowledge to action to prevent injury and protect the population. Additionally, information on the burden of the problem, costs associated with action or inaction, and options for policy formulation are all important to include (Jilcott, Ammerman, Sommers, & Glasgow, 2007; Pollack et al., 2010).

Tomson et al. (2005) reported on the usefulness of research evidence in implementing a national drug policy in the Lao People's Democratic Republic. Their research concluded that a close interaction between the researchers and the policymakers and attention to broad dissemination of results is important to acceptance of new evidence for drug policies, but that more research is needed to understand the interaction necessary between researchers and decision makers.

In 2005, the Congress passed legislation as part of the Deficit Reduction Act that requires the Secretary of Department of Health and Human Services through the Center for Medicare and Medicaid Services (CMS) to identify health care conditions among admitted patients to the hospital that are (a) high cost, high volume, or both; (b) result in the assignment of a case to a diagnosis-related group that has a higher payment when present as a secondary diagnosis, and (c) could reasonably have been prevented through the application of evidence-based guidelines (http://www.cms.gov/HospitalAcqCond/06_Hospital-Acquired _Conditions.asp). The new law was applicable to 3,500 acute care hospitals reimbursed by Medicare. On July 31, 2008, CMS identified 12 categories of conditions that met the three criteria stated previously and were selected for this hospital-acquired condition (HAC) payment provision in the fiscal year 2009 final rule:

1. Foreign object retained after surgery
2. Air embolism
3. Blood incompatibility
4. Stage III and IV pressure ulcers
5. Falls and trauma, including fractures, dislocations, intracranial injuries, crushing injuries, burns, and electric shock
6. Manifestations of poor glycemic control, such as diabetic ketoacidosis, nonketotic hyperosmolar coma, hypoglycemic coma, secondary diabetes with ketoacidosis, and secondary diabetes with hyperosmolarity
7. Catheter-associated urinary tract infection (UTI)
8. Vascular catheter-associated infection
9. Surgical site infection following (a) coronary artery bypass graft (CABG); (b) bariatric surgeries such as laparoscopic gastric bypass, gastroenterostomy, and laparoscopic gastric restrictive surgery; and (c) orthopedic procedures of the spine, neck, shoulder, and elbow
10. Deep vein thrombosis (DVT)/pulmonary embolism (PE) following total knee or hip replacement

Medicare will no longer pay hospitals at higher rates for the increased costs of care if any of these 10 conditions that have been determined to be reasonably preventable by following generally accepted evidence-based practice guidelines are acquired during the hospitalization.

This policy, using evidence-based practice guidelines based on the translation of research to practice and now to policy, is important to standardizing and improving access to appropriate treatment for patients. The benefits should be significant to health care (White, 2008).

The transitional care model (TCM), developed by researchers at the University of Pennsylvania and funded by the National Institutes of Health, is another example of a translation of an evidence-based strategy into a practice delivery model. The model uses advanced practice registered nurses with specialized training to care for older adults with multiple chronic conditions and support their family caregivers (Naylor et al., 2004; Naylor et al., 2009). The TCM has had significant and sustained outcomes including: avoiding hospital readmissions and emergency room visits for primary and coexisting conditions; improvements in health outcomes after discharge; enhancement in patient and family caregiver satisfaction; and reductions in total health care costs (Naylor & Sochalski, 2010). This success of the TCM has positioned it for translation into national health care policy. Aetna has adopted the TCM to achieve better outcomes for its older adult enrollees with multiple chronic problems. American Association of Retired Persons (AARP) has recommended expansion of the services of the TCM to its members. The National Quality Forum has endorsed the deployment of evidence-based transitional care, such as the TCM, as one of 25 national preferred practices for care coordination. Lastly, the Patient Protection and Affordable Care Act of 2010, President Obama's health care reform legislation, includes support for design, measurement, and payment innovation around evidence-based transitional care.

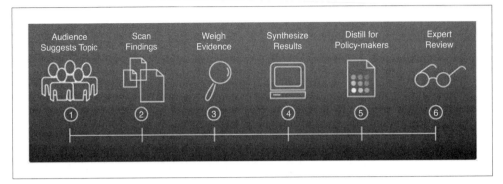

FIGURE 8.1   The RWJF Synthesis Project Framework. Retrieved from
http://www.rwjf.org/pr/synthesisabout.jsp.

The Robert Wood Johnson Foundation (RWJF) Synthesis Project (Figure 8.1) was started to give policymakers access to reliable information, develop insights into complex policy decisions, and produce briefs and reports that synthesize research findings on perennial health policy questions . The project started with a question: "Why aren't research results more useful to policymakers?" (Colby, Quinn, Williams, Bilheimer, & Goodell, 2008) Policymakers answered and identified three needs for use of research evidence in the development of policy: clear translation, accessible and easy-to-use information, and relevance to the policy context (Colby et al., 2008). They explained that policymakers are besieged with information, but results are not translated for policy decisions; research does not address pressing policy questions; journal articles and research reports are written for researchers not policymakers; and policymakers have little time to stay abreast of current research (http://www.rwjf.org/pr/synthesisabout.jsp). The RWJF Synthesis initiative developed products to address policymakers' requests for short, skim-able, and policy-focused information, focusing on the findings, not the methods (Colby et al., 2008). They developed policy briefs, research synthesis reports, and data charts. These project deliverables are structured around policy questions, rather than research issues, they distill and weigh the strength of research evidence in a rigorous and objective manner, and they draw out the policy implications of findings (http://www.rwjf.org/pr/synthesisabout.jsp). Finally, they attempt to tell a "synthesis story" that addresses four questions: (a) Why is this of interest to policymakers? (b) What "story" does the evidence tell? (c) What choices does the evidence suggest would be most effective? and (d) What are the implications for policymakers (Colby et al., 2008)?

■ STRATEGIES TO INCREASE THE UPTAKE OF RESEARCH TO POLICY

The literature abounds with discussion of strategies to increase the uptake of evidence into policy or lessons learned from an attempt to translate research into policy. As has been said about moving evidence into practice, there is a similar need to move from knowing to doing (Nutley, Walter, & Davies, 2003). Lavis et al. (2002) concludes that careful attention must be paid to where we look for research use, what we are looking for, the conditions under which the research is used and not used and, most importantly, the way in which research is used and its use in the context of other competing influences in the policymaking process. Brownson et al. (2006) suggest several actions to bridge the research policy chasm, but all are aimed at the researcher: understand the complexity and drivers in decision making; find a way to understand and be involved in the policy process; communicate information more effectively; make better use of analytic tools; educate staffers on science; develop systems for policy surveillance; conduct policy research; improve training and educational programs for scientists; build appropriate, transdisciplinary teams; and cultivate political champions. Likewise, policymakers have responsibility to bridge this chasm also.

Mercer et al. (2010) wrote a case study examining the lessons learned from translating evidence on the effectiveness of laws to lower the legal blood alcohol limit for drivers. They reported that the successful translation of evidence into policy was related to the following: (a) salience of the health problem and policy intervention, in addition to the compelling relationships between the health problem, policy intervention, and health outcomes; (b) use of systematic review methods to synthesize the full body of evidence; (c) use of a recognized, credible, and impartial process for assessing the evidence; (d) development of evidence-based policy recommendations by an independent, impartial body; (e) ability to capitalize on readiness and teachable moments; (f) active participation of key partners and intended users throughout all stages of the process; (g) use of personalized channels, targeted formats, and compelling graphics to disseminate the evidence; (h) capacity to involve multiple stakeholders in encouraging uptake and adherence; and (i) attention paid to addressing sustainability.

The literature discusses many ways to facilitate the uptake of research to policy, yet it is widely recognized that it is still a difficult challenge (Dickson & Flynn, 2009; Hinshaw & Grady, 2011). However, experience has taught that there are several key strategies that will increase the likelihood that policy makers will use evidence in their decision making for policy development. First, and most importantly, is to develop effective two-way communication with the policy maker. This should begin ahead of the policy question reaching the public agenda. An open dialogue between the research community and the policy makers about health care issues of concern in real time will increase the likelihood that each communicates their needs in the research and policy making processes. Second, it is important that researchers take the time to ensure that the research is perceived as timely, relevant, and of high quality.

In today's environment, the inclusion of effectiveness data as evidence is a key to success to inform choices that both clinicians and patients are confronting. New evidence that affects comparative effectiveness should be reviewed and incorporated when relevant and appropriate (Coopey, James, Lawrence and Clancey, 2008).

Finally, provide a synthesis of the relevant evidence to inform policies. As discussed previously, RWJF suggests the use of the "Synthesis Story." There are two other valuable techniques that are used to synthesize data and evidence for policy makers. The policy brief, often referred to as the "two pager," is written by those trying to influence or impact a policy maker or a decision. The purpose of a policy brief is to assist the policy maker to evaluate policy options on a specific issue. Policy briefs offer policy options informed by evidence with rationale and consequences for choosing each option. The brief usually makes a recommendation for a preferred and specific course of action. See Box 8.1, How to Write a Policy Brief.

The other technique is to do a systematic review of the evidence (Dobbins, 2010; Dobbins et al, 2001). A systematic review is the application of explicit scientific methods that appraise and summarize evidence. A systematic review reduces a large amount of evidence on

BOX 8.1

How to Write a Policy Brief – The Two Pager

Components of a Policy Brief

1. **Executive Summary or Abstract**—The executive summary or abstract should be a short summary of approximately 150 words that states clearly and succinctly the purpose of the policy brief and its recommendations.

2. **Statement of the Issue/Problem**—The statement of the issue is the first section of the policy brief and is a short statement of the problem with a clear description of definition of the issue. Sometimes the statement of the issue is phrased as a question that requires a decision.

3. **Background Section**—The background section describes the background and history of the issue. Be clear, precise, and succinct. This section should include only the essential facts that a decision maker "needs to know" to understand the context of the problem. There are usually reams of information that can be included in this section, however, consider that your job is to filter all the possible information about this issue and what do you think the policy maker really needs to read. For example, discuss any pre-existing policies, any policy options that have been considered in the past, or merely describe what has taken place in the past or been done by others for and against this issue. It is important to note that the absence of action in the past may be considered a policy decision.

4. **Statement of your organization's interests in the issue**—The statement of your organization's interest in the issue is important to remind the policy maker or reader of why the issue matters for that organization, group or the country.

5. **Policy Options**—The policy options section of the policy brief delineates the possible courses of action or inaction. Usually the decision maker is given at least three potential courses of action. Those three courses of action include the status quo, maximum change and some policy option in between no action and maximum change. Sometimes there are more than one choice in between which then increases the number of policy options and the complexity of decision making. Include the advantages and disadvantages of each policy option.

6. **Recommendation**—In the recommendation section, state what your recommendation is for action. This is usually done by prioritizing the relative pros and cons of the options presented and then making a recommendation of one option.

7. **Sources or consultations**—Include and references, sources of information and interviews or consultations conducted with experts on the issue.

BOX 8.2

What Is a Systematic Review?

A systematic review is a summary of the literature that uses explicit methods to perform a comprehensive literature search and critical appraisal of individual studies. This critical appraisal reviews for strength, quality and consistency of the evidence. The review may also use appropriate statistical techniques to combine these valid studies (Straus, Richardson, Glasziou, and Haynes, 2005). A systematic review provides a mechanism to identify studies with strong and weak designs and limit the bias of the weaker designs that might overestimate the effects or benefits of the evidence.

 For policy making, the systematic review uses specific and reproducible search strategies to generate evidence to answer a specific policy question. The systematic review provides the strongest type of evidence that is available on the policy issue, both published and unpublished. A review of the strength and quality is conducted on all of the existing evidence on that policy topic/question. The review of the evidence is then combined into a single analysis where explicit methods are used to limit bias and to evaluate the quality of the evidence.

Websites that house current systematic reviews of evidence include:

www.cochrane.org

www.joannabriggs.edu.au

www.ahrq.gov OR www.ngc.gov

---

an issue of concern to a report that determines the quality, quantity, and consistency of that evidence. As part of the scientific methods, the systematic review attempts to limit bias and improve the reliability of any recommendations.

The combination of the information from many studies on a specific issue can increase the strength of the overall evidence than any one study result could yield, increasing its power.

See Box 8.2, What Is a Systematic Review?

■ SUMMARY

This chapter has discussed the importance of translating new evidence not only into practice, but also for policymaking. For evidence to be used in the policymaking arena, there is a critical need that evidence be of high quality, yet, understandable and accessible to policymakers. Lavis, Posada, Haines, and Osei (2004) suggest using systematic reviews to summarize new evidence and answer three simple questions for policymakers: (a) could it work, (b) will it work or what will it take to make it work, and (c) is the balance of risk and benefit worth it?

However, politics will always have a role in policymaking. When it comes to the translation of research into health care policy, attention must be directed to recognizing the importance of the current health care policy agenda and how problems or issues got on and off the policy agenda. This also means regularly interacting with policymakers to understand what is currently making news, what is of interest to all of the audiences that they have to contend with (consumers, policymakers, and practitioners alike), and finding out what the policy questions are that they need data to answer. This would create a perfect world where policy is informed with evidence and that policy could be directed to improve health and reduce health inequalities in our health care system.

■ REFERENCES

Anderson, J. E. (2011). *Public policymaking: An introduction* (7th ed.). Boston, MA: Wadsworth Cengage Learning.

Brownson, R. C., Chriqui, J. F., & Stamatakis, K. A. (2009). Understanding evidence-based public health policy. *American Journal of Public Health, 99*(9), 1576–1583.

Brownson, R. C., & Jones, E. (2009). Bridging the gap: Translating research into policy and practice. *Preventive Medicine, 49*(4), 313–315.

Brownson, R. C., Royer, C., Ewing, R., & McBride, T. D. (2006). Researchers and policymakers: Travelers in parallel universes. *American Journal of Preventive Medicine, 30*(2), 164–172.

Caplan, N. (1979). The two-communities theory and knowledge utilization. *American Behavioral Scientist, 22*(3), 459–470.

Caplan, N. S., Morrison, A., & Stambaugh, R. J. (1975). *The use of social science knowledge in policy decisions at the national level: A report to respondents.* Ann Arbor, MI: University of Michigan.

Colby, D. C., Quinn, B. C., Williams, C. H., Bilheimer, L. T., & Goodell, S. (2008). Research glut and information famine: Making research evidence more useful for policymakers. *Health Affairs, 27*(4), 1177–1182.

Coopey, M., James, M. D., Lawrence, W., & Clancey, C. M. (2008). The challenge of comparative effectiveness: Getting the right information to the right people at the right time. *Journal of Nursing Care Quality, 23*(1), 1–5.

Department of Health and Human Services, Center for Medicare and Medicaid Services (2011). Hospital-acquired conditions. Baltimore, MD: Authors. Retrieved from http://www.cms.gov/HospitalAcqCond/06_Hospital-Acquired_Conditions.asp

Dickson, G., & Flynn, L. (2009). *Nursing policy research: Turning evidence-based research into health policy.* New York: Springer Publishing.

Dobbins, M. (2010). Dissemination and use of research evidence for policy and practice. In J. Rycroft-Malone, & T. Bucknall, Eds., *Models & frameworks for implementing evidence-based practice.* UK: John Wiley & Sons.

Dobbins, M., Cockerill, R., & Barnsley, J., (2001). Factors affecting the utilization of systematic reviews: A study of public health decision makers. *International Journal of Technology Assessment in Health Care, 17*(2), 203–214.

Dobbins, M., Ciliska, D., Cockerill, R., Barnsley, J., & DiCenso, A. (2002). A framework for the dissemination and utilization of research for health-care policy and practice. *The Online Journal of Knowledge Synthesis for Nursing, 9*, 7.

Gold, M. (2009). Pathways to the use of health services research in policy. *Health Services Research*, *44*(4), 1111–1136.

GRADE* Working Group. (2004). Grading quality of evidence and strength of recommendations. *British Medical Journal*, *328*(7454), 1490–1494

Green, A., & Bennett, S. (Eds.). (2007). *Sound choices: Enhancing capacity for evidence-informed health policy.* Geneva: World Health Organization.

Hinshaw, A. S., & Grady, P., Eds. (2011). *Shaping health policy through nursing research.* New York: Springer Publishing.

Innvaer, S., Vist, G., Trommald, M., & Oxman, A. (2002). Health policy-makers' perceptions of their use of evidence: A systematic review. *Journal of Health Services Research & Policy*, *7*(4), 239–244.

Irvin, C. B., Afilalo, M., Sherman, S. C., Stack, S. J., Huckson, S., Kaji, A., & Eskin, B. (2007). The use of health care policy to facilitate evidence-based knowledge translation in emergency medicine. *Academic Emergency Medicine*, *14*(11), 1030–1035.

Jacobson, N., Butterill, D., & Goering, P. (2003). Development of a framework for knowledge translation: Understanding user context. *Journal of Health Services Research & Policy*, *8*(2), 94–99.

Jadad, A. R., Moore, R. A., Carroll, D., Jenkinson, C., Reynolds, D. J., Gavaghan, D. J., & McQuay, H. J. (1996). Assessing the quality of reports of randomized clinical trials: Is blinding necessary? *Controlled Clinical Trials, 17*(1), 1–12.

Jilcott, S., Ammerman, A., Sommers, J., & Glasgow, R. E. (2007). Applying the RE-AIM framework to assess the public health impact of policy change. *Annals of Behavioral Medicine*, *34*(2), 105–114.

Kamien, M., & Schwartz, N. (1975). Market structure and innovation: A survey. *Journal of Economic Literature*, *13*, 1–37.

Kingdon, J. W. (2003). *Agendas, alternatives, and public policies* (2nd ed.). New York, NY: Addison-Wesley Educational Publishers.

Lavis, J. N. (2006). Research, public policymaking, and knowledge-translation processes: Canadian efforts to build bridges. *The Journal of Continuing Education in the Health Professions*, *26*(1), 37–45.

Lavis, J. N., Lomas, J., Hamid, M., & Sewankambo, N. K. (2006). Assessing country-level efforts to link research to action. *Bulletin of the World Health Organization*, *84*(8), 620–628.

Lavis, J. N., Posada, F. B., Haines, A., & Osei, E. (2004). Use of research to inform public policymaking. *Lancet*, *364*(9445), 1615–1621.

Lavis, J. N., Robertson, D., Woodside, J. M., McLeod, C. B., & Abelson, J. (2003). How can research organizations more effectively transfer research knowledge to decision makers? *The Milbank Quarterly*, *81*(2), 221–248.

Lavis, J. N., Ross, S. E., Hurley, J. E., Hohenadel, J. M., Stoddart, G. L., Woodward, C. A., & Abelson, J. (2002). Examining the role of health services research in public policymaking. *The Milbank Quarterly*, *80*(1), 125–154.

Lynch, T., & Gregor, S. (2003). Technology-push or user-pull? The slow death of the transfer-of-technology approach to intelligent support systems development. In S. Clarke, E. Coakes, M. G. Hunter, & A. Wenn (Eds.), *Socio-technical and human cognition elements of information systems.* Hershey, PA: Information Science Publishing.

Mason, D., Chaffee, M., & Leavitt, J. (2011). *Policy & politics in nursing and health care* (6th ed.). St. Louis, MO: Elsevier Saunders.

Mercer, S. L., Sleet, D. A., Elder, R. W., Cole, K. H., Shults, R. A., & Nichols, J. L. (2010). Translating evidence into policy: Lessons from the case of lowering the legal blood alcohol limit for drivers. *Annals of Epidemiology, 20*(6), 412–420.

Naylor, M., & Sochalski, J. A. (2010). Scaling up: Bringing the transitional care model into the mainstream. *Commonwealth Fund, 103*, 1–12.

Naylor, M. D., Brooten, D. A., Campbell, R. L., Maislin, G., McCauley, K. M., & Schwatz, J. S. (2004). Transitional care of older adults hospitalized with heart failure: A randomized, controlled trial. *Journal of the American Geriatrics Society, 52*(5), 675–684.

Naylor, M. D., Feldman, P. H., Keating, S., Koren, M. J., Kurtzman, E. T., Maccoy, M. C., & Krakauer, R. (2009). Translating research into practice: Transitional care for older adults. *Journal of Evaluation in Clinical Practice, 15*(6), 1164–1170.

Nieva, V. F., Murphy, R., Ridley, N., Donaldson, N., Combes, J., Mitchell, P., . . . Carpenter, D. (2005). From science to service: A framework for the transfer of patient safety research into practice. *Advances in Patient Safety, 2*.

Nutley, S., Walter, I., & Davies, H. (2003). Moving from knowing to doing: A framework for understanding the evidence-into-practice agenda. *Evaluation, 9*(2), 125–148.

Pollack, K. M., Samuels, A., Frattaroli, S., & Gielen, A. C. (2010). The translation imperative: Moving research into policy. *Injury Prevention, 16*(2), 141–142.

Rütten, A., Lüschen, G., von Lengerke, T., Abel, T., Kannas, L., Rodríguez Diaz, J. A., . . . van der Zee, J. (2003). Determinants of health policy impact: A theoretical framework for policy analysis. *Sozial- und Präventimedizin, 48*(5): 293–300.

Schmid, T. L., Pratt, M., & Witmer, L. (2006). A framework for physical activity policy research. *Journal of Physical Activity and Health, 3*(Suppl. 1), S20–S29.

Sorian, R., & Baugh, T. (2002). Power of information: Closing the gap between research and policy. *Health Affairs, 21*(2), 264–273.

Straus, S. E., Richardson, W., Glasziou, P., & Haynes, R. (2005). *Evidence-based medicine: How to practice and teach evidence-based medicine* (3rd ed.). London, United Kingdom: Elsevier.

Tomson, G., Paphassarang, C., Jönsson, K., Houamboun, K., Akkhavong, K., & Wahlström, R. (2005). Decision-makers and the usefulness of research evidence in policy implementation— a case study from Lao PDR. *Social Science & Medicine, 61*(6), 1291–1299.

Weinick, R. M. & Shin, P. W. (2003). Monitoring the health care safety net: Developing data-driven capabilities to support policymaking. Washington, DC: Agency for Healthcare Research and Quality.

Weiss, C. (1979). The many meanings of research utilization. *Public Administration Review, 39*(5), 426–431.

White, K. M. (2008). The new CMS payment system: Too much, too soon? *Nursing Management, 39*(10), 38–42.

CHAPTER NINE

Information Technology: A Foundation and Enabler for Translation of Evidence Into Practice

Barbara B. Frink

■ INTRODUCTION

Information technology is a critical component of the translation of evidence to clinical practice. It plays a pivotal role in all aspects of the process: from scientific discovery, through knowledge dissemination, practice guideline creation, clinical decision support and electronic health record (EHR) systems, and the use and reuse of data for generations of new knowledge/evidence for practice or research. Information technology infrastructure is fundamental to evidence-based practice today, and future developments in generating new knowledge are dependent on it. Information technology is not just about technology. In the context of evidence-based practice, equally critical aspects of the information infrastructure are the cultures and collaboration of stakeholders, and the policies that govern and give meaning to individual and population health care.

The reader will be introduced to the role of information technology in the process of translating evidence to clinical practice from three perspectives: (a) translation of biomedical research evidence knowledge to practice; (b) introduction of evidence knowledge to the processes of care; and (c) generating practice-based evidence and research evidence from the processes of care.

One of the fundamental questions for patients and families, providers of care, and payers of care is: What is the most effective care or treatment for this patient at this point in time, with what expected risks, benefits, and outcomes? To answer this question, the available knowledge—or evidence—is applied to a specific clinical situation. Although this may appear to be a straightforward process, the application of evidence to practice requires complex decision processes as well as an infrastructure of multiple health care entity relationships. Examples of such entities are: (a) the biomedical research enterprise, (b) the national quality and patient safety infrastructure, (c) the national and professional society practice guidelines, (d) the health advocacy organizations, (e) the clinical health information technology infrastructure, (f) the health beliefs and culture of patients and families, (g) and the practice patterns of individuals and groups of clinicians. Information technology is fundamental to carrying out the work of these entities. Each entity has a role in the generation, testing, and application of evidence to clinical care; however, efforts are often isolated or not directly "translatable" from one group or endeavor to another. There can be many challenges for clinicians in making the transition from informal anecdotal social network and colleague connections to use of formalized databases and knowledge repositories as a part of the clinical workflow (Pravikoff, Tanner, & Pierce, 2005; Tanner, Pierce, & Pravikoff, 2004). Assisting and directing the cultural changes that will support clinicians in making these adjustments are the key areas of focus for clinical information technology professionals and clinical informatics professionals.

Much has been written about the translation of research knowledge to clinical practice, and gaps between the existence of clinical evidence and adoption of best practices based on that evidence to care and treatment decisions. *Crossing the Quality Chasm* (Institute of Medicine [IOM], 2001) addressed some of the challenges facing U.S. health care in this area which were attributed to increasing complexity of science and technology; rise in chronic illness incidence; poorly organized health care delivery systems; and lack of critical information technology. This was amplified by a 2003 study that reported that evidence-based care is delivered only 55% of the time in the United States (McGlynn et al., 2003). To address these challenges, several major programs and initiatives have been developed to support the need for translation, development, dissemination, and adoption of evidence to practice. These include national quality measures, guideline development and testing, research agendas, knowledge content providers, and health information technology decision support applications (Agency for Healthcare Research and Quality [AHRQ], translating research into practice [TRIP] I, II, 2004; AHRQ, 2010; Bakken & McArthur, 2001). The focus for this chapter is highlighting key areas in which health information technology supports the translation of evidence to practice.

As can be seen from the diverse number of stakeholders involved, information technology is a necessary, but not sufficient, enabler of translation of evidence to practice. Additional components are presented in other chapters of this text. Understanding the role of information technology in evidence-based practice requires both a granular view of individual patient encounters, and a high level perspective that includes the influence of public policy and the aggregation and analysis of vast amounts of clinical data captured at the point of care. The chapter begins with a brief introduction of what might be considered to be a futuristic vision: the potential of information technology to transform data captured at the point of care into new practice-based evidence—new knowledge—that can be applied in clinical practice. The chapter sections that follow consider the role of information technology in the translation of biomedical research knowledge to practice from several perspectives: a vision of generating new knowledge from practice-based evidence; policy perspectives of translating research evidence to practice and discovering knowledge from the process of patient care; a practice perspective of introducing evidence into the process of care, including clinical decision support; and the role of information technology in generating new language.

■ THE VISION: GENERATING NEW KNOWLEDGE—PRACTICE-BASED EVIDENCE

The convergence of innovation and development in information technology with developments in dissemination of scientific evidence is transforming the potential for both evidence-based clinical practice and the generation of new knowledge from clinical practice. Dr. Elias Zerhouni, former director of the National Institutes of Health (NIH), has characterized this convergence as the health care era of the four Ps: predictive, personalized, preemptive, and participatory medicine (Zerhouni, 2007). In this era, patients and families become full participants in health care decisions and have access to knowledge from scientific studies as well as from the results of new discoveries based on practice evidence and personalized health data.

> The translation of scientific evidence into clinical practice is a fundamental issue in the generation and application of knowledge in health care. That translation process has traditionally followed specific guidelines and conformed to an evidence hierarchy. It is becoming increasingly clear that practice-related questions cannot always be answered effectively with current methods of inquiry . . . new data sources will be required. . . . Through the use of integrated data networks and data repositories of clinical care transactions, health information technology provides an opportunity to answer such questions in a more timely and cost effective manner. . . . Leveraging health care information technology and reusing the associated clinical data will produce a new source of study information that will likely disrupt the hierarchy of evidence. Nevertheless, the scale and the richness of these data sets will become a powerful aid in new discovery. (Frink & Dhar, 2011, p. 332)

Dr. Carolyn Clancy, director of the AHRQ, articulated the relationship between investment in health information technology and potential for this new level of knowledge generation:

> Anticipated growth in investments in health IT across the health care sector now offers an unprecedented opportunity for redefining the possibilities of observational studies, accelerating and targeting the uptake of relevant information, and providing feedback to the biomedical enterprise itself. (Clancy, 2006, p. 591)

Despite the scientific and health care communities' support of evidence-based approaches to care and futuristic visions of informatics-generated practice knowledge, there is recent evidence of consumer skepticism about evidence-based practice in health care. In a 2010 qualitative study (Carman et al., 2010), researchers found the following: "The key finding from focus groups, interviews, and the online survey is that there is a fundamental disconnect between the central tenets of evidence-based health care and the knowledge, values, and beliefs held by many consumers" (p. 3). Such findings offer clarifying information and challenge for both health care information technology professionals, as well as clinicians, because the vision for a new era of evidence-based practice enabled by information technology is embraced. Because the ultimate goal of evidence-based care is improved health of the population, understanding the perspectives of consumers is a critical component of the process. As each of the chapter sections demonstrates, for the potential of this vision to be realized, there are many complex and important challenges to be addressed, and new areas of discovery that must underpin the application, use, and mining of health information technology.

■ POLICY PERSPECTIVE: TRANSLATION OF RESEARCH EVIDENCE TO PRACTICE

"Reliable evidence is essential to improve health care quality and to support efficient use of limited resources" (Tunis, Stryer, & Clancy, 2003, p. 1624). In both public and scientific media, much rhetoric and print has been devoted to the "under performance" of the U.S.

health care system. Although the scope of the entire biomedical research enterprise in the United States is substantial (NIH Fiscal Year [FY] 2007 budget was $28.6 billion; pharmaceutical industry budget in 2005 was $51.3 billion; Loscalzo, 2006), it represents only a small percentage of the 2 trillion total investment in U.S. health care. Questions pertaining to the effectiveness of clinical interventions and treatments, which fall under the umbrella of evidence-based practice, represent less than 1% of the biomedical research investment. Even given the relatively small investment in evidence-based practice research, there remain severe gaps in the application of that evidence into practice (Liang, 2007).

This is a topic of continued focus for the national medical science agenda. In the American Recovery and Reinvestment Act of 2009 (ARRA; see http://www.recovery.gov), the NIH received $400 million for comparative effectiveness research, and an additional $1 billion (3.2%) was proposed in the FY 2011 president's budget. Dr. Francis Collins, director of the NIH, stated:

> Research ought to do something to tell us what works. If you have multiple ways of approaching a particular medical problem that are all being used out there by some patients and some physicians, it would be nice to know which of those approaches actually has the greatest benefit. This is an opportunity to provide the evidence that health care reform needs in order to design a system that offers to people interventions that are actually well-validated that you know are going to be beneficial. (Evans, 2010, p. 1)

The rise of evidence-based medicine, first described in 1991, began to change the paradigm of clinical practice from individual clinical observation and inference, to one of discovery of the best available evidence accompanied by critical appraisal of study methods, and determination of the validity of results (Evidence-Based Medicine Working Group, 1992; Montori & Guyatt, 2008). In no small measure, this change was enabled by the availability and accessibility of the Internet and the development of tools for search and retrieval. Table 9.1 provides a listing of the information technology developments that have enabled both access to evidence-based knowledge and the dissemination of evidence-based practice tools and resources.

The product of scientific research is new knowledge; however, that knowledge is not immediately available for application in practice for several reasons. First, the study is likely to have been conducted under controlled conditions, and the same outcomes may not occur under noncontrolled practice situations. Second, a single study does not necessarily result in evidence; it is the generation of consistent results across multiple studies that results in sufficient and valid evidence for practice. Third, findings from scientific studies may not be directly applicable to practice; interventions may need to be adapted for use in practice; and the practice of multiple disciplines may be affected by the new knowledge (Keckley & Frink, 2009b). The complexity of the translation of evidence into practice presents challenges at both the technological and organizational levels (Stetler, Ritchie, Rycroft-Malone, Schultz, & Charns, 2009).

The development and availability of knowledge repositories of systematic reviews and evidence syntheses are invaluable to both scientists and clinical practitioners. These online resources provide varying degrees of evidence documentation and may have a specific or general focus on content. Several examples of such reviews, which include the Cochrane Review, the Joanna Briggs Institute, Cumulative Index to Nursing and Allied Health Literature (CINAHL), and Google Scholar are presented in Table 9.2. In addition, resources such as the

TABLE 9.1 Developments in Knowledge Access and Dissemination Supporting Evidence-Based Practice

Source of Evidence	Tool Development and Web Developers	Examples	Dissemination Strategy
Publication databases	Search engines • National Library of Medicine • Google • Microsoft Bing	• Medline database • PubMed • OVID, Wolters Kluwer Health • CINAHL Plus-EBSCO Publishing	"Pull" technology: the user searches, selects from choices, and "pulls" the information for use.
Publication resources	Publishers, proprietary developers such as • Google, Microsoft • McMaster Premium Literature Service (PLUS) • Agency for Healthcare Research and Quality (AHRQ)	• ACP Journal Club PLUS— Highlights articles of exceptional research/evidence quality. Abstracts included allowing user evaluation of evidence. • AHRQ—evidence-based practice centers	"Push" technology: the user requests that information matching certain criteria be "pushed" to user electronically.
Systematic review database	Compilation of systematic reviews of the evidence on specific clinical topics	Cochrane Database—over 300 systematic reviews	Push or pull technology: user preference
Electronic textbooks	• Health care text publishers • Website driven • Embedded in software applications	• British Medical Journal (BMJ) clinical evidence • Physicians' Information and Education Resource (PIER)	Pull technology: users select the website and the content desired. Push technology: the evidence is embedded in the software application as part of the electronic health record (EHR).
Decision support systems	Knowledge management systems and evidence-based EHR applications	• Zynx Health, Inc.—nursing, medical, allied health, plus evidence center • Hearst • Clin-eguide, Wolters Kluwer Health • EHR vendors include links to best practice knowledge resources, and/or provide best practice alerts and reminders.	Push or pull technology: If links are provided, then users select reference information; if alerts and reminders (based on best practice guidelines) are automated with the care process, they are pushed to the clinical user.

Note. ACP = American College of Physicians; CINAHL = Cumulative Index to Nursing and Allied Health Literature. Adapted from Montori, V. M., & Guyatt, G. H. (2008). Progress in evidence-based medicine. *Journal of the American Medical Association, 300*(15), 1814–1816. doi: 10.1001/jama.300.15.1814

TABLE 9.2 **Examples of Evidence-Based Search Resources**

Name	Website	Description	Access
The Cochrane Collaboration Cochrane Reviews	http://www2.cochrane.org/reviews/	An international network that publishes the Cochrane reviews on health policy issues, research methodology, and health advocacy topics. Strong advocates for evidence-based decision making and systematic methods for evidence reviews in health care. International leadership seat on WHO World Health Assembly as of January 2011.	Subscription membership and license fees by institution or individual for online and/or DVD-ROM access to the Cochrane library (http://www2.cochrane.org/reviews/clibaccess.htm). Many systematic reviews are available for free. (http://www2.cochrane.org/reviews/)
Joanna Briggs Institute	http://www.joannabriggs.edu.au	Developed by the faculty of health sciences in Australia. Promotes and supports evidence-based health care.	Subscription membership is required. Targets nursing, midwifery, medicine, and allied health professionals.
JBI Clinical Online Network of Evidence for Care and Therapeutics (COnNECT)—Subset of Joanna Briggs Institute	http://www.jbiconnect.org	International scope, web-based resource. Provides users with "resources and tools to search, appraise, summarise, embed, utilise, and evaluate evidence-based information." (From Website Introduction)	Open search through the NIH or National Library of Medicine until October 2010 (http://nihlibrary.nih.gov/Features/Pages/jbiconnect.aspx). Other services require membership in COnNECT or the Joanna Briggs Institute. Targets health care professionals, health care service providers, and consumers.

CINAHL—EBSCO Host Publication	http://ebscohost.com/cinahl	Web-based resource. Point of care references based on research and knowledge utilization.	Available for integration within EHRs or as search repository. Fee-based service.
Google Scholar	http://scholar.google.com	Web-based search engine resource for scholarly literature of all types. Ranks search documents based on level of evidence.	Open access: Targets scholarly communities across many disciplines, including health care.
EMBASE Elsevier Publishers	http://www.embase.com	Database of over 20 million indexed references from 7,000 peer-reviewed biomedical journals.	Online subscription access: Available to institutions and organizations.
Translating Research into Practice (TRIP) I and TRIP II. AHRQ sponsored	http://www.ahrq.gov/research/trip2fac.htm	Online resource of studies supporting and demonstrating the results of translating research into practice. One phase is focused on the use of health information technology.	Open access. Targets health care researchers and health care providers.

Note. AHRQ = Agency for Healthcare Research and Quality; CINAHL = Cumulative Index to Nursing and Allied Health Literature; EHR = electronic health record; WHO = World Health Organization.

National Guidelines Clearinghouse—a publicly available resource for evidence-based guidelines for clinical practice—ensure that guidelines meet specific criteria and are not based on individual experiential data or loosely defined consensus. It provides expert commentary for providers as well as syntheses of guidelines for clinical practice (AHRQ, 2010).

Several factors influence the clinical evidence continuum, not the least of which is the level of the evidence produced by research methodology. A brief review of that continuum is presented in Figure 9.1.

Note that the continuum is both traditional and futuristic in that data from clinical practice adoption is viewed as informing new research and evidence. In a recent publication of the American Medical Informatics Association (AMIA; Bloomrosen & Detmer, 2010), they refer to a "dynamic and collaborative evidence continuum" (p. 116). They contend that the current evidence to practice model is "top down"—knowledge flows from the research community, to translators, to disseminators, and eventually to clinical practitioners. However, a new continuum model is emerging that is based on shared accountability and information exchange. That is, as knowledge is generated from multiple data sources, including practice-based research, clinical data repositories, and modeling and simulation, continuous feedback on the effectiveness of evidence in practice should be made available. The use of innovative technologies such as implantable devices with informatics components, geographic

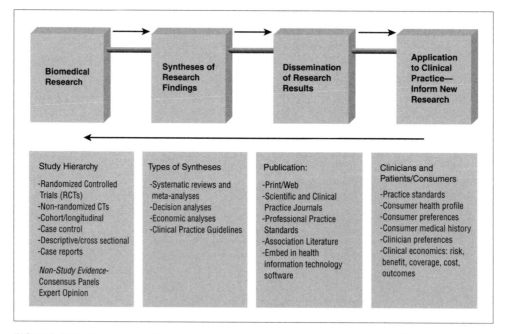

FIGURE 9.1   Levels of evidence on the continuum of research into practice. Adapted from Bloomrosen, M., & Detmer, D. E. (2010). Informatics, evidence-based care, and research; implications for national policy: A report of an American Medical Informatics Association health policy conference. *Journal of the American Medical Informatics Association, 17*(2), 115–123. doi: 10.1136/jamia.2009.001370. Keckley, P. H., & Frink, B. B. (2009a). Comparative effectiveness: A strategic perspective on what it is and what it may mean for the United States. *Journal of Health and Life Sciences Law, 3*(1), 53–90. Keckley, P. H., & Frink, B. B. (2009b). Comparative effectiveness: Perspectives for consideration (pp. 1–36). Deloitte Center for Health Solutions.

information systems, and technology sensors/recording devices, add to the evidence-based continuum by providing real-time contextual data from practice to the clinical decision process. Such innovation adds new complexity and evidence that has not before been available (Keckley, Dhar, & Underwood, 2009; Keckley & Frink, 2009a).

Mediated through information technology, access to new knowledge, and the opportunity to apply and evaluate the effectiveness of that knowledge in practice is leading to new ways of planning and delivering care. Fundamental to transforming care delivery are the design, adoption, and meaningful use of information technology in the form of EHRs throughout the health care system.

■ POLICY PERSPECTIVE: KNOWLEDGE DISCOVERY FROM THE PROCESS OF PATIENT CARE

The IOM, in a 2007 roundtable on evidence-based medicine (Olsen, Aisner, McGinnis, 2007), was the first to challenge the health care system to become a "rapid learning system," by accelerating the rate at which new knowledge is generated, applied, and evaluated in practice. The goal and vision of the IOM is reflected in the following statement:

> We seek the development of a learning health care system that is designed to generate and apply the best evidence for the collaborative health care choices of each patient and provider; to drive the process of discovery as a natural outgrowth of patient care; and to ensure innovation, quality, safety, and value in health care. . . . Our vision is for a health care system that draws on the best evidence to provide the care most appropriate to each patient, emphasizes prevention and health promotion, delivers the most value, adds to learning throughout the delivery of care, and leads to improvements in the nation's health. Goal: By the year 2020, 90 percent of clinical decisions will be supported by accurate, timely, and up-to-date clinical information, and will reflect the best available evidence. (Olsen, Aisner, McGinnis, 2007, p. ix)

To accomplish this vision, the IOM identified several requirements, three of which are directly related to information technology: clinical decision support systems (CDSS), universal EHRs, and tools for linking databases, data mining, and use of data. Although the practice of applying deliberative database analytics for answers to questions of interest (data mining) is not new, the continual expansion of computing capacity is enabling not only the "mining" of data for new patterns of relationships among variables, it is also enabling the prediction of patterns and relationships among variables. For example:

> Collecting, organizing, and analyzing individual genetic and health information, and comparing those data to population-based health outcomes data will illuminate subpopulations with patterns of risk and disease that have not as yet been evident. Establishing large scale data repositories of actual clinical outcomes will enable observational studies for clinical interventions not necessarily appropriate for randomized trials. (Frink & Dhar, 2011, p. 338)

Another major policy influence in the use of health information technology to improve health care came in 2009, with the enactment of the American Recovery and Reinvestment Act of 2009 (ARRA). A portion of this act, known as Health Information Technology for Economic and Clinical Health (HITECH) act, provides significant investment (more than $19 billion) as incentives for both physician practices and health care provider organizations to more rapidly adopt systems that will enable them to demonstrate the "meaningful use" of health information technology. Meaningful use has three components: (a) certified use of an EHR in a meaningful way; (b) use of certified EHR technology for the electronic exchange of health information that improves quality of health care; and (c) the use of certified EHR technology to submit quality data and other measures. This national program is proceeding in three stages. For Stage 1, two regulations were released in 2010 for implementation in 2011 and 2012: the first is the definition of meaningful use objectives that providers and practices must meet to qualify for reimbursement payments, and the second is the technical qualifications for certification of electronic health record technology (see http://healthit.hhs.gov/portal/server.pt/community/healthit_hhs_gov__meaningful_use_announcement/2996). For Stage 2, definition of meaningful use of EHRs regulations are expected in mid-2011, to be implemented in 2013. Finally, for Stage 3, definitions are expected to be implemented in 2015; although the final definition of meaningful use has not been published as of this writing, the definition has received an extensive public comment and is being incorporated into a Centers for Medicare and Medicaid Services (CMS) ruling (see CMS, 2010; https://www.cms.gov/EHRIncentivePrograms/30_Meaningful_Use.asp#BOOKMARK1). Health information policy groups have been influential and involved in public comment on meaningful use. For a comparison of meaningful use definitions, as proposed by three health informatics policy organizations (Health Information Management and Systems Society, Markle Foundation, AMIA), visit http://www.aamc.org/members/gir/hit/meaningfulusecomparison.pdf.

Summary public comments submitted by the AMIA to the U.S. Department of Health and Human Services (DHHS), Secretary Kathleen Sibelius reflect the importance of health information technology to evidence-based practice:

> Three principles are essential to achieving meaningful use of certified electronic health record (EHR) technology: (a) we must invest in people, as well as technology; (b) Users need EHR systems that provide cognitive support and evidence-based functionalities; and (c) Adoption of EHR systems requires a balancing of benefits and burdens that users will accept. (Shortliffe, 2010, p. 2)

The focus of the next section of this chapter is on the EHR, including CDSS as health information technology tools that enable the introduction of evidence to the processes of care.

■ THE PRACTICE PERSPECTIVE: INTRODUCING EVIDENCE INTO THE PROCESS OF CARE

Electronic Health Records

In the context of translating evidence to practice, the EHR is a fundamental link in the continuum. EHRs, which have been in existence for several decades, are in a continual state of development, refinement, and adoption. An EHR is the electronic version of an individual's health and treatment history, usually maintained by a clinician or health care provider organization. Common functional components of an EHR include clinical and administrative patient data, health history, medication history, laboratory data, pathology data, radiology images and reports, progress notes, clinical problem lists, plans of care, vital signs, procedure reports, physician and other clinician orders, and clinical documentation of clinical care processes and outcomes. In 2003, the International Organization for Standardization identified the eight components of a fully functional EHR: (a) health information and data, (b) results management, (c) order entry management, (d) decision support, (e) electronic communication and connectivity, (f) patient support, (g) administrative processes, and (h) reporting and population health management. By contrast, minimally functional or core EHRs were defined as those having patient health information, terminology, reference data such as drugs, and patient identification information (ISO/Technical Committee, 2003). Such minimally functional systems provide basic patient data that are useful in an administrative or clinical reference context.

EHRs exist in almost all types of clinical practice settings: outpatient/ambulatory care, physician practices, hospitals, specialty hospitals, long-term care, home health care, health systems, and integrated practice models such as Kaiser Permanente or the Mayo Clinic.

EHRs were initially designed as transactional systems, beginning with reporting of clinical results such as laboratory tests. As the technology became more sophisticated, transactions became highly complex algorithms and began to include complex clinical workflows. EHRs also provided a "lifetime" clinical record, which meant that patient data no longer resided in paper records but within an always retrievable form from clinical data repositories. All EHRs are not created equal; there are fundamental differences in the degree of integration between and among components, in usability for clinicians, in data presentation, and in clinical workflows. Although EHR systems must meet national and international technology standards, they are often built on proprietary architectures by multiple vendors; thus, interoperability between and among systems rarely exists without the design and building of interfaces, which require ongoing maintenance and may not result in full interoperability. The degree of variation in use of common data standards, languages, syntaxes, taxonomies, and terminologies in software and clinical application also affect the seamless transmission or common understanding of data.

Surrounding the EHR is an information infrastructure that has received national health policy attention with the founding of the Office of the National Coordinator for Health Information Technology in 2004 (http://www.healthit.hhs.gov/portal/server.pt). This office now sets national health information technology policy and has established two national advisory committees: the Health Information Technology (HIT) Policy Committee and the HIT Standards Committee. For further information, see the Office of the National Coordinator resources in Table 9.3.

TABLE 9.3 **Office of the National Coordinator Committees**

Health Information Technology Policy Committee

See the policy recommendations at:
http://healthit.hhs.gov/portal/server.pt?open=512&objID=1815&parentname=CommunityPage&parentid=37&mode=2&in_hi_userid=11673&cached=true

Health Information Technology Standards Committee

See the standards recommendations at:
http://healthit.hhs.gov/portal/server.pt?open=512&objID=1818&parentname=CommunityPage&parentid=34&mode=2&in_hi_userid=11673&cached=true

Although it is not the focus of this chapter, both standards and policies are critical underpinnings to a national health information infrastructure (Kuperman et al., 2010). If evidence is to be applied to practice and enabled through information technology and the EHR, then that evidence must be encoded and communicated in such a way that it is semantically clear, interoperable between systems, retrievable, and secure (Office of the National Coordinator for Health Information Technology, 2010). Bakken (2001) described components of informatics infrastructure that are essential to support evidence-based practice, both the application of evidence to practice and the building of evidence from practice: "standardized terminologies and structures, digital sources of evidence, data exchange standards, informatics processes, and informatics competencies" (Bakken, 2001, p. 201). Standardized terminologies and data structures are key to building an information infrastructure, as well as providing standards for query and research in establishing evidence. As a professional discipline, nursing has a relatively short history in the development of taxonomies, classifications, and nomenclatures. Resources for further investigation in this area are provided in Table 9.4.

EHR adoption and use are necessary, but not sufficient, to enable evidence-based practice. "To attain EHR's full potential, its adoption and implementation should be treated as a means of facilitating redesign of outdated, inefficient, and error-prone care processes and a vehicle for organizational change . . . "(Brokel & Harrison, 2009, p. 82). Both the reduction of clinical errors and the use of clinical guidelines in practice have been touted as major benefits of EHR adoption (Bates, 2002; Bates & Gawande, 2003). However, study findings from ambulatory care practices show that results are mixed in regard to direct relationships between EHR use and improved quality (Linder, Ma, Bates, Middleton, & Stafford, 2007; Simborg, 2008; Welch et al., 2007). Similarly, there have been challenges in inpatient environments because of interruptions in clinical workflow and unintended consequences of EHR adoption.

TABLE 9.4   **Nursing Classifications and Taxonomies Examples**

International Classification for Nursing Practice (ICNP)
   http://www.icn.ch/pillarsprograms/international-classification-for-nursing-practicer

Nursing Interventions Classification (NIC)
   http://www.nursing.uiowa.edu/excellence/nursing_knowledge/clinical_effectiveness/nic.htm

Nursing Outcomes Classification (NOC)
   http://www.nursing.uiowa.edu/excellence/nursing_knowledge/clinical_effectiveness/
   nocoverview.htm

North American Nursing Diagnosis Association (NANDA)
   http://www.nanda.org

Home Health Care Classification (HHCC)
   http://www.nursingworld.org/MainMenuCategories/ANAMarketplace/ANAPeriodicals/OJIN/
   TableofContents/Volume72002/No3Sept2002/ArticlesPreviousTopic/HHCCAnOverview.aspx

International Journal of Nursing Terminologies and Classifications
   http://www3.interscience.wiley.com/journal/118516889/home

Note. All URLs were accessed on June 12, 2010.

Several studies report the challenges and the potential risk consequences of EHR adoption (Chaudhry et al., 2006; Han et al., 2005; Harrison, Koppel, & Bar-Lev, 2007; Keene et al., 2007; Koppel et al., 2005; Metzger, Welebob, Bates, Lipsitz, & Classen, 2010; Wears & Berg, 2005). Studies of EHR adoption that have positively affected aspects of quality, clinical workflow improvements, and clinical transformation have also been reported (Brokel & Harrison, 2009; Kaushal & Bates, 2002; Kaushal, Shojania, & Bates, 2003; Poon et al., 2010; Schulman, Kuperman, Kharbanda, & Kaushal, 2007; Zhou et al., 2009). However, results continue to be uncertain or varied (DesRoches et al., 2010; McCullough, Casey, Moscovice, & Prasad, 2010; Metzger et al., 2010), demonstrating a continuing need for studies focused on risks and benefits of EHR adoption. A systematic literature review of 94 primary electronic patient record (EPR) studies and 24 systematic reviews of EPR studies (Greenhalgh, Potts, Wong, Bark, & Swinglehurst, 2009) supports the view that findings of EHR implementation and use are mixed and uncertain.

> The metanarrative method has shown that "conflicting" findings in this large and heterogeneous literature can be fruitfully expressed as tensions and paradoxes relating to the nature of the EPR, the context in which it is implemented and used, and the way success in an EPR program is defined and pursued. (p. 771)

Greenhalgh and colleagues (2009) drew additional conclusions from this extensive systematic review: (a) there will always be a need for human intervention in EHRs to provide context (or recontext) to knowledge; (b) EHRs may cause inefficiencies in primary clinical workflow while adding efficiency to secondary administrative work such as billing, audits, research; and (c) smaller EHR systems may be more efficient and effective than larger EHR systems.

These studies demonstrated that EHRs are not panaceas for solving health care delivery and quality of care challenges. The selection, implementation, and adoption of EHRs in clinical settings require considerable human and capital resources during each phase of this multistage process. Often, primary emphases and resources are placed during the early phases of implementation and adoption of EHRs, with far fewer resources devoted to evaluation of the effectiveness of use, and results of incorporating evidence into the processes of care. The need for continued research is clear, with investigations that include the complexity of multiple EHR stakeholders, as well as policy, process, practice, and technology. As the ARRA HITECH investment takes effect in 2011, there will be increased national focus on not only what constitutes meaningful use of EHR, but the demonstration of that use on quality and health outcomes in all practice areas of health care delivery.

The fully functional EHR system incorporates evidence into the clinical process workflow. However, many health care organizations have minimally functional or no EHRs. The findings of a 2007 national survey of 1,392 nurses showed that less than one in five registered nurses (RNs) work in settings (both inpatient and ambulatory) that use even minimally functional EHRs (DesRoches, Donelan, Buerhuas, & Zhonghe, 2008). Survey respondents who reported using EHRs reported more organizational involvement with quality improvement activities than those who do not have use of EHRs. See Table 9.5 for a summary of these quality improvement activities results by EHR type. These survey results indicate that only a small percentage of nurses and other clinicians have access to fully functional EHRs; thus, the level at which evidence can be linked to practice (through such functions as clinical decision support including guidelines, best practices, alerts, and reminders) for those practitioners is limited at best.

TABLE 9.5   **Selected Factors Affecting Acceptance of Clinical Decision Support**

Availability Factors Affecting CDSS Use	Acceptance Factors
Adequate hardware	Endorsed by colleagues
Adequate training	Little threat to professional autonomy
Adequate support	No compromise to physician/patient relationship
Integration into clinical workflows	Perceived threats to professional privacy
Relevance/Timeliness of messages and alerts	

Note. CDSS = clinical decision support systems. Adapted from Moxey, A., Robertson, J., Newby, D., Hains, I., Williamson, M., & Pearson, S. A. (2010). Computerized clinical decision support for prescribing: Provision does not guarantee uptake. *Journal of the American Medical Informatics Association, 17*(1), 25–33. doi: 10.1197/jamia.M3170

A unique partnership among a health care delivery organization, a university, and a health care information technology vendor is testing the process and outcome of "identifying, embedding, using, acquiring, and analyzing knowledge-based data into an intelligent information system" to provide nursing decision support and improve nursing sensitive care outcomes (Lang, 2008; Lang et al., 2006). Such pioneering work not only demonstrates the complex processes involved in knowledge management and translation, but also the complex stakeholder relationships that are critical to providing new levels of collaboration and learning.

■ CLINICAL DECISION SUPPORT SYSTEMS

The purpose of computerized CDSS is to provide individual patients, clinicians, or other health care providers with both timely knowledge and person-specific information to improve clinical decision making and health care. Underpinning the CDSS is a central knowledge repository, usually in the form of a database. The repository may contain medical reference material, citations, national clinical guidelines, order sets for clinical conditions, diagnostic information, and drug data (Berner, 2009). If CDSS are designed to provide patient-specific information, then a mechanism to provide patient-specific information is designed into the system. For example, an interface may be built between an EHR and a knowledge repository, so that patient-specific information may be filtered against the knowledge base. Algorithms built into the software generate reports, recommendations, alerts, or reminders to the clinician. Bakken, Stone, and Larson (2008) describe the process and components of a CDSS designed for nursing, and remind us that to be successful, CDSS must be designed consistent with nursing workflow. Consider a simple example: In an inpatient clinical unit, through a use of a falls risk assessment, a patient has been declared at risk for falling. An EHR nursing application may be designed to automatically generate a falls prevention protocol as a result of the risk assessment. It is important to ascertain the clinical workflow around fall prevention before designing the automation of the protocol. For example, do other departments or services need notification, and in what sequence? Do supplies need to be ordered? What are the implications for patient and family member education? Is there an evidence-based policy or other reference material that should be available to the nurse in regard to implementing this protocol? How and where (in the EHR) these activities are communicated and documented can greatly influence both the efficiency and effectiveness of automating this aspect of care. Considering the complexity of care, guidelines, protocols, and interdisciplinary clinical practice, one can quickly see that incorporating evidence and automating aspects of the clinical workflow can be a challenging process. In addition, it is not sufficient to design and implement the process; there must be continual review and evaluation of both processes and the outcomes realized from the automation. Maintaining competency in informatics and evidence-based practice is critical for all clinicians to realize the benefits of CDSS (Bakken et al., 2008; McBride & Detmer, 2008).

CDSS may be stand-alone systems or may be integrated with the EHR or other clinical information systems. The process for design and implementation of even one guideline translation into CDSS is iterative, complex, and usually multidisciplinary. However, if effectively designed and implemented, CDSS can make a significant contribution to the translation and consistent use of best practices in clinical environments (Trafton et al., 2010). Multiple computer platforms are used in providing CDSS information to clinicians and/or patients, such as the internet, personal computer software, and networked applications such as EHRs or handheld smartphone devices (Berner, 2009). Garg and colleagues (2005) conducted a systematic review of clinical trials conducted to test the effects of CDSS use. One hundred studies (randomized and nonrandomized) that compared CDSS assisted care with non-CDSS care on patient outcomes or practitioner performance were included in the systematic review. The authors report that the more recently the trial was conducted, the greater was the methodological quality. See Table 9.6 for a description of types of CDSS included in the systematic review and selected summary findings. The primary conclusions of this systematic review are that CDSS have been demonstrated to improve clinician performance; however, the effect of CDSS use on patient outcomes is not always included in study design, and even when included, yields inconsistent results.

Although the primary intent of CDSS is to provide appropriate knowledge at the point of care, and thereby improve care decisions and/or reduce errors, there is no consistent availability of these systems to health care providers, and when systems are available, they are not necessarily used or used effectively. For example, health care technology EHR vendors usually include clinical decision support capability within their clinical software applications and, in addition, may partner with a third party clinical content provider to enrich their CDSS application. However, each vendor approaches the CDSS in a proprietary manner, as do content providers, resulting in variation between and among EHR systems in regard to CDSS. In addition, the health care organization that is purchasing the EHR often has considerable latitude to work with their vendor to design a unique CDSS tailored to their particular clinical populations. In recognition of these issues, in 2006, the Office of the National Coordinator (ONC) for Health Information Technology at the Department of Health and Human Services (DHHS) funded a contract to develop a roadmap for national action on clinical decision support (Osheroff et al., 2007). The roadmap authors identified three pillars of knowledge for CDSS:

- The best knowledge is available when needed—organized in such a manner that knowledge is stored, transmitted, and delivered to the clinical decision process.
- CDSS have high adoption rates and are used effectively—must be broadly implemented and used to add clinical value, as well as operational and financial value.
- CDSS must undergo continuous improvement in both content and methods using feedback, evaluation, experience, and data.(Osheroff et al., 2006, pp. 4–5)

TABLE 9.6 **Types of Computerized Clinical Decision Support Systems**

Type of CDSS	Systematic Review	Results
Diagnosis systems	10 trials	• All trials measured clinician performance—only 40% (four) of studies showed improved clinician performance. • Five trials assessed patient outcomes. No trial demonstrated improvement in outcomes.
Prevention reminder systems	21 trials	• All trials measured clinician performance—76% (16) of studies showed improved clinician performance. • Most trials in ambulatory care; one hospital system tested. • One trial assessed patient outcomes. No improvement demonstrated.
Disease management systems	40 trials	• Thirty-seven trials measured clinician performance—62% (23) of studies showed improved clinician performance. • Twenty-seven trials assessed patient outcomes—18% (five) of the trials demonstrated outcome improvements.
Drug dosing and prescribing systems	29 trials	• Single drug dosing improved clinician performance by 62% (24 studies). • Eighteen trials assessed patient outcomes. Two trials reported improved patient outcomes.

Note. CDSS = clinical decision support system. Adapted from Garg, A. X., Adhikari, N. K., McDonald, H., Rosas-Arellano, M. P., Devereaux, P. J., Beyene, J., . . . Haynes, R. B. (2005). Effects of computerized clinical decision support systems on practitioner performance and patient outcomes: A systematic review. *Journal of the American Medical Association, 293*(10), 1223–1238. doi: 10.1001/jama.293.10.1223

With additional funding from the commonwealth fund and strategic actions based on the pillars, the work of promoting comprehensive CDSS in the context of meaningful use of EHRs continues.

One of the key hallmarks of excellent health information technology systems is that they provide CDSS (Bates, 2002). If CDSS can be effectively integrated into clinician workflows, there is potentially a direct effect on quality, safety, and cost of care. Using the falls protocol example—connecting the risk assessment with the automatic launching of an interdisciplinary falls protocol—clinicians are simultaneously notified of a patient risk, and appropriate actions and documentation requirements are added to the clinician workflow. Such actions, when implemented appropriately and with critical thinking, should have a direct effect on quality, safety, and costs associated with patients who are at risk for falling.

Several studies and systematic reviews have been conducted to determine the evidence that supports CDSS functions and clinician acceptance/use of CDSS (Moxey et al., 2010; Patterson et al., 2005; Schedlbauer et al., 2009; Sittig, Krall, Dykstra, Russell, & Chin, 2006). Although there has been considerable progress in the field, the findings are inconsistent. It is clear that providing appropriate knowledge in a usable format is only one aspect of effective decision support. In a review of 58 studies for CDSS for prescribing, many other factors contributed to acceptance and use of CDSS. See Table 9.7 for factors affecting adoption of CDSS.

TABLE 9.7 **Minimally Functional Electronic Health Record Use by Registered Nurses: Reported Quality Improvement Activities**

Routine Use: Minimally Functional EHR	Zero Components of EHR
Formal quality improvement program: 78%	Formal quality improvement program: 48%
Increase focus on recognizing nursing excellence: 69%	Increase focus on recognizing nursing excellence: 52%
Physician–nurse teamwork encouraged: 61%	Physician–nurse teamwork encouraged: 50%

Note. EHR = electronic health record. Adapted from DesRoches, C., Donelan, K., Buerhuas, P., & Zhonghe, L. (2008). Registered nurses' use of electronic health records: Findings from a national survey. *Medscape Journal of Medicine, 10*(7), 164.

A study conducted on the effective use of HIV clinical reminders found that workload was a primary contributor to not using clinical reminders. Other factors included the time needed to document why the reminder did not apply or was inappropriate to the clinical situation and inadequate training in the use of reminder system (Patterson et al., 2005; Saleem et al., 2005).

There continues to be considerable attention to CDSS development and use at a national policy level. Current challenges include the accommodation of CDSS to support personalized medicine, that is health care delivery that is informed by an individual's unique clinical information: "genetic, genomic, molecular, biological, and environmental" (Downing, Boyle, Brinner, & Osheroff, 2009, p. 2). Future CDSS may be designed to include the application of evidence-based guidelines in the context of individual genetic and genomic data. Such applications will link EHR resources with other reference data sets to support clinical decision making; thus, expanding the concept of CDSS well beyond the structure or design of current EHRs.

■ POSSIBILITY PERSPECTIVE: THE ROLE OF INFORMATION TECHNOLOGY IN GENERATING NEW KNOWLEDGE

Electronic health records and the application of CDSS will continue to play a pivotal role in the generation of new knowledge and evidence for practice. The concept of rapid learning health care systems is predicated on the use of multiple EHR databases as tools for rapidly advancing knowledge about clinical care as actually delivered across the nation. A formal rapid learning system network might include multiple EHR databases, sponsors of other data repositories, research networks, registries, and data banks pertaining to age, geography, or extensive longitudinal research such as the National Children's Study (Etheredge, 2007; Slutsky, 2007). However, rapid learning health care systems are not just networks, databases, and knowledge content; they must also include the human infrastructure that supports collaborative clinical decision making based on a "culture of shared responsibility" among health care providers, patients and their families, and researchers (Bloomrosen & Detmer, 2010).

In contrast to randomized controlled trials (RCTs), which are still the gold standard for research, EHR database research can create "real-time" learning across millions of patients' health care treatments and encounters. The combination of the cost of RCTs coupled with gaps that exist between biomedical discovery, translation of discovery to practice innovation, and determination of effectiveness of practice innovations creates a compelling case for harvesting clinical practice data in the context of a rapid learning environment, and of combining some of the best characteristics of observational studies as well as RCTs, (Frink & Dhar, 2011; Keckley & Frink, 2009a; Perlin & Kupersmith, 2007; Stewart, Shah, Selna, Paulus, & Walker, 2007). Additional potential benefits of use of EHR systems for rapid learning are to use the EHR repository for evaluating the effects of (a) monitoring the effectiveness of drugs and treatment longitudinally for populations and subpopulations; (b) rapidly diffusing new evidence through integration of guidelines and decision support tools into EHRs; and (c) using EHRs to provide the tools and evidence in formats that provide efficient clinician workflow, and enable incorporating evidence-use at the point of care (Liang, 2007).

If such EHR data and tools were broadly available, results for safety, effectiveness, and outcomes could be determined in real-life clinical environments. Two examples are the building of clinical case registries from clinical data (Backus et al., 2009) and national quality data sets derived from multiple provider organizations (Dunton & Montalvo, 2009). The issue of interoperability between systems, as well as the design of robust integrated data networks, is key to effective use of real-life clinical data. Additional attention must be paid to communication between and among broad constituencies, who have different needs and uses for clinical and scientific data. To support the effective use of real-life clinical data, changes to the health information infrastructure must occur simultaneously with the application of data standards and standards that safeguard both the privacy and security of health care information. However, methodological and privacy issues need to be addressed in a comprehensive framework because practice data, collected for delivery of care documentation, are accessed through operational systems and networks for other purposes (Diamond, Mostashari, & Shirky, 2009; Frink & Dhar, 2011; Keckley & Frink, 2009a; Stewart, et al., 2007).

Despite the value of aggregated health data to the goals of the U.S. health system, there is no fully defined national framework for the use of health data. The AMIA, based on health data use conferences in 2006 and 2007, identified "reuse of health data" as the definition for the use of personal health data for purposes other than those for which they were originally collected. The first conference focused on the perspectives of the consumer; patient safety, quality, and research; public health; and industry (Safran et al., 2007). The conferees identified several conflicting objectives inherent in reuse of health data: health system needs versus individual patient or clinician needs; public safety versus privacy of personal health information; best practices and medical-legal, ethical issues versus practical demands; and technology advancements versus traditional data use. One of the methods described to deal with these conflicts is data stewardship (Bloomrosen & Detmer, 2008).

> Data stewardship encompasses the responsibilities and accountabilities associated with managing, collecting, viewing, storing, sharing, disclosing, or otherwise making use of personal health information. Principles of data stewardship apply to all the personnel, systems, and processes engaging in health information storage and exchange within and across organizations. (p. 718)

In light of the policy challenges surrounding the reuse of health data, one of the 2006 conference recommendations was to explore establishing a voluntary compliance process for health data stewardship, such as the Certification Commission for Healthcare Information Technology (CCHIT; http:/www./cchit.org).

Technology advances and innovations in both business systems and networks also influence the development of health care knowledge generation. Advances in "cloud" computing (more a new business model than a new technical model; Rosenthal et al., 2010) and other network methodologies add to the possibilities for mining aggregated health data. Research networks and grid technologies already support major biomedical research endeavors, with their large data sets, multiple owners, and archives (Szolovits, 2007). Lessons learned from collaborative research efforts such as the Cancer Biomedical Informatics Grid (caBIG; https://www.cabig.nci.nih.gov) and the Biomedical Informatics Research Network (BIRN; http://www.birncommunity.org) may help to guide more broadly based health data networks.

The technology-enabled possibilities for continued development in the translation of evidence to—and from—practice are outpacing our ability to transform our clinical work and clinical care environments. By harnessing, with appropriate policies, standards, and safeguards, the power of information technology, we should be able to demonstrate the value of applying evidence at the point of care and generating evidence from clinical practice.

■ SUMMARY

Information technology is vital to the translation of evidence to clinical practice, and the potential for generation of knowledge from clinical practice. The complex biomedical research enterprise and the challenges of translating scientific discovery and innovation to practice require the mediation of information technology, most frequently in the form of clinical decision support and EHR systems. Aggregation of disparate health data sources, enabled by network technologies and data standards, are beginning to demonstrate the potential for generating knowledge from clinical practice data. This creates the possibility of bridging the gaps that exist between results of clinical trials and observational studies. The creation of new evidence, including links with personalized genetic/genomic data, hold the potential for addressing some of the health care system's greatest challenges, managing the cost and improving the quality of health care for the population. For the clinician, maintaining competencies in evidence-based care and informatics will support the use of evidence in practice: the most effective care for the individual at the appropriate time, with understanding and disclosure of both risks and benefits.

Although this chapter has presented the role of health information technology as an enabler of translating scientific evidence into clinical practice and generating new evidence from practice in a sequential manner, the processes are not linear. Certain aspects of information technology, such as an EHR, must exist before you can automate aspects of the care process; however, the development of health information technology is concurrent: in the policy arena, the practice environment, and the research and clinical consortia devoted to generating new knowledge from large scale data mining of practice data. Each of these areas require continuing study and development for determining the best practices to achieve both short and long-term goals of translating scientific evidence into clinical practice. It should be clear, that although considerable progress has been achieved, there remain many areas of uncertainty and gaps in knowledge. When new knowledge is tested in clinical practice and generated from clinical practice, there must be a continuous focus on translation of the new evidence into meaningful use of health information technology to support the health needs of the population.

■ ACKNOWLEDGMENTS

The author wishes to thank Anne Wake, PhD and Suzanne Feetham, PhD, RN, FAAN, for reviewing this manuscript.

■ REFERENCES

Agency for Healthcare Research and Quality (2004). The TRIP initiative. Retrieved from http://www.ahrq.gov/research/trip2fac.htm#Initiative

Agency for Healthcare Research and Quality. (2010). National guidelines clearinghouse. Retrieved from http://www.guideline.gov/

Agency for Healthcare Research and Quality. (2010). National quality measures clearinghouse. Retrieved from http://www.qualitymeasures.ahrq.gov/hhs/hhs.index.aspx

American Recovery and Reinvestment Act, 111 U. S. C. § 1553. (2009)

Backus, L. I., Gavrilov, S., Loomis, T. P., Halloran, J. P., Phillips, B. R., Belperio, P. S., & Mole, L. A. (2009). Clinical case registries: Simultaneous local and national disease registries for population quality management. *Journal of the American Medical Informatics Association, 16*(6), 775–783. doi: 10.1197/jamia.M3203

Bakken, S. (2001). An informatics infrastructure is essential for evidence-based practice. *Journal of the American Medical Informatics Association, 8*(3), 199–201. doi: 10.1136/jamia.2001.0080199

Bakken, S., Currie, L. M., Lee, N. J., Roberts, W. D., Collins, S. A., & Cimino, J. J. (2008). Integrating evidence into clinical information systems for nursing decision support. *International Journal of Medical Informatics, 77*(6), 413–420. doi: 10.1016/j.ijmedinf.2007.08.006

Bakken, S., & McArthur, J. (2001). Evidence-based nursing practice. *Journal of the American Medical Informatics Association, 8*(3), 289–290. doi: 10.1136/jamia.2001.0080289

Bakken, S., Stone, P. W., & Larson, E. L. (2008). A nursing informatics research agenda for 2008–18: Contextual influences and key components. *Nursing Outlook, 56*(5), 206–214.

Bates, D. W. (2002). The quality case for information technology in healthcare. *BMC Medical Informatics and Decision Making, 2*, 7.

Bates, D. W., & Gawande, A. A. (2003). Improving safety with information technology. *The New England Journal of Medicine, 348*(25), 2526–2534. doi: 10.1056/NEJMsa020847

Berner, E. S. (2009). *Clinical decision support systems: State of the art.* (AHRQ Publication No. 09-0069-EF). Rockville, MD: Agency for Healthcare Research and Quality.

Bloomrosen, M., & Detmer, D. E. (2008). Advancing the framework: Use of health data—A report of a working conference of the American Medical Informatics Association. *Journal of the American Medical Informatics Association, 15*(6), 715–722. doi: 10.1197/jamia.M2905

Bloomrosen, M., & Detmer, D. E. (2010). Informatics, evidence-based care, and research; implications for national policy: A report of an American Medical Informatics Association health policy conference. *Journal of the American Medical Informatics Association, 17*(2), 115–123. doi: 10.1136/jamia.2009.001370

Brokel, J. M., & Harrison, M. I. (2009). Redesigning care processes using an electronic health record: A system's experience. *Joint Commission Journal on Quality and Patient Safety, 35*(2), 82–92.

Carman, K. L., Maurer, M., Yegian, J. M., Dardess, P., McGee, J., Evers, M., & Marlo, K. O. (2010). Evidence that consumers are skeptical about evidence-based health care. *Health Affairs, 29*(7), 1400–1406. doi: 10.1377/hlthaff.2009.0296

Chaudhry, B., Wang, J., Wu, S., Maglione, M., Mojica, W., Roth, E., . . . Shekelle, P. G. (2006). Systematic review: Impact of health information technology on quality, efficiency, and costs of medical care. *Annals of Internal Medicine, 144*(10), 742–752.

Clancy, C. M. (2006). Getting to "smart" health care. *Health Affairs, 25*(6), w589–w592. doi: 10.1377/hlthaff.25.w589

CMS. (2010). CMS EHR Meaningful Use Overview. Retrieved from http://www.cms.gov/ EHRIncentivePrograms/30_meaningful_Use.asp#BOOKMARK1

DesRoches, C. M., Campbell, E. G., Vogeli, C., Zheng, J., Rao, S. R., Shields, A. E., . . . Jha, A. K. (2010). Electronic health records' limited successes suggest more targeted uses. *Health Affairs, 29*(4), 639–646. doi: 10.1377/hlthaff.2009.1086

DesRoches, C., Donelan, K., Buerhuas, P., & Zhonghe, L. (2008). Registered nurses' use of electronic health records: Findings from a national survey. *Medscape Journal of Medicine, 10*(7), 164.

Diamond, C. C., Mostashari, F., & Shirky, C. (2009). Collecting and sharing data for population health: A new paradigm. *Health Affairs, 28*(2), 454–466. doi: 10.1377/hlthaff.28.2.454

Downing, G. J., Boyle, S. N., Brinner, K. M., & Osheroff, J. A. (2009). Information management to enable personalized medicine: Stakeholder roles in building clinical decision support. *BMC Medical Informatics and Decision Making, 9*, 44.

Dunton, N., & Montalvo, I. (Eds.). (2009). *Sustained improvement in nursing quality: Hospital performance on NDNQI indicators, 2007–2008.* Silver Spring, MD: American Nurses Association.

Etheredge, L. M. (2007). A rapid-learning health system. *Health Affairs, 26*(2), w107–w118. doi: 10.1377/hlthaff.26.2.w107

Evans, J. (2010, April). NIH Chief Francis Collins: Medical research "ought to tell us what works." *Kaiser Health News.* Retrieved from http://www.kaiserhealthnews.org/Checking-In-With/ francis-collins-comparative-effectiveness.aspx

Evidence-Based Medicine Working Group. (1992). Evidence-based medicine. A new approach to teaching the practice of medicine. *Journal of the American Medical Association, 268*(17), 2420–2425. doi: 10.1001/jama.1992.03490170092032

Frink, B. B., & Dhar, A. (2011). Transforming care: Discovery enabled by health information technology. In M. J. Ball, J. V. Douglas, & P. Hinton Walker (Eds.), *Nursing informatics: Where technology and caring meet* (4th ed., pp. 331–341). Guilford-Surrey, United Kingdom: Springer-Verlag.

Garg, A. X., Adhikari, N. K., McDonald, H., Rosas-Arellano, M. P., Devereaux, P. J., Beyene, J., . . . Haynes, R. B. (2005). Effects of computerized clinical decision support systems on practitioner performance and patient outcomes: A systematic review. *Journal of the American Medical Association, 293*(10), 1223–1238. doi: 10.1001/jama.293.10.1223

Greenhalgh, T., Potts, H. W., Wong, G., Bark, P., & Swinglehurst, D. (2009). Tensions and paradoxes in electronic patient record research: A systematic literature review using the meta-narrative method. *Milbank Quarterly, 87*(4), 729–788.

Han, Y. Y., Carcillo, J. A., Venkataraman, S. T., Clark, R. S., Watson, R. S., Nguyen, T. C., . . . Orr, R. A. (2005). Unexpected increased mortality after implementation of a commercially sold computerized physician order entry system. *Pediatrics, 116*(6), 1506–1512. doi: 10.1542/peds.2005–1287

Harrison, M. I., Koppel, R., & Bar-Lev, S. (2007). Unintended consequences of information technologies in health care—An interactive sociotechnical analysis. *Journal of the American Medical Informatics Association, 14*(5), 542–549.

Institute of Medicine. (2007). *The learning healthcare system: Workshop summary*. In L. Olsen, D. Aisner, & J. M. McGinnis (Eds.). Washington, DC: National Academies Press.

International Organization for Standardization/Technical Committees. (2003, August). *ISO/TC 215 Technical report. Electronic health record definition, scope, and context* (2nd draft, pp. 1–33).

Joanna Briggs Institute. (2011). Website Introduction User Guide. Retrieved from http://www .jbiconnectplus.org/Help/ConnectPlusUserGuide.pdf

Kaushal, R., & Bates, D. W. (2002). Information technology and medication safety: What is the benefit? *Quality and Safety Health Care, 11*(3), 261–265.

Kaushal, R., Shojania, K. G., & Bates, D. W. (2003). Effects of computerized physician order entry and clinical decision support systems on medication safety: A systematic review. *Archives of Internal Medicine, 163*(12), 1409–1416.

Keckley, P., Dhar, A., & Underwood, H. (2009). *The ROI for targeted therapies: A strategic perspective assessing the barriers and incentives for adopting personalized medicine* (pp. 1–32). Deloitte Center for Health Solutions. Retrieved from http://www.deloitte.com/assets/Dcom-UnitedStates/ Local%20Assets/Documents/us_chs_ROIforTargetedTherapies_January2009(1).pdf

Keckley, P. H., & Frink, B. B. (2009a). Comparative effectiveness: A strategic perspective on what it is and what it may mean for the United States. *Journal of Health and Life Sciences Law, 3*(1), 53–90.

Keckley, P. H., & Frink, B. B. (2009b). *Comparative effectiveness: Perspectives for consideration* (pp. 1–36). Deloitte Center for Health Solutions.

Keene, A., Ashton, L., Shure, D., Napoleone, D., Katyal, C., & Bellin, E. (2007). Mortality before and after initiation of a computerized physician order entry system in a critically ill pediatric population. *Pediatric Critical Care Medicine, 8*(3), 268–271.

Koppel, R., Metlay, J. P., Cohen, A., Abaluck, B., Localio, A. R., Kimmel, S. E., & Strom, B. L. (2005). Role of computerized physician order entry systems in facilitating medication errors. *Journal of the American Medical Association, 293*(10), 1197–1203. doi: 10.1001/jama.293.10.1197

Kuperman, G. J., Blair, J. S., Franck, R. A., Devaraj, S., Low, A. F. & NHIN Trial Implementations Core Services Content Working Group. (2010). Developing data content specifications for the nationwide health information network trial implementations. *Journal of the American Medical Informatics Association, 17*(1), 6–12. doi: 10.1197/jamia.M3282

Lang, N. M. (2008). The promise of simultaneous transformation of practice and research with the use of clinical information systems. *Nursing Outlook, 56*(5), 232–236.

Lang, N. M., Hook, M. L., Akre, M. E., Kim, T. Y., Berg, K. S., Lundeen, S. P., . . . Ela, S. (2006). Translating knowledge-based nursing into referential and executable applications in an intelligent clinical information system. In C. A. Weaver, C. W. Delaney, P. Webber, & R. L. Carr (Eds.), *Nursing and informatics for the 21st century: An international look at practice, trends, and the future* (pp. 291–303). Chicago, IL: Healthcare Information and Management Systems Society.

Liang, L. (2007). The gap between evidence and practice. *Health Affairs, 26*(2), w119–w121. doi: 10.1377/hlthaff.26.2.w119

Linder, J. A., Ma, J., Bates, D. W., Middleton, B., & Stafford, R. S. (2007). Electronic health record use and the quality of ambulatory care in the United States. *Archives of Internal Medicine, 167*(13), 1400–1405. doi: 10.1001/archinte.167.13.1400

Loscalzo, J. (2006). The NIH budget and the future of biomedical research. *New England Journal of Medicine, 354*(16), 1665–1667. doi: 10.1056/NEJMp068050

McBride, A. B., & Detmer, D. E. (2008). Using informatics to go beyond technologic thinking. *Nursing Outlook, 56*(5), 195–196. doi: 10.1016/j.outlook.2008.04.001

McCullough, J. S., Casey, M., Moscovice, I., & Prasad, S. (2010). The effect of health information technology on quality in U.S. hospitals. *Health Affairs, 29*(4), 647–654. doi: 10.1377/hlthaff.2010.0155

McGlynn, E. A., Asch, S. M., Adams, J., Keesey, J., Hicks, J., DeCristofaro, A., & Kerr, E. A. (2003). The quality of health care delivered to adults in the United States. *New England Journal of Medicine, 348*(26), 2635–2645. doi: 10.1056/NEJMsa022615

Metzger, J., Welebob, E., Bates, D. W., Lipsitz, S., & Classen, D. C. (2010). Mixed results in the safety performance of computerized physician order entry. *Health Affairs, 29*(4), 655–663. doi: 10.1377/hlthaff.2010.0160

Montori, V. M., & Guyatt, G. H. (2008). Progress in evidence-based medicine. *Journal of the American Medical Association, 300*(15), 1814–1816. doi: 10.1001/jama.300.15.1814

Moxey, A., Robertson, J., Newby, D., Hains, I., Williamson, M., & Pearson, S. A. (2010). Computerized clinical decision support for prescribing: Provision does not guarantee uptake. *Journal of the American Medical Informatics Association, 17*(1), 25–33. doi: 10.1197/jamia.M3170

Office of the National Coordinator for Health Information Technology. (2010). Retrieved from http://health.hhs.gov

Olsen, L., Aisner, D., & McGinnis, J. M. (Eds.). (2007). *The Learning Healthcare System: Workshop Summary* (IOM Roundtable on Evidence-Based Medicine). Washington, DC: National Academies Press.

Osheroff, J. A., Teich, J. M., Middleton, B. F., Steen, E. B., Wright, A., & Detmer, D. E. (2006). A roadmap for national action on clinical decision support. Bethesda, MD: American Medical Informatics Association.

Osheroff, J. A., Teich, J. M., Middleton, B., Steen, E. B., Wright, A., & Detmer, D. E. (2007). A roadmap for national action on clinical decision support. *Journal of the American Medical Informatics Association, 14*(2), 141–145. doi: 10.1197/jamia.M2334

Patterson, E. S., Doebbeling, B. N., Fung, C. H., Militello, L., Anders, S., & Asch, S. M. (2005). Identifying barriers to the effective use of clinical reminders: Bootstrapping multiple methods. *Journal of Biomedical Informatics, 38*(3), 189–199. doi: 10.1016/j.jbi.2004.11.015

Perlin, J. B., & Kupersmith, J. (2007). Information technology and the inferential gap. *Health Affairs, 26*(2), w192–w194. doi: 10.1377/hlthaff.26.2.w192

Poon, E. G., Wright, A., Simon, S. R., Jenter, C. A., Kaushal, R., Volk, L. A., . . . Bates, D. W. (2010). Relationship between use of electronic health record features and health care quality: Results of a statewide survey. *Medical Care, 48*(3), 203–209.

Pravikoff, D. S., Tanner, A. B., & Pierce, S. T. (2005). Readiness of U.S. nurses for evidence-based practice. *American Journal of Nursing, 105*(9), 40–51.

Rosenthal, A., Mork, P., Li, M. H., Stanford, J., Koester, D., & Reynolds, P. (2010). Cloud computing: A new business paradigm for biomedical information sharing. *Journal of Biomedical Informatics, 43*(2), 342–353. doi: 10.1016/j.jbi.2009.08.014

Safran, C., Bloomrosen, M., Hammond, W. E., Labkoff, S., Markel-Fox, S., Tang, P. C., . . . Expert Panel. (2007). Toward a national framework for the secondary use of health data: An American Medical Informatics Association white paper. *Journal of the American Medical Informatics Association, 14*(1), 1–9.

Saleem, J. J., Patterson, E. S., Militello, L., Render, M. L., Orshansky, G., & Asch, S. M. (2005). Exploring barriers and facilitators to the use of computerized clinical reminders. *Journal of the American Medical Informatics Association, 12*(4), 438–447.

Schedlbauer, A., Prasad, V., Mulvaney, C., Phansalkar, S., Stanton, W., Bates, D. W., Avery, A. J. (2009). What evidence supports the use of computerized alerts and prompts to improve clinicians' prescribing behavior? *Journal of the American Medical Informatics Association, 16*(4), 531–538. doi: 10.1197/jamia.M2910

Schulman, J., Kuperman, G. J., Kharbanda, A., & Kaushal, R. (2007). Discovering how to think about a hospital patient information system by struggling to evaluate it: A committee's journal. *Journal of the American Medical Informatics Association, 14*(5), 537–541.

Shortliffe, E. H. (2010). Final AMIA comments to secretary HHS on meaningful use. Retrieved from https://www.amia.org/files/shared/Final__AMIA_Comments_Meaningful_Use_03_09_10.pdf

Simborg, D. W. (2008). Promoting electronic health record adoption. Is it the correct focus? *Journal of the American Medical Informatics Association, 15*(2), 127–129.

Sittig, D. F., Krall, M. A., Dykstra, R. H., Russell, A., & Chin, H. L. (2006). A survey of factors affecting clinician acceptance of clinical decision support. *BMC Medical Informatics and Decision Making, 6*, 6.

Slutsky, J. R. (2007). Moving closer to a rapid-learning health care system. *Health Affairs, 26*(2), w122–w124. doi: 10.1377/hlthaff.26.2.w122

Stetler, C. B., Ritchie, J. A., Rycroft-Malone, J., Schultz, A. A., & Charns, M. P. (2009). Institutionalizing evidence-based practice: An organizational case study using a model of strategic change. *Implementation Science, 4*(1), 78.

Stewart, W. F., Shah, N. R., Selna, M. J., Paulus, R. A., & Walker, J. M. (2007). Bridging the inferential gap: The electronic health record and clinical evidence. *Health Affairs, 26*(2), w181–w191. doi: 10.1377/hlthaff.26.2.w181

Szolovits, P. (2007). What is a grid? *Journal of the American Medical Informatics Association, 14*(3), 386–386. doi: 10.1197/jamia.M2351

Tanner, A., Pierce, S., & Pravikoff, D. (2004). Readiness for evidence-based practice: Information literacy needs of nurses in the United States. *Students in Health Technology and Informatics, 107*(Pt. 2), 936–940.

Trafton, J. A., Martins, S. B., Michel, M. C., Wang, D., Tu, S. W., Clark, D. J., . . . Goldstein, M. K. (2010). Designing an automated clinical decision support system to match clinical practice guidelines for opioid therapy for chronic pain. *Implementation Science, 5*, 26.

Tunis, S. R., Stryer, D. B., & Clancy, C. M. (2003). Practical clinical trials: Increasing the value of clinical research for decision making in clinical and health policy. *Journal of the American Medical Association, 290*(12), 1624–1632. doi: 10.1001/jama.290.12.1624

Wears, R. L., & Berg, M. (2005). Computer technology and clinical work: Still waiting for Godot. *Journal of the American Medical Association, 293*(10), 1261–1263. doi: 10.1001/jama.293.10.1261

Welch, W. P., Bazarko, D., Ritten, K., Burgess, Y., Harmon, R., & Sandy, L. G. (2007). Electronic health records in four community physician practices: Impact on quality and cost of care. *Journal of the American Medical Informatics Association, 14*(3), 320–328. doi: 10.1197/jamia.M2125

Zerhouni, E. (2007). The promise of personalized medicine. *NIH Medline Plus, 1*–3. Retrieved from http://www.nih.gov/about/director/interviews/NLMmagazinewinter2007.pdf

Zhou, L., Soran, C. S., Jenter, C. A., Volk, L. A., Orav, E. J., Bates, D. W., & Simon, S. R. (2009). The relationship between electronic health record use and quality of care over time. *Journal of the American Medical Informatics Association, 16*(4), 457–464. doi: 10.1197/jamia.M3128

PART TWO

Methods for Translation

CHAPTER TEN

Creating a Culture That Promotes Translation

Joyce Williams

■ INTRODUCTION

Evidence-based practice (EBP) establishes the basic tenets with respect to knowledge translation (KT) and continues step by step to improve the path from awareness to adherence. This includes remodeling and closing the knowledge to evidence practice gaps. To achieve a positive outcome, presenting clear definitions of the concept lessens any misunderstanding.

EBP is an established problem-solving approach to clinical decision making within a health care organization that integrates the best available scientific evidence with the best available experiential (patient and practitioner) evidence (Newhouse, Dearholt, Poe, Pugh, & White, 2007). Moving beyond EBP and building the model to understand and implement KT among health care practitioners necessitates sensitivity within the organization. Innovation must incorporate new knowledge and new technology and create a team to manage resources and knowledge (Gray, 2001).

Defining the culture is the initial phase to rollout and sharing the strategy to improve outcomes in patient care. Organizational culture is recognized as the basic pattern of attitudes, beliefs, and values that model the operation. Along with these are the shared assumptions that members of the organization hold (Denhardt, 1999). Each organization has its own DNA; core values shape the purpose of the environment and provide a powerful cornerstone for developing capacities and behaviors (Osborne & Plastrik, 1997).

The cultures within health organizations may jeopardize implementation of new ideas, unless a realistic approach is used. Taking a fresh approach by explaining the worth of the organization, including its beliefs and what the core values stand for, can be powerful to quash the assumptions that have become embedded in the institutional culture or when providers have become stagnant or fear improving and learning of new methods. This will eliminate the old saying, "we've always done it this way" or ". . . the way things are done around here." It is understandable that some fear advancement because they prefer to remain deep-rooted in their practice methods. Changing paradigms involves a strategy in which needs are identified to improve current therapies and reach outcomes that will be positive for consumers and underscore the importance of sustained advancements in care.

■ CULTURE

Organizations, by their very nature, possess essential goals that are intrinsic, built into the system and witnessed in protocols and procedures, and contribute to the social component of the system. The success of any organization is because of its culture; it is one of the most important and predictable aspects but is the hardest to change. Open communication provides trust as well as shared knowledge. One solution to use when attempting change is allowing for feedback with immediate response.

Staff that is comfortable in an institution may become complacent. They become stuck in a rut, with little or no creativity, which leads to poor morale and an unhealthy atmosphere. Any organization with a controlling management and little flexibility will be challenged to adapt satisfactorily to innovations. Staff members who appreciate progress need to identify the barriers to overcome when coworkers are resistant to change and develop ways to remain positive.

Culture is the vehicle by which the organization shares modes of behavior. Value is a major link between culture and action. Causal effects of any organization are demonstrated in strategic plans where the beliefs and assumptions influence the cohesion and unity among staff.

Structure and culture collectively guide the internal workings of organizational systems, and are the conduits that lead to output by individuals and produce successful outcomes. Explicit knowledge created by researchers is highly valued. The entire organization must focus on learning. Essential to learning, according to Peter Senge, are clarifying the vision and objectives, creating an organizational model and what it stands for, building shared visions from leaders to the whole organization, learning in teams, and linking each element into a cohesive existence (Gray, 2001).

■ PARADIGMS

Change can be looked at in terms of paradigms. This involves knowing the identity of an organization. Paradigms are found in the unwritten rules and manifest between peers and supervisors, employees and consumers. They advise us in actions and what is understood. Shifting a paradigm is crucial to changing a culture and, thus, the assumptions and perceptions that embody the establishment. This requires knowledge of obstacles in the current methodology. One must identify the gap between those who "know" and those who "implement" to eliminate the "know–do" gap. This enables practitioners to reach beyond current care models and provide comprehensive evidence-based approaches to health care that will influence the socioeconomic determinants of health and well-being (Havemann, 2008). Improvements to EBP are founded in scientific research and may require shifting paradigms by articulating an action plan and providing concrete benchmarks and buffers to aid in the process. Sometimes, it may be easier to work within existing paradigms and remodel them for research to move current standards forward.

There is the occasional fashionable or trendy paradigm. When these are present, they require a robust examination of the process to determine if the desired outcome will be achieved. Notable leaders often create new paradigms to add a fresh outlook in an organization and to revitalize stagnant groups with the hope of improvement in evaluative end-results.

This transitional period is not always easy, but as time goes on, individuals become accustomed to the new blueprint and let go of the old model. Changing the habits of employees is more efficient when meeting them halfway. This is accomplished by using a design in which all are encouraged to learn and participate, followed by offering opportunities and workouts, where the redesign is shared and short group exercises follow. Good knowledge management offers time for listening, enables free flow of ideas and emotional commitments, thus, forming a connection between leaders and staff. This develops the capacity to create, find, appraise, use, and store evidence basic to informative decision-making.

■ ORGANIZATIONAL CULTURE

Patterns of shared basic assumptions that groups learn by solving problems of external adaptation and internal integration are considered valid and, therefore, to be taught to new members as the best way to perceive, think, and feel (Schein, 1993, pp. 373–374), and helps integrate individuals to work effectively as a whole within the organization. The comparison can be made that the purpose, incentive, accountability, and power of organization culture are the DNA designers seek to change (Osborne & Plastrik, 1997).

When one looks at organizational cultures, an examination identifies the existing process to facilitate an understanding of the variables that are major elements of the system. Knowledge of the factors that shape a culture allows leaders and staff to introduce new ideas and promote growth within the practice. There is interdependency in the system beginning with the core operations, leading to outcomes for the users that are based on strategic plans. Important to shaping the culture are objectives where accountability is strong and positive results are achieved.

Culture is collective in nature and evolves over time through interaction, development, and sharing of common beliefs and values (Bowditch & Buono, 1997). Within each organization are individual and self-governing characteristics that shape the ways staff perform and work together and strategize toward common goals. The promotion of evidence-based decision-making responsibilities is shared by leaders and staff alike and encompasses behavior and language. The interaction among these groups is an evolutionary process among interrelated professionals to convey EBP and translation into practice.

■ ORGANIZATIONAL CULTURE VERSUS CLIMATE

Organizations receive the resources necessary to function from its environment. In the past, approaches emphasized efficiency and control but current transformation seeks openness to change and the capacity to adapt as significant elements in organizational survival. This may cause turbulence for a time; however, involving practitioners as well as leaders in the decision-making process promotes equity and involvement.

Barriers to effective adoption of practice development include the dual approach of scientific methodology, meaning the laboratory versus the clinical environment. Movement from established routines to new guidelines calls for a gradual transformation beginning with attitude change and emotional release, especially in the first phases. This is followed by feedback and continual reorganization, leading to progressive acceptance. The developmental process of application of the science, systematic connections to EBP, and teamwork provides balance for success of KT concepts.

■ NORMS, VALUES, AND BASIC ASSUMPTIONS OF AN ORGANIZATION

An organization's underlying system of beliefs and values must be transformed for change to be sustainable (Schein, 1997; Senge, 1990; Denhardt, 1999). Values and beliefs are the essence of the organization's philosophy for achieving success. They reflect "the way things should be" (Bowditch & Buono, 1997, p. 292), and direct acceptable behaviors in clinical care. Karl Popper's (1958) principle of making scientific progress through explicit attempts to refute, refine, and, thus, improve fundamental principles and theories (http://www.newmindsets.com/resources/2ndGenELearning.pdf) remains significant in EBP and KT. Promoting an evidence-based management matrix includes the three main topics: inform, change, and monitor (Gray, 2001) with the patient as the center of implementation of care.

Value statements are part of the checks and balance system that holds leadership responsible and aids in consistency. They reflect commitment to professionalism, integrity, service, and quality. Sharing values from the top down is one means of disseminating and collaborating for best practice and provides the link between ideas and actions. When value is not recognized or supported, formative processes are stunted.

Cultures develop as organizations learn to cope with the problems of external adaptation and internal integration (Hann, Bower, Campbell, Marshall, & Reeves, 2007). Personal attitudes and beliefs are integral to clinicians and impacts patient care. This can be seen in outcomes-based and results-driven care. Maintaining a therapeutic relationship between patient and clinician supports trusting relationships. Furthermore, partnerships among practitioners correlate with the underpinnings of capacity building, and build opportunities for evaluation and research within the organization. Standards in the workplace set the quality and are predicated on the conceptualization of knowledge transfer, the process that influences EBP interventions.

Socialization within the organization is reflected in the attitude of employees. How the employee views the organizational purpose may differ from leaders and coworkers. Equating the goals of administration with the individuals in the organization requires communication to articulate shared thinking. Theoretical constructs and scientific analysis in health care has led to EBP initiatives. Decoding the phenomena of an employee's perception within the culture contributes to the environment of culture and climate.

Collaboration and communication help identify systems within health care organizations and trace the energy exchange in provision of care. Von Bertalanffly described a model of open system theory. Using this premise, relationships depend on the external environment (Shafritz & Hyde, 1997). We can deduct that knowledge and experience sharing reflects positively on the organization and leads to homeostasis and equilibrium in the structure.

Organizational processes are viewed as organic where flexibility and spontaneity are dominant, as opposed to mechanistic where control or stability prevails. Another aspect important in the organization is activities that ensure smooth functioning where internal components relate to the outside world. This is in contrast to the external view where competition is notable.

Bosch, Dijkstra, Wensing, van der Weijden, & Grol (2008) describe independent factors that measure the organizational culture. They feel that more than one culture is found and plays a part in the overall institution. The mix of cultures is organized into internal and external or stable versus flexible. Further delineation produces at least four types of cultures. One group value consists of teamwork, cohesiveness, and sharing. Developmental culture provides innovative promotion, risk taking, and growth stimulation. A rational culture strives for achievement; these use champions to achieve goals whereas hierarchical cultures exhibit rules, regulations, stability, and coordination (Bosch et al.). Procedures are used to collect and record outcome measurements. Within the environment, the following characteristics are used to predict and validate quality of care such as participation which demonstrates safety of decision making, support for innovation, discussion and review of procedures, quality monitoring, clarity of objectives, and teamwork (Hann et al., 2007).

■ IMPORTANCE OF ORGANIZATIONAL CULTURE AND CLIMATE

Organizational climate is frequently viewed as an environment of information sharing (Hann et al., 2007). Core problems within organizations are the lack of integration, collaboration, and adaption. Power distribution and breakdown confront the very culture of contemporary organizations. Tension among staff plus ambiguous control and coordination are predictors of unstable environments and lead to uncertainty and necessitate rapid changes in values and goals within the process culture (Shafritz & Hyde, 1997).

Certain aspects of organizational culture (little or no value for individual responsibility) and climate (rigid leadership styles and poor communication channels) are associated with lower rates of worker morale, higher levels of work stress, higher accident rates, and higher rates of adverse events. Several features within the environment can reduce barriers and promote optimal cultures and climates. Interdependency along with work values increase motivation in adaptive structures.

Capacity building provides skills and a learning environment that will engage stakeholders to produce and share knowledge, thus, promoting accountability, inclusion, participation, and cohesions (Havemann, 2008). The opportunity for KT and health care is enriched with robust training environments (Estabrooks et al., 2009). Training and learning improves employee motivation. Leaders must be role models for transformation. Efforts to maintain identity throughout the process increases tolerance and collaboration, and fosters a willingness to participate in change.

Identification and theory development across disciplines, designing, integrating, and resolving conceptual problems produce effective KT strategies where organizations can advance the understanding of the effects of KT. Teamwork fosters vision, interaction, commitment, and cooperation to develop new ideas. Perceived team effectiveness and the balance among culture values affect participation achievement, openness to innovation, and adherence to rules. Quality of care depends on the balance between flexibility and control and how opportunities are measured and improved, using protocols and teamwork (Bosch et al., 2008). Beliefs are formed, maintained and transformed by the organization; knowing them is primary before they can be communicated openly. Leadership may have additional or differing ideas from staff; however, it is the fusion of both levels that articulates the common ground and values demonstrated in the organization. Recognition of the culture and practicing its norms exemplifies value and acceptance by those which again are reflected in the core values.

The workplace atmosphere is evident in the various layers in the organization. Social interaction and communication reflect positively or negatively. Leadership, staff and support personnel promote a certain camaraderie which is apparent in the morale of groups and individuals. A perspective new employee may find an artificial feeling during the initial interview and on further interactions will be able to identify the bonds and connection between staff. Understanding individual behaviors is helpful to ascertain the right fit for a new employee. Promoting value toward members and emphasizing rich modes of communication enhance the landscape for new employees and show a best fit strategy.

Communication is a process whereby information is exchanged and interpreted. The methodology is diverse ranging from behavioral exchange such as eye contact, body language, gestures to spoken words, and writing and drawing recognized as symbolic. Important to the message is conveyance of understanding the intended message. Interpretation rests on the information itself and the context. This interactive process is based on clarity, information, motivation, and expression (Bowditch & Buono, 1997). Providing these components during interpersonal communications influences and elicits commitment to values and goals.

Barriers to effective communication result in people talking at each other or not listening, which interrupt the understanding necessary for recognition of the meaning of the transaction. An excess of data clogs the potential for information to enter and be interpreted as intended. The overload reduces the capacity for commitment often seen today with contemporary technology. Allowing adequate attention to communicative approaches minimizes disruption, limits defensive attitudes, and improves the overall communication effort. This direct approach provides clear and active support for people in organizations.

Another fundamental aspect of communication is networking, which is dominant in productive organizations. Innovation, socialization, and development are incorporated in this focus. The overall objectives and structure of any organization establishes the strength and ease of communication with each other.

■ ORGANIZATIONAL GOALS

Both culture and climate are important determinants of health care performance (Hann et al., 2007). Three determinants are appropriate in assessing organization effectiveness. These are goals that are clear, measurable and consensual (Bowditch & Buono, 1997). Appropriate goal setting is reflected by the mission and the operational practices on a day-to-day basis. Successful outcomes are noted in the morale of the employees and the passion observed as work is conducted.

Health Care Organizations Possess Discernable Cultures That Affect Quality and Performance

The strength of an organization is promulgated in shared beliefs and existing values. Cohesiveness among staff can be viewed as solid and strong when collective values dominate. Likewise, bendable relationships yield weakness and offer little effect to the overall philosophy in institutions. Bosch and colleagues (2008) described teamwork as elementary in sharing common goals, distribution of work, training, and communication for improvement in patient care. Historically, positive associations in teams demonstrate improved outcomes in clinical performance. Support for teamwork and quality of care is effective and results in achieving high levels of success, and is associated with organization culture and performance.

Primary care organizations may have group cultures that tend to be "inward looking" (Bowditch & Buono, 1997). These lack flexibility, sharing, and collaboration. Acquiring the appropriate balance between control-oriented and flexible cultures provides continuous measurement, improvement, and teamwork to reach desired outcomes. Lack of protocols limits the effectiveness, whereas openness to innovation is associated with team worth.

■ CHANGE

Restructuring requires constructive thinking to change the process in hopes of reaching optimal outcomes and to maintain established strong commitments. Change becomes arduous when the tasks, external environment, and traditions are assessed. Updates to the strategic vision precede changes to systems, structures, and processes if the adaptation is to stick. Successful adaptation should be phased in gradually. Creating the concept for transition and providing an open exchange of ideas controls potential defensive attacks and fosters a participatory willingness among groups. It is increasingly important to facilitate transformation by sharing information. The greater the degree of sharing by individuals, the more synergy is released. In general, the organization is responsible for its way of life and how programs are executed to achieve success.

Actions of people are tangible. Their causes can be traced to factors attributed to personal and situational behaviors. Significant to this theory is what is perceived to be the underlying cause, not to be confused with assumptions that can differ extensively among people. Conflict arises when interpretations in a given situation oppose each other. To alleviate this potential, open communications serve as conduits in combination with education modules to focus on differences prevalent among individuals. Communication known as the 360-degree feedback describes structured evaluation processes specific to the whole team for performance evaluations (Hoffman in Bowditch & Buono, 1997, p. 68).

Positive changes are instituted to align with the accepted goals to benefit the organization. Disruption occurs when changes are not in sync with the desired outcome and reflect in less than optimal morale. To combat any negativity, options are needed for leaders when communication is effective to demonstrate the significance of the outcome and why this opportunity will be advantageous for the group.

Major Dimensions in the Assessment of Organizational Culture or Climate

Organizational success or failure is predicated on the quality of the leaders (Boone & Bowen, 1987, p. 302). Leader behavior and effectiveness are directly correlated with staff performance. Leadership is a method where influence is directed toward individuals and groups to attain specific goals (Bowditch & Buono, 1997). Organizational heroes or role models are identified as those that clarify the values and beliefs essential for success.

Leaders can exert power and use it for prestige, reward, or to control groups. Referent power attracts individuals to identify with their characteristics where they dominate in the organization. A combination of these types of leaders is known as emergent leadership, which is ideal for optimal culture and climate in most organizations. The effectiveness of leaders is demonstrated in their motivation and the ways in which they use power. The ability to inspire speaks to the culture and climate because without this talent, groups will not engage and provide the permission to lead (Bowditch & Buono, 1997). This power is measured slowly through proposals, assessments, relationships, vision, building networks, open communication, and sensitivity.

Effective groups demonstrate high group loyalty, defend efficiency, communication and respect for each other, and welcome support that contributes to performance goals. Within these organizations, interlocking groups communicate allegiance, favorable attitudes, and trust. Communications are sensitive, efficient, and effective (Boone & Bowen, 1987). The characteristics integral to effective KT are principles that support problem-solving activities with optimal standards. Consistent with relationships are those individuals that possess great knowledge and insight, providing opportunity to influence the advancement of practice common among leaders. Conveying essential information permits strong bonds within group relationships.

Effective weapons for organizational communication consist of maintaining perspective, involving employees in the model, selection of pioneers to promote the idea and commitment for the duration. Maintaining these communication skills helps employees to see the value in the recognized need, understand the execution of the need, and facilitate the implementation of the need. Culture change is continuous, challenging, and powerful.

Quality of work life (QWL) was introduced in the late 1960s as a means of a holistic wellness approach to the employee in the long term. It encompasses the physical and mental health of the person, including the social and behavioral aspects of a person's being. Prospective knowledge expansion, worker safety, and protection of rights, differentiating accountability are all aspects included in QWL. Breaking this down further, one looks at how effective employees are within the organization, open communications between management and subordinates to improve or resolve issues, and collaborative incentive programs for improvement in outcomes.

Anticipated health care worker outcomes are belief in the system and synergistic relationships to support the culture and climate in the organization. Important to the philosophy are wellness and whole-person QWL, integration and communication, and optimizing substantive goals within the environment. Secondary objectives are openness to practice ideals, opportunities for research and organizational resources with appropriate compensation for services. Linkages and partnerships afford opportunities for skill and knowledge development, minimize staff turnover, and create balance—enhancing worker outcomes.

■ COMPETING VALUES FRAMEWORK

Competing values speak to the philosophy of the organization and are the essence for success. "Interpretive frameworks" (Jelinek in Bowditch & Buono, 1997, p. 292), despite the various dimensions, emerge as somewhat universal. Some organizations have different cultures and subcultures that muddy opportunities for maintaining strong values.

Within each organization, cultures emerge and are viewed in connection to imagery, symbols, events, values, and beliefs. A friendly and social environment promotes a clannish culture. The contrast to this would be a market culture where product is outcome-oriented. Additional components of culture include the hierarchical characteristics, which mean the flexibility or not of the organization, its structure, and whether it is process driven. This particular aspect of culture restricts autonomy and empowerment. The creation or evolution of cultures is known as developmental culture where learning is conducive and begins with setting short and long-term goals.

The competing values framework (CVF) of organizational culture is a 4-quadrant model of value systems within 2 axes, reflecting different value orientations (Scott-Cawiezell, Jones, Moore, & Vojir, 2005). One path is flexibility versus control where determinants influence organizational structure. The second axis is concerned with internal and external focus. Choices must be made that include concentration and integration or separation and distribution. Most organizations function on multiple cultures that have merged over time, with certain aspects dominating the others.

Six content dimensions are used to frame the questions for the assessment. These dimensions consider the dominant organizational characteristic, administration, management style, organizational "glue," strategic emphasis, and criteria for success (Scott-Cawiezell et al., 2005). The valuation makes obvious both positive or negative cultures and the components linked to their values and beliefs.

Knowledge Transfer and the Role of Culture

KT and culture are important concepts, but their use depends on how well they are received by an organization. Research gaps exist where the data support change, but achieving this in an organization is contingent on the culture and the environment of the organization. Several factors account for this from technical issues to governance, funding, and operationalization. Clarification of the culture strategy stimulates leadership and challenges management practices.

Care That Is Supported by Current Scientific Evidence

Challenges exist from significant underuse of established therapies to the application of EBP and the development of innovative approaches to translating this evidence (Lang, Wyer, & Haynes, 2007). Reasons that hinder informative and well-substantiated clinical research are countless and multifaceted, and the result is inefficiency and a reduction in both quantity and quality of life (Straus, Tetroe, & Graham, 2009a). Delivery of care that is supported by science improves quality of care, reduces risk of adverse events, and will close the gaps in translating knowledge to practice.

Optimizing Knowledge Translation

KT, the application of knowledge, from a theoretical perspective is a comprehensive compilation of exchange, synthesis, and the ethically sound applications of research findings. Furthermore, it accelerates the knowledge cycle, and is a natural transformation of knowledge into use (Armstrong, Waters, Roberts, Oliver, & Popay, 2006). Once research is identified and supportive of an innovation, it can transfer more easily for adoption.

Evidence

Ample evidence exists in clinical practice. It is how this knowledge is implemented that strategically influences change in practice. The fact that research studies have been identified, conducted, and published resulting in support for EBP; the degree of incorporation into practice is inconsistent. Many challenges are apparent from research to implementation.

Get Evidence Straight

Getting the evidence straight is the first approach of a 2-part plan toward KT once the evidence model is created. The second part of the plan is to get the evidence used. This interconnected system can be clarified by a pyramid figure describing a hierarchic scheme for understanding different forms of presenting published research evidence (Haynes in Lang et al., 2007). They further describe getting the evidence used through a graphic of an evidence to practice pipeline.

Using these principles in a systematic approach provides for a seamless amalgamation, beginning with the research to determine optimal evidence and ending with therapeutic interventions. This workflow is ideal in the practice arena.

Clinical assessments are being conducted day after day, and KT takes that body of evidence and turns it into a decision-making opportunity whereby EBP is optimized by incorporating validated evidence into patient care.

Social factors determine how clinicians listen and interpret what is said. Terminology is understood differently by individuals, whether they are from the same region or different countries. The differences can be decreased by explanations and further descriptions of what materials are being expressed.

Clarity of information is not always what it seems to be. Use of slang or jargon can be misconstrued, thus, necessitating full explanations to limit misinterpretation of the stated message.

Motivational factors useful in the development of KT are synergistic in the culture, especially while beginning the transition of EBP into an organization. Obtaining buy-in from groups is critical in the entire process when a new course of action is being incorporated. Working within the domains of knowledge, attitude, and behavior, the clinician will bring about positive changes and reduce potential barriers or undesired effects. Change is a complex process that calls for an evaluation of the entire health care organization (Sudsawad, 2007). Tools and products demonstrating best quality knowledge are synthesized into practice guidelines to facilitate patient decisions or algorithms (Straus et al., 2009b).

Implementing change in the organization requires a systematic approach. The course of action can be positioned by first identifying key elements/factors in the process.

Core Competencies for Health Care Education (Health Professions Educational Summit)

The Institute of Medicine (IOM) has recommended that health care stand committed to patient-centered care and meeting patient's needs. To meet this charge, teams must work in collaboration that engages professionals from medicine, nursing, psychology, radiology, rehabilitation, and so on. Using joint efforts improves the holistic approach and implements best practice plans for the patient. The IOM further states that the education of health professionals should focus on delivery of patient-centered care by members of a diverse health care team that underscores EBP, quality improvement, and use of information technology. Each of these core competencies reflects forward thinking and guides health care for future advancement.

EBP is a response to the problematic divergence between questions surfacing in the clinical area and a responsive pathway to locate indicated answers. The compiled research is then used to provide optimal care. EBP is not in itself the end of the process. Quality improvement is part of the check-and-balance system that provides an opportunity to measure and test the hypothesis for validity. This step is designed to meet the rigor necessary for quality evidence by the ability to replicate the method and reach similar conclusions for implementation. Support for this procedure is predicated on support from technological information and management, which is a conduit to communication and knowledge development.

Before implementation of a change in practice can be initiated, an assessment of the environment and culture must take place in the organization. Examining the mission, vision, and core values will inform those interested in the transformation. Beyond this action is knowledge of the leadership and management tier, plus those responsible for the education and training. Do they display the commitment necessary to push this movement forward? And are they capable and diverse to work with staff to support the team on all levels? Lastly, do the educators comprehend EBP knowledge and skills, have the additional resources and access to technological methodologies (computers, internet, and databases), information science professionals, and integrated health system information systems as well as library access to augment the training and workshops needed to customize and share the path toward change?

The change process can begin once the assumptions have been carefully examined for the organization. These include the value and belief system of the organization and the connectedness of the professionals about to make the transition. Intrinsic to the process is robust leadership which steps forward and leads by example, demonstrating the positive components of EBP, and facilitates the exchange of information each step of the way. Introducing the change in phases limits the hurdles because large drastic changes are harder to tolerate, whereas incremental modifications are less contested. Using this philosophy reinforces affirmative trust and creates further interest in the concept. When executing a change among great numbers in an organization, it is often prudent to divide the efforts and transition from one area to another if possible. This can be done by starting with one unit and following a systematic path, moving from one location to another until all areas have been approached.

Elements for Successful Change

Change is an integral part of any organization's culture. The process follows an incremental progression and follows redirection of pathways to care. All establishments should have well-delineated visions and goals, describing the tenets that support the mission. The most effective way to create and transfer knowledge is through development of a comprehensive plan to educate, followed by evaluation tools and methods along with collaboration and experience to reach desired outcomes.

Management must demonstrate confidence in the plan and have a well-thought-out protocol to change the landscape (i.e., maintain consistency of terms and data definitions). This shift has to be persistent, include the potential barriers that might hinder the progression of the movement and dispel and fears of misperceptions germane to EBP. There is overwhelming support for shifting the current paradigm to one that contributes effective to patient-centered care. Defining the concept within the organization and communicating this vision contained in the strategic plan will compel professionals to come on board with energy, using teamwork and synergy to reach optimal outcomes. Case studies are also an innovative way to report on progress toward a specific objective or cluster objectives on a particular topic.

Clear goals articulate what needs are shared, the training needed, and advanced communication portals to conduct and contribute to improvement to the vision of the organization. Additionally, structural changes lead to quality improvement that contributes to high-quality care. An organization is not complete without its resources and administrative support. These individuals are those people that make the work of groups manageable. They also help organize workflow, receive reports, and provide the behind-the-scenes continuity possible. There will always be resistance somewhere in the process, but this can usually be managed by individual or small group assistance. Optimism is highly recommended to achieve buy-in from everyone.

Creating a Culture for Translation

To build the infrastructure, it is necessary to close the quality chasm between current practices and optimal standards (Bosch et al., 2008).

The process of culture change involves a shift in philosophy and practice toward patient-directed, consumer-driven health promotion and quality of life (White-Chu, Graves, Godfrey, Bonner, & Sloane, 2009). During remodeling, it is helpful to identify the resources that will contribute to efficiency throughout the process. Some of the potential resources are leaders who develop opportunities and educational programs for staff, create communication networks and forums where good discussion can take place and where people become engaged in issues that shed light on their skills, and share personal expertise and skills. Other tangible resources are timelines, libraries with a bank of information pertinent to translational knowledge and change, case examples, access to technological equipment and experienced professionals. Building the infrastructure requires evaluations at regular intervals to measure and track achievement of targets.

Champions

Within the subset of infrastructure are organizational heroes who are role models who personify the cultural value system and define the organization's concept in tangible ways. These individuals may be leaders or practitioners, and they represent and reinforce the values of culture by underscoring models of improvement in outcomes of patient care; thus, providing a standard of performance while motivating organizational members (Greiner & Knebel,

2003, p. 129). This is in direct contrast to those that circulate myths, thus, undermining the cultural values. This cultural network does not support the organization's needs and creates dysfunction. Stopping this behavior and cultivating a positive environment by featuring champions, dispels, and creates a joint effort toward positive change.

Mentors

Capacity-building measures also include mentorships that incorporate designing protocols, analysis of results, journal clubs that introduce relevant literature-noting gaps, and, finally, creating linkages within the clinical arena (Verhoef, Mulkins, Kania, Findlay-Reece, & Mior, 2010). Another form of advisement is the use of knowledge brokers (KB) who work closely with leaders and staff to facilitate systems change and establish connections between researchers and users (Dobbins et al., 2009). KBs facilitate a decision-making culture and stress the value of EBP to energize KT strategies.

Leaders

Changes in health care require strong leadership to help staff move good evidence into practice and optimize patients' outcomes (Gawlinski & Rutledge, 2008). A strategy begins with creating forums for discussions that will set the stage and provide the organizational structure, roles and responsibilities of the group, and a timeline for the process. The agenda will reflect items such as the team goals, potential models for evaluation, discussion of the models, resource materials, ongoing communication forums, and future meetings. Strong leaders model behaviors and attitudes throughout processes and understand that good ideas come from everywhere, and they provide encouragement and support to everyone to reach the objective.

Technical Resources

A strong component of any organization is data mining and information technology. The informatics system must be able to yield appropriate surveillance and collection of trends internally and externally, with the ability to locate reports on disease treatment protocols to determine what works and what does not. Additionally, access to outside web-based resources via the internet will connect medical information resources locally, regionally, nationally, and internationally. This opportunity provides the necessary means to remain connected to other professionals and also translates well to future publications and media newsbytes.

Stakeholder awareness is one of the critical components in the global response to KT and buy-in. To provide the best EBP and translate it to the patient population, acknowledgement of and working with partners facilitates the desired outcomes. Partnerships exist to strengthen, produce, and manage that narrows the know–do gap caused by structured forms of cooperation and multisectoral actions (Havemann, 2008). Care must be continuous, customized, and personalized to meet the needs of the patient. KT is making users aware of knowledge and facilitating the use of it. It closes the gap between what we know and what we do, and moves knowledge into action (Graham & Tetroe, 2009). Health professionals support patient care through knowledge acquisition and use of EBP guidelines. Safe care is a priority and prevention of errors that interfere with identified patient outcomes. Transparency in the decision process of patient care while acknowledging the needs of the patient promotes the central worth of the patient. None of this can be accomplished without collaboration, communication, delegation of responsibilities, and exchange of information in coordination of care (IOM, 2003). These principles relate to the importance of stakeholder involvement in the care of the patient.

Professionalism is cultivated through excellent informal and formal communication. Providing a culture and environment conducive to innovative practice stimulates practitioners to offer patient-centered care. EBP and KT focuses on transdisciplinary, holistic, global partnerships in research, knowledge generation, translation, and action (Shahab & Ghaffar, 2008). Engagement of the team of care givers and using established good EBP methodology endorses robust networks that are valuable to all. Evaluative criteria is demonstrated by documenting "progress" in assessments and changes from baseline measures toward the targeted outcomes and often results in cost-effectiveness.

■ CONCLUSION

Health care has moved from a model in which researchers disseminate, to one in which there is acknowledgment of the reciprocity needed to practice evidence-informed care (Armstrong et al., 2006). The common denominator of KT research develops with leaders who practice and model behavior where the patient is the center of care and practitioners unite to work effectively and efficiently to common goals in a culture of caring. Dagenais, Riddle, Laurendeau, & Souffez (2009) describes KT as "the exchange, synthesis, and ethically sound application of knowledge—within a complex system of interactions among researchers and users—to accelerate the capture of the benefits or research" to improve health. Engineering change in health care systems and groups (Straus et al., 2009) is interrelated in the culture cycle in organizations. Integrating knowledge from research and linking this exchange among researchers and practitioners is the aim and practice of KT in organizations.

■ REFERENCES

Armstrong, R., Waters, E., Roberts, H., Oliver, S., & Popay, J. (2006). The role and theoretical evolution of knowledge translation and exchange in public health. *Journal of Public Health, 28*(4), 384–389.

Boone, L. E., & Bowen, D. D. (1987). *The great writings in management and organizational behavior* (2nd ed.). Boston, MA: McGraw-Hill.

Bosch, M., Dijkstra, R., Wensing, M., van der Weijden, T., & Grol, R. (2008). Organizational culture, team climate, and diabetes care in small office-based practices. *BMC Health Services Research, 8*, 180–188.

Bowditch, J. L., & Buono, A. F. (1997). *A primer on organizational behavior* (4th ed.). New York, NY: John Wiley & Sons.

Dagenais, C., Riddle, V., Laurendeau, M. C., & Souffez, L. (2009). Knowledge translation research in population health: Establishing a collaborative research agenda. *Health Research Policy and Systems, 7*, 28. Retrieved from http://www.health-policy-systems.com/content/7/1/28

Denhardt, R. B. (1999). *Public administration: An action orientation* (3rd ed.). Fort Worth, TX: Harcourt Brace College.

Dobbins, M., Hanna, S. E., Ciliska, D., Manske, S., Cameron, R., Mercer, S., . . . Robeson, P. (2009). A randomized controlled trial evaluating the impact of knowledge translation and exchange strategies. *Implementation Science*, *4*, 61. Retrieved from http://www.implementation science.com/content/4/1/23

Estabrooks, C. A., Hutchinson, A. M., Squires, J. E., Birdsell, J., Cummings, G. G., Degner, L., . . . Norton, P. G. (2009). Translating research in elder care: An introduction to a study protocol series. *Implementation Science*, *4*, 51. Retrieved from http://www.implementationscience.com/content/4/1/51

Gawlinski, A., & Rutledge, D. (2008). Selecting a model for evidence-based practice changes: A practical approach. *AACN Advanced Critical Care*, *19*(3), 219–300.

Graham, I. D., & Tetroe, J. M. (2009). Getting evidence into policy and practice: Perspective of a health research funder. *Journal of the Canadian Academy of Child and Adolescent Psychiatry*, *18*(1), 46–50.

Gray, J. A. M. (2001). *Evidence-based health care: How to make a health policy and management decisions* (2nd ed.). London, England: Churchill Livingstone.

Greiner, A. & Knebel, E. (Eds). (2003). *Health professions education: A bridge to quality*. Washington DC: The National Academies Press.

Hann, M., Bower, P., Campbell, S., Marshall, M., & Reeves, D. (2007). The association between culture, climate, and quality care in primary health care teams. *Family Practice*, *24*(4), 323–329. Retrieved from http://fampra.oxfordjournals.org/cgi/reprint/cmm020v1

Havemann, K. (2008). The changing landscape of research for health. *Global Forum Update for Health*, *5*, 59–63. Retrieved from http://www.globalforumhealth.org/Media-Publications/Publications/Global-Forum-Update-on-Research-for-Health-Volume-5-Fostering-innovation-for-global-health/Global-Forum-Update-on-Research-for-Health-Volume-5-Fostering-innovation-for-global-health-Individual-articles

Institute of Medicine. (2003). The learning healthcare system: Workshop summary (IOM Roundtable on Evidence-Based Medicine). Retrieved from http://books.nap.edu/catalog.php?record_id=11903

Lang, E. S., Wyer, P. C., & Haynes, R. B. (2007). Knowledge translation: Closing the evidence-to-practice gap. *Annals of Emergency Medicine*, *49*(3), 355–363.

Newhouse, R., Dearholt, S., Poe, S., Pugh, L. C., & White, K. (2007). *Johns Hopkins nursing evidence-based practice model and guidelines*. Indianapolis, IN: Sigma Theta Tau International.

Osborne, D., & Plastrik, P. (1997). *Banishing bureaucracy: The five strategies for reinventing government*. Reading, MA: Addison-Wesley Publishing.

Popper, K. (1958). *The logic of scientific discovery*. London: Hutchinson.

Schein, E. (1997). Organizational culture and leadership. Retrieved from http://www.tnellen.com/ted/tc/schein.html

Schein, E. (1993). Organizational culture and leadership. In J. Shafritz & J. S. Ott (Eds.), *Classics of organizational theory* (pp. 373–374). Forth Worth, TX: Harcourt College Publishers.

Scott-Cawiezell, J., Jones, K., Moore, L., & Vojir, C. (2005). Nursing home culture: A critical component in sustained improvement. *Journal of Nursing Care Quality*, *20*(4), 341–348.

Senge, P. (1990). The fifth discipline: The art and practice of the learning organization. Retrieve from http://www.infed.org/thinkers/senge.htm

Shahab, S., & Ghaffar, A. (2008). Strengthening the base: Innovation and convergence in climate change and public health. *Global Forum Update on Research for Health*, *5*, 36–40.

Shafritz, J. M., & Hyde, A. C. (1997). *Classics of public administration* (4th ed.). Fort Worth, TX: Harcourt Brace College Publishers.

Straus, S. E., Tetroe, J., & Graham, I. (2009a). Knowledge translation is the use of knowledge in health care decision making. *Journal of Clinical Epidemiology, 61*(1), 6–10. doi: 10.1016/j.jclinepi.2009.08.016

Straus, S. E., Tetroe, J., & Graham, I. D., Eds. (2009b). *Knowledge translation in health care: Moving from evidence to practice.* Hoboken, NJ: Blackwell Publishing.

Sudsawad, P. (2007). *Knowledge translation: Introduction to models, strategies, and measures.* Austin, TX: Southwest Educational Development Laboratory, National Center for the Dissemination of Disability Research. Retrieved from http://www.ncddr.org/kt/products/ktintro/ktintro.pdf

Verhoef, M. J., Mulkins, A., Kania, A., Findlay-Reece, B., & Mior, S. (2010). Identifying the barriers to conducting outcomes research in integrative health care clinic settings—a qualitative study. *BMC Health Services Research, 10,* 14. Retrieved from http://www.biomedcentral.com/1472-6963/10/14

White-Chu, E. F., Graves, W. J., Godfrey, S. M., Bonner, A., & Sloane, P. (2009). Beyond the medical model: The culture change revolution in long-term care. *Journal of the American Medical Directors Association, 10*(6), 370–378.

CHAPTER ELEVEN

Challenges and Barriers in Translation

Sharon Dudley-Brown

■ INTRODUCTION

We know that there are many challenges and barriers in translation of evidence, evidenced by the lag time in adoption and the general lack of translation of evidence in health care. According to McGlynn and colleagues (2003), only one-half of evidence reaches widespread use.

To translate evidence into practice, a cascade framework can be used—an adaptation of a knowledge translation cascade by the World Health Organization (WHO; Tugwell, Robinson, Grimshaw, & Santesso, 2006). First, is the identification of barriers and facilitators; second, is the prioritization of the barriers; third, is choosing a model for translation to address key barriers; fourth, is using that model and developing appropriate interventions to address the barriers; fifth, is the evaluation of the translation; and sixth is the dissemination of the translation. This chapter will address steps one through four because the last two steps are covered in later chapters.

■ IDENTIFICATION OF BARRIERS RELATED TO EVIDENCE TRANSLATION

The identification of barriers and facilitators is suggested to be completed a priori any translation project. Both challenges and barriers can be broken down through those described by Funk, Champagne, Wiese, and Tornquist (1991a) and Funk, Tornquist, and Champagne (1995) as barriers to research utilization. However, one can argue that these are the same categories of barriers when exploring those related to evidence translation. These include the characteristics of the adopter, the characteristics of the innovation, the characteristics of the communication, and the characteristics of the organization or institution. These categories were initially developed from a factor analysis of the BARRIERS scale, developed by Funk and colleagues (1991a) and Funk, Tornquist, and Champagne (1995). Characteristics of the adopter are essentially the characteristics of the individual who will adopt the evidence, or the nurse. This category takes into consideration the nurse's knowledge, skills, and awareness of the evidence, as well as the nurse's willingness to change or try new ideas. The second category is the characteristics of the organization, which addresses the organization's role in the translation process. This includes authority to make changes, administrative support for implementation, facilities, and time for implementation. The third category, characteristics of the innovation, is the qualities of the evidence and prior research. This also includes the "innovation," to borrow from Rogers's (1983) work on diffusion of innovations, which is defined as the idea, practice, or object that is new to the potential adopter. The last category focuses on the characteristics of the communication (another category borrowed from Rogers's work). This includes the accessibility of the evidence and channels of communication.

Use of BARRIERS Scale

A recent systematic review of the BARRIERS scale (Funk, Champagne, Wiese, & Tornquist, 1991b; Funk, Tornquist, & Champagne, 1995) explored the state of knowledge resulting from use of the scale and to make recommendations about the future use of the scale. Authors included 63 studies, most of which were cross-sectional design, but of weak to moderate quality. The scale was found to be reliable, as assessed by internal consistency. However, validity of the scale to accurately capture barriers was lacking. One possible contributory factor is the fact that the scale was developed in the late 1980s to early 1990s, and the health care environment and the nursing profession have changed over the past 30 years. For example, patient participation in decision making has increased, and patients' preferences and opinions may present a barrier to research utilization. The initial scale did not contain any questions related to patients' opinions; however, Greene (1997) added this to their scale and measured barriers toward pain management in oncology. In that study, the item "patients will not take medication or follow the recommendations" was ranked as the third highest barrier by nurses.

The main barriers reported from this systematic review were related to the setting and the presentation of research findings. Overall, despite varying geographic locations, sample size, response rate, study setting, and assessment of study quality, identified barriers were consistent. Of the top 10 barriers, the items "there is insufficient time on the job to implement new ideas," "the nurse does not have time to read research," "the nurse does not have enough authority to change patient care procedures," "the statistical analyses are not understandable," together with "the relevant literature is not compiled in any place," were the most frequently reported. Six of the top 10 barriers belonged to the setting subscale. Few studies reported associations between reported research use and perceptions of barriers to research utilization.

Other Scales of Use

While Funk and colleagues' BARRIERS scale has been used to explore reasons why nurses do not use research (Funk et al., 1991a; Funk, Tornquist, & Champagne, 1995) there have been more recent studies looking at barriers and facilitators to use evidence-based practice (EBP). Leasure, Stirlen, and Thompson (2008) specifically wanted to identify the presence or absence of provider and organizational variables associated with use of EBP among nurses. Using a researcher-developed instrument on perceived internal and external organizational processes related to implementation of EBP changes. Questionnaires were mailed to nurse executives who then gave the questionnaires to staff nurses. Results from 119 nurses revealed the following facilitators: reading journals that publish original research, journal club, nursing research committee, a facility research committee, and facility access to the Internet. Barriers found included lack of staff involvement in projects, no communication of projects that were completed, no knowledge on outcomes, and the fact that most job descriptions did not include a research component. Although a methodological flaw (bias) of sending the questionnaires first to nurse managers who distributed them to their staff, the findings are similar to those of Funk and colleagues' (1991a, 1995).

Glasgow and Emmons (2007) cite four categories of barriers to translation, which include characteristics of (a) the intervention, (b) the target settings, (c) the research or revaluation design, and (d) the interactions among the first three categories (Exhibit 11.1).

The Promoting Action on Research Implementation in Health Services (PARIHS) framework was developed to represent essential determinants of successful implementation of research into clinical practice (Kitson, Harvey, & McCormack, 1998) and can be dually used to explore challenges and barriers in translation. The PARIHS framework posits three core elements that determine the success of research implementation:

1. Evidence—the strength and nature of the evidence as perceived by multiple stakeholders;
2. Context—the quality of the context or environment in which the research is implemented, and
3. Facilitation—processes by which implementation is facilitated

Each of these three core elements, in turn, comprise multiple, distinct components (see Chapters 2 and 3 on frameworks for translation). Because of its focus on those three areas critical in translation, it can be used to determine a priori, potential barriers to translation.

Meijers's Work on Contextual Factors

Exploring contextual factors and research utilization, Meijers and colleagues (2006) conducted a systematic review exploring the relationship between contextual factors and research utilization, and mapped to the PARIHS model. In 10 papers, six contextual factors were identified as having a statistically significant relationship with research use, namely the role of the nurse, multifaceted access to resources, organizational climate, multifaceted support, time for research activities, and provision of education. The contextual factors could successfully be mapped to the dimensions of context in the PARIHS framework (context, culture, leadership), with the exception of evaluation. However, the authors found that few studies were found of sufficient quality because of methodological limitations, and the results in reviewed studies were mixed. They concluded that the strength of the relationship between the six contextual factors and research utilization by nurses is still largely unknown; however, findings do provide support of the PARIHS framework for better understanding of the impact of context on research use.

Facilitators to Translation of Evidence

Although challenges and barriers are both individual and institutional, facilitators to translation of evidence largely depend on the organization or institution. Cummings, Estabrooks, Midodzi, Wallin, and Hayduk (2007) developed and tested a theoretical model of organizational

EXHIBIT 11.1

Barriers of Dissemination/Translation (Glasgow & Emmons, 2007)

1. Characteristics of the intervention
   a. High cost
   b. Intensive time demands
   c. High level of staff expertise required
   d. Difficult to learn or understand
   e. Not packaged or "manualized"
   f. Not developed considering user needs
   g. Not designed to be self-sustaining
   h. Highly specific to particular setting
   i. Not modularized or customized

2. Situation of intended target settings
   a. Competing demands
   b. Program imposed from outside
   c. Financial/organizational stability
   d. Specific needs of clients and setting
   e. Limited resources
   f. Limited time
   g. Limited organizational support
   h. Prevailing practices work against innovation
   i. Perverse incentives or regulations
   j. Challenges implementing interventions with quality

3. Research design
   a. Not relevant or representative: sample of patients, sample of setting, sample of clinicians
   b. Failure to evaluate cost
   c. Failure to evaluate reach
   d. Failure to evaluate setting adoption
   e. Failure to assess implementation
   f. Failure to evaluate maintenance
   g. Failure to evaluate sustainability

4. Interactions among three other barrier types
   a. Because of participation barriers, the program reach or participation is low
   b. Interventions are not flexible
   c. Intervention is not appropriate for the target population
   d. Staffing pattern does not match intervention needs
   e. Organization and intervention philosohphies are not aligned
   f. Organization is unable to implement intervention adequately

influences on research use, based on the PARIHS framework, and assess the influence of less positive to more positive contexts on research use. Findings of hospital characteristics that positively influenced research use by nurses were staff development, opportunity for nurse-to-nurse collaboration, and staffing and support services. Increased emotional exhaustion led to less-reported research use and higher rates of nurse and patient-reported events. Nurses working in contexts with more positive culture, leadership, and evaluation reported significantly more research use, staff development, and lower rates of patients and staff adverse events. The authors conclude that the findings highlight the combined importance of culture, leadership, and evaluation to increase research use and improve patient safety. Findings also strengthen the PARIHS framework and its use to guide research into practice and translation (Cummings et al., 2007).

Foxcroft and Cole (2000) conducted a Cochrane review to determine to what extent organizational infrastructures are effective in promoting the implementation of research evidence on the promotion of evidence-based nursing practice. The authors found no studies rigorous enough to be included, finding seven case studies. They concluded that conceptual models on organizational processes to promote EBP need to be better evaluated, and suggested time series designs to further explore this topic. Clearly, although organizational infrastructure is important, there are no clear guidelines on its implementation in terms of the promotion of EBP.

Newhouse and colleagues (2007) explored ways institutions could build infrastructure to support EBP. These include leadership, establishing a structure for building and sustaining EBP, such as shared governance committees, development of an EBP skill set with the availability of EBP experts and mentors, development of material resources, setting expectations (revising job descriptions), collaborating with a school of nursing, and continuing to revise and update tools.

Mohide and Coker (2005) also described their organizational interventions to increase the rate of research dissemination and uptake. They used an evidence-based nursing (EBN) committee as an organizational strategy to shift the culture toward scholarship. Specific strategies and activities included organizational commitment to EBP, strategic positioning of the EBN committee within nursing's administrative structure, articulation of a mission, conceptualization of a model for EBN practice, learning on the job, selection and adoption of an evidence-based model for implementing change, and marketing for a change in culture toward clinical scholarship.

■ PRIORITIZATION OF BARRIERS

After identification of barriers and facilitators, one must prioritize the barriers. One way to prioritize has been proposed by Tugwell and colleagues (2006), by prioritizing across the six P's: public/community, patient, press, practitioner, policy maker, and private sector (as discussed in Chapter 12). Barriers "must be prioritized as to whether they are modifiable, which are 'mission critical,' and how to address them" (Tugwell et al., 2006, p. 646). Tugwell and colleagues (2006, p. 646) go on to describe how to identify key barriers based on three criteria: modifiability, available interventions, and "bottleneck issues," but stating that barriers need to be prioritized based on local settings and relevant stakeholders.

■ CHOOSING A MODEL FOR TRANSLATION

Models for translation, such as the PARIHS framework, can be used not only to explore and assess challenges and barriers to translation, but also can be used to address the challenges and barriers found. This is the next step in the above-mentioned cascade framework for translation. For example, the category of context, which includes culture, leadership, and evaluation, is important in translation. Although culture can be assessed and described (see Chapter 10), evaluation (see Chapter 14) and assessment of leadership (see Chapter 6) are also important. Leadership can be used to address any barriers or challenges found in assessment. In addition to leadership, in addressing barriers to translation, is an organization's readiness to change.

An Organizational Readiness to Change Assessment instrument (ORCA), organized according to the core elements and subelements of the PARIHS framework, was developed (Helfrich, Li, Sharp, & Sales, 2009). The instrument comprises three major scales corresponding to the core elements of the PARIHS framework: (a) Strength and extent of evidence for the clinical practice changes represented by the quality improvement (QI) program, assessed with four subscales; (b) quality of the organizational context for the QI program, assessed with six subscales; and (c) capacity for internal facilitation of the QI program, assessed with nine subscales. Each subscale comprised between three and six items, assessing a common dimension of the given scale. Although the authors found general support for the reliability and factor structure of the ORCA, there was poor reliability among measures of evidence, and factor analysis results for measures of general resources and clinical champion role did not conform to the PARIHS framework. Additional validation is needed, including criterion validation.

■ DEVELOP APPROPRIATE INTERVENTIONS TO ADDRESS THE BARRIERS

The aforementioned strategies for assessing and acting on challenges and barriers to translation of evidence have primarily focused on organizations. From the perspective of an individual provider, one can use Pathman's pipeline (Pathman, Konrad, Freed, Freeman, & Koch, 1996; Diner et al., 2007; Glasziou & Haynes, 2005) to move evidence into action, and to assess and address potential challenges and barriers. This pipeline, linear in fashion, focuses on translation of knowledge and includes the following: clinician awareness, acceptance, applicability, ability, act on, agreement, and then adherence to the evidence. Specifically, these are provider-oriented and patient-focused strategies to assist in translation of evidence into practice. Although the initial proposed pipeline was to address physician adherence to guidelines, Pathman and colleagues (1996) described four stages from evidence to action: the clinician needs to be aware, then agree, then adopt, and then adhere. Diner and colleagues (2007) later proposed a revised Pathman's pipeline, and an adaptation of Glasziou and Haynes' (2005), to address the path to optimal patient outcomes, moving from evidence to practice. Diner and colleagues' adaptation includes the "leaks" along the pipeline. The leaks, the droplets of water, provide illustrative examples of information loss, misuse, or inapplicability at each level. The first five leaks deal with the physician and health care team, whereas the last two leaks are specific to the patient's environment. This model addresses how to "slow the leaks" and, thus, improve the flow of information from high-quality, clinically relevant evidence to the achievement of optimal patient outcomes. Unlike previous models, this is more individually than institutionally based.

Diner and colleagues (2007) also addressed barriers to change of practice, also for the individual practitioner. These include self-motivation and incentives that reinforce old behavior, the environment (budget, liability, peer group influence), recommendations that contradict previously accepted standards of care, and competing nonprovider influences such as pharmaceutical marketing, hospital administration, concern over costs, and joint commission mandates. Removing barriers to translation to an individual practitioner may indeed prove more difficult than addressing those barriers from an institutional perspective. Individual concerns, values, and motivation may be more difficult to change; and strategies in the literature are scarce.

Kulier, Gee, and Khan (2008) described five steps to guide implementation of new research findings into practice, using the pipeline metaphor, adapted from Glasziou and Haynes (2005).

- Step one, *knowledge and awareness*—is for the clinician to be aware of new clinically useful and applicable evidence. They suggest such institutional interventions such as journal club meetings and ward rounds.
- Step two, *acceptance and persuasion*—focuses on persuading the clinician about the potential benefit for the patient. One proposed intervention strategy is the use of key opinion leaders, and providing information from multiple sources.
- Step three, *decision making*—involves the choice about implementing research findings. The authors again suggest more institutional strategies such as the use of clinical directors, or persons in a position of power to bring about change within the organization. It is here, in the decision-making phase that truly depends on the individual, and here is where values and motivation are important to bring about any change.
- Step four, *implementation*—focuses on all the variables needed to actually implement a change. Here, the authors suggest such interventions as the use of clinical protocols and clinical practice guidelines.
- Step five, *continuation*—focuses on maintenance of the change. This can occur through regular monitoring, audits, and ongoing feedback.

Although assessment of challenges and barriers in translation is acknowledged by many, it is the unforeseen challenges and barriers that occur during translation that may pose more of a challenge, and may be difficult to overcome. It is with knowledge, through frameworks, that can assist the translation by identifying and addressing as many barriers in advance.

Another challenge in translation of evidence rests with the consumer. Carman and colleagues (2010, p. 2) explored how making health care decisions based on evidence of effectiveness could be translated into language that consumers would understand and embrace, as part of the development of a "communication toolkit" to help consumers communicate more effectively about evidence-based health care. Using focus groups, interviews, and an online survey with health care consumers, the researchers found many beliefs, values, and knowledge to be at odds with what policy makers prescribe as evidence-based health care. Few consumers understood terms such as "medical evidence" or "quality guidelines," and many believed that more health care and newer care meant higher quality, better care. Thus, translation of evidence-based health care into understandable concepts and activities that support and motivate consumers must occur at the provider level, the institutional level, as well as with employers, health plans, and policy makers.

■ CONCLUSION

In summary, the translation of evidence is fraught with challenges and barriers, although the imperative is strong. The translation of knowledge has been promoted by the Institute of Medicine (IOM) and has been linked to health care quality. The translation of knowledge has been linked to the concept of a paradigm shift of Thomas Kuhn, in that, science does not progress linearly, but periodically undergoes paradigm shifts. Now is the time for a paradigm shift. However, barriers still exist to the application of knowledge, specifically in the area of risk versus benefit, comfort with current practice versus outcomes, cost, rewards, lack of experience, values, contexts, and others. As individual practitioners, we need to acknowledge and address these challenges and barriers, and institutions must also promote translation and address both individual and institutional barriers.

■ REFERENCES

Carman, K. L., Maurer, M., Yegian, J. M., Dardess, P., McGee, P., Evers, M., & Marlo, K. O. (2010). Evidence that consumers are skeptical about evidence-based health care. *Health Affairs, 29*(7), 1400–1406.

Cummings, G. G., Estabrooks, C. A., Midodzi, W. K., Wallin, L., & Hayduk, L. (2007). Influence of organizational characteristics and context on research utilization. *Nursing Research, 56*(4 Suppl.), S24–S39.

Diner, B. M., Carpenter, C. R., O'Connell, T., Pang, P., Brown, M. D., Seupaul, R. A., . . . KT-CC Theme IIIa Members (2007). Graduate medical education and knowledge translation: Role models, information pipelines, and practice change thresholds. *Academic Emergency Medicine, 14*(11), 1008–1014.

Foxcroft, D., & Cole, N. (2000). Organizational infrastructures to promote evidence-based nursing practice. *Cochrane Database of Systematic Reviews,* (3), CD002212.

Funk, S. G., Champagne, M. T., Wiese, R. A., & Tornquist, E. M. (1991a). Barriers to using research findings in practice: The clinician's perspective. *Applied Nursing Research, 4*(2), 90–95.

Funk, S. G., Champagne, M. T., Wiese, R. A., & Tornquist, E. M. (1991b). BARRIERS: The barriers to research utilization scale. *Applied Nursing Research, 4*(1), 39–45.

Funk, S. G., Tornquist, E. M., & Champagne, M. T. (1995). Barriers and facilitators of research utilization. An integrative review. *Nursing Clinics of North America, 30*(3), 395–407.

Glasgow, R. E., & Emmons, K. M. (2007). How can we increase translation of research into practice? Types of evidence needed. *Annual Review of Public Health, 28,* 413–433.

Glasziou, P., & Haynes, B. (2005). The paths from research to improved health outcomes *Evidence-Based Nursing, 8*(2), 36–38.

Greene, P. E. (1997). Diffusion of innovations in cancer pain management and barriers to changing practice: A study of office practice oncology nurses. Unpublished doctoral dissertation, Georgia State University, School of Nursing—Georgia.

Helfrich, C. D., Li, Y. F., Sharp, N. D., & Sales, A. E. (2009). Organizational readiness to change assessment (ORCA): Development of an instrument based on the Promoting Action on Research in Health Services (PARIHS) framework. *Implementation Science, 4*, 38.

Kitson, A., Harvey, G., & McCormack, B. (1998). Enabling the implementation of evidence based practice: A conceptual framework. *Quality in Health Care, 7*(3), 149–158.

Kulier, R., Gee, H., & Khan, K. S. (2008). Five steps from evidence to effect: Exercising clinical freedom to implement research findings. *British Journal of Obstetrics & Gynecology, 115*(10), 1197–1202.

Leasure, A. R., Stirlen, J., & Thompson, C. (2008). Barriers and facilitators to the use of evidence-based best practices. *Dimensions of Critical Care Nursing, 27*(2), 74–82.

McGlynn, E. A, Asch, S. M., Adams, J., Keesey, J., Hicks, J., DeCristofaro, A., & Kerr, E. A. (2003). The quality of health care delivered to adults in the United States. *New England Journal of Medicine, 348*(26), 2635–2645.

Meijers, J. M., Janssen, M. A., Cummings, G. G., Wallin, L., Estabrooks, C. A., & Halfens, R. Y. G. (2006). Assessing the relationships between contextual factors and research utilization in nursing: Systematic literature review. *Journal of Advanced Nursing, 55*(5), 622–635.

Mohide, E. A., & Coker, E. (2005). Toward clinical scholarship: Promoting evidence-based practice in the clinical setting. *Journal of Professional Nursing, 21*(6), 372–379.

Newhouse, R. P., Dearholt, S., Pugh, L. C., & White, K. M. (2007). Organizational change strategies for evidence-based practice. *Journal of Nursing Administration, 37*(12): 552–557.

Pathman, D. E., Konrad, T. R., Freed, G. L., Freeman, V. A., & Koch, G. G. (1996). The awareness-to-adherence model of the steps to clinical guideline compliance. The case of pediatric vaccine recommendations. *Medical Care, 34*(9), 873–889.

Rogers, E. M. (1983). *Diffusion of innovations.* New York: The Free Press.

Tugwell, P., Robinson, V., Grimshaw, J., & Santesso, N. (2006). Systematic reviews and knowledge translation. *Bulletin of the World Health Organization, 84*(8), 643–51.

CHAPTER TWELVE

Legal and Ethical Issues in Translation

Sharon Dudley-Brown
Cynda Hylton Rushton

Whether evidence is translated into clinical practice is contingent on the overarching social, legal, ethical, and political climate (Larkin et al., 2007). Researchers and clinicians alike must address questions of legal risk and fairness in translation of evidence. This chapter will discuss the legal and ethical issues in the translation of evidence into practice.

■ LEGAL ISSUES IN TRANSLATION

Legal considerations in the translation of evidence include Food and Drug Administration (FDA) regulations, patent laws, the tort system, and the current malpractice environment. The FDA has specific regulations for investigational new drugs and devices, which widen the evidence-to-practice gap by potentially delaying the use of newer drugs and devices that may improve outcomes. Along the same line is the potential delay for a patented treatment that may produce better outcomes than what is standard. The tort system, which varies from state to state in the United States, may delay translation as well. The standard of care can be used to show actual practice patterns, or how a standard was violated.

Clinical Practice Guidelines as the Standard of Care

The issue of standard of care and development and use of clinical practice guidelines (CPGs) are at the center of malpractice issues in translation. An adversarial legal milieu promotes clinical inertia and delays translation because early adoption of evidence often seems as a deviation from the prevailing standard of care. However, ignorance of evidence may promote inertia, but many people do not practice according to guidelines because of worries of deviation from them, even if based on patient- and situation-specific issues that should be taken into consideration. Because the prevailing standard of care is based on what care is customary in a given place and time, providers are lulled into complacency that may result in a delay in translation of evidence into practice (Larkin et al., 2007). Practicing clinicians typically respond to threats to malpractice over adherence to CPGs.

CPGs have been developed, disseminated, and used to the advance of evidence-based practice. CPGs have been defined as "systematically developed statements to assist practitioner and patient decisions about appropriate health care for specific clinical circumstances" (Field & Lohr, 1990). However, CPGs are a double-edged sword. Whereas they can guide clinicians in the diagnosis and management of a particular problem, they can be, and are, used by third-party payors, regulatory bodies, and courts in the determination of whether care was appropriate and adequate (Rosoff, 2001).

Expert Witness Testimony: CPGs Versus Customary Practice

The use of expert testimony is frequently used to deal with quality-of-care issues that arise in the courts. The main issues calling for expert testimony are (a) applicable standard of care, (b) causation, and (c) the assessment of damages, which often involves (d) medical prognosis (Rosoff, 2001). Whereas the type of issue dictates the nature and scope of the expert witness' testimony, the last three issues (causation, assessment of damages, and prognosis) usually requires the expert witness to apply his or her expertise directly to the question at hand, whereas in the first issue, the standard of care is different. In this situation, the expert witness does not testify to what he or she thinks is the proper way to treat the case but, rather, to what others in the profession commonly could do in such a situation. Thus, the expert witnesses' contribution is his or her knowledge of how professional peers commonly handle similar situations. The issue of whether CPGs are evidence-based and whether they are synonymous with customary practice still remains to be seen.

However, newly developed CPGs may differ substantially from prevailing practice, and, thus, if *customary practice* is the legal standard, CPGs would not be used extensively in the legal system. However, according to Rosoff (2001), whereas CPGs have been used as evidence of customary practice, they have also been used as evidence of a respectable majority, evidence of reasonable prudence, evidence of acceptable practice, and as a legal standard of care. Usually, the existence of a duty to care is straightforward. Most actions of medical negligence hinge on questions of standard of care or in determination of causation. CPGs, thus, may affect both of these elements of negligence. However, standards of care can vary greatly geographically, and a CPG can be either a minimum or maximum standard of care. Both negligence and causation are issues in U.S., Canadian, and U.K. laws (Hurwitz, 1994; McDonagh and Hurwitz, 2003; Rosoff, 2001).

The Debate: CPGs as a Sword or a Shield for the Practitioner

As Rosoff (2001) states, CPGs can be used as a sword or a shield. Used as a sword, a CPG can be used by a patient-plaintiff, using a CPG to place blame by establishing that there was a guideline that the defendant should have used or followed but did not. In contrast, a defendant (the provider) can use it as a shield by showing that he or she acted in conformity with an established guideline. Rosoff (2001) goes on to state that CPGs are more commonly used by plaintiffs. Certain states (Minnesota, Maine) have adopted laws that provide only for defensive use of a CPG, and the American Medical Association (AMA) has declared that there is insufficient evidence to show that CPGs can be developed specifically enough to be used as a defense in medical liability litigation (American Medical Association, 1993). Thus, the AMA opposes direct adoption of CPGs as a legal standard and urges that they should be used as evidence of *standards of practice* and that their degree of authority depends on their degree of acceptance among peers.

Whether CPGs are accepted as standards of evidence among peers is debated. According to Tanenbaum (1994) who has conducted research on how physicians reason about their clinical care, learn from their experiences, and pass information along to colleagues, she believes that physicians have two different ways of processing information: deterministic reasoning, which searches out mechanisms of illness based on the sciences and probabilistic reasoning draws of past experiences. She concludes that a clinician's decisions are not likely to be influenced by outcomes research and, thus, skepticism about the information that forms the basis of evidence-based medicine. "The probabilistic plays the odds, while the determinists imagine the process" (Tanenbaum, 1994, p. 30–31).

The Debate: CPGs and the Provider's Autonomy

Another pressing issue in the use of CPGs is the potential for it being in conflict with provider judgment and autonomy, either individual or collective autonomy of professional groups. In addition to erosion of autonomy, there is a greater risk of liability and how relevant are CPGs to an individual's practice.

The law has two functions: litigation, the settlement of disputes, which is retrospective in orientation; and regulation, which is prospective and more forward-looking. The law's regulatory function is more compatible with the notion of evidence-based practice, which is more probabilistic. Regulation, which deals with what might happen, a probabilistic notion, rather than trying to determine what actually did happen in a spat incident, is the focus of litigation (Rosoff, 2001).

In terms of legal issues, most center around the individual provider, and much of that has focused on CPGs. However, on an institutional and organizational basis, legal issues in translation center around policies and procedures. Issues such as the evidence used to develop policies and procedures, when the policies and procedures are updated, and who should follow them, are all pertinent.

■ ETHICAL ISSUES IN TRANSLATION

> Ethical and educated providers must look to their patients' interests and their own conscience, not legal dicta or malpractice fears, as the ideal moral compass for getting the right knowledge into practice for the right patient, at the right place, for the right price, and at the right time. (Larkin et al., 2007)

Translation of scientific evidence into clinical practice involves the balancing of important ethical values and principles to provide ethically sound clinical care. Embedded in translation are questions regarding autonomy (of both the patient/family and clinicians), how to balance the benefits and potential burdens of the innovation or new practice, and how to fairly allocate the innovation to those who can benefit from it while taking into account issues of access, cost, and social and economic consequences.

An Ethical Framework for Translation of Evidence Into Practice

The ethical principles of respect for persons (including autonomy, veracity, and fidelity), beneficence (doing good or providing benefit), nonmaleficence (avoiding or minimizing harms or burdens), justice, and integrity undergird the process of translating scientific evidence into clinical practice. These ethical principles are closely aligned with the ethical principles that inform the conduct of research (Beauchamp & Childress, 2009).

Respect for Persons

According to Rushton (2007), respect for persons is a broad ethical principle that encompasses autonomy (self-determination), veracity (truth telling), fidelity (keeping promises), and privacy (maintaining confidentiality). Each of these aspects is relevant to translation of evidence into practice.

Autonomy

The ethical principle of autonomy refers to a person's self-determination and freedom of choice. It requires that priority be given to honoring the choices made by patients or their designated surrogates when they (a) possess decision-making capacity, (b) have been fully informed and understand the consequences of their decisions, and (c) are able to make choices freely and without coercion. The legal and ethical standard for informed consent is an extension of the principle of respect for persons. Informed consent is also the legal standard by which permission is sought for medical treatment of an individual. Informed decisions are made with full knowledge of that which needs to be done and why. Similarly, they reflect the values and goals of the person who is making the decision. This interplay of values and choices is necessarily informed by the relevant data, experience, and recommendations of the clinician. The values of the scientific and medical community regarding scientific evidence or treatment options may not necessarily reflect the values of the patients and families served through medical and nursing care, thereby, causing conflicts or misunderstandings.

Patient autonomy may be extended to gathering independent research or data about treatment options and asking their clinicians to prescribe them. Patients and families may pursue other avenues such as complementary therapists, community resources, neighbors, or friends, to learn about and decide about their treatment options. Increasingly, patients are looking to the Internet for the latest information, often without guidance about the reliability, validity, or interpretation of the information in their particular circumstance. Discerning the nuances of the information and evaluating the data is enhanced by collaboration with clinicians or other knowledgeable persons. Likewise, understanding the decision-making preferences of patients and families and the boundaries of their requests of clinicians for specific therapies should be made transparent.

Autonomy is also relevant to clinician decision making. Clinicians, as autonomous agents, are also free to choose the therapies they offer to patients or their surrogates and to determine their own framework and process for balancing benefits and burdens of certain therapies or innovations. Their autonomy is, however, necessarily constrained in certain ways (described in the legal section) and influences the process of decision making and communication with patients, families, and other clinicians. The autonomy of the clinician is also relevant when considering patient requests for certain therapies that clinicians either do not believe will be beneficial, may cause harm, or are otherwise inappropriate. Clinicians have an obligation to preserve their own integrity within the context of their relationships with patients and families. In some cases, clinicians are justified in refusing to prescribe treatments that undermine their professional integrity.

Veracity

The ethical obligation to be honest and truthful applies to the translation of evidence into practice. Clinician recommendations regarding the use of a new or innovative therapy is predicated on the reliability, honesty, and integrity of the data on which it is based. Often, there is uncertainty about the effectiveness, safety, or applicability of a specific intervention. In such cases, disclosure of what is known and unknown, along with mechanisms for ongoing monitoring of effect and responding to adverse events, is necessary. Safeguards to assure that data or other information has been adequately and accurately assessed are needed to create confidence by all parties. Similarly, clinicians need to be honest about the boundaries of their willingness to consider or recommend treatments without sufficient scientific evidence to support their adoption. Clinicians also have an obligation to disclose any real or perceived conflicts of interest that may be related to their recommendations for therapies or innovations (Sugarman & McKenna, 2003).

Fidelity

Promise keeping or fidelity is central to the principle of respect for persons. Keeping promises is foundational to building trust between clinicians, patients, and their surrogates (Rushton, Reina, & Reina, 2007). Discerning how patients or their surrogates prefer to participate in health care decision making and treatment, their values regarding quality of life, tolerance for ambiguity and uncertainty, and expectations regarding their relationships with clinicians and the treatments they undertake is foundational to the principle of fidelity. Each of these dimensions is relevant to translational practice.

Clinicians must similarly be transparent and clear about the boundaries of their roles, decision-making process, and conflict resolution. Making explicit what promises they are making to patients and what expectations they have for their relationships help to support understanding and collaboration. When translating evidence into practice, it is essential that promises about how the clinician and the patient will consider various therapies and resolve any differences of opinion can help to avoid conflicts. Frequently, implicit promises do not become explicit until there is a perceived breach of them. Discovering unexpressed expectations by proactively inquiring about them can be essential in avoiding or mediating conflicts.

Balancing Benefit and Burden: Beneficence and Nonmaleficence

Based on the principles of beneficence and nonmaleficence, health care professionals seek to promote the well-being of their patients and to reduce or alleviate harm (Beauchamp & Childress, 2009). When promoting goods such as health, relief from pain and suffering, and the prevention of illness, clinicians may seek answers to questions such as: How to determine what is "good" in a specific situation? Can circumstances or certain types of evidence alter what is considered "good"? What is the threshold of benefit that is needed to justify adoption of new practices? How much harm, known or unknown, is justified when innovating or adopting new practices?

Choices among treatments should benefit the person, and clearly outweigh the associated burdens and harms. Weighing of benefits and burdens occurs within a framework of patient/family goals and preferences, treatment goals, possible outcomes, and the probability and degree of certainty about the benefits and burdens. Decision making is more complicated when the prospect of successful outcome is less certain, the outcome of the treatment is expected to be of marginal usefulness, or the degree of burden is high. Clinicians relying on empirical or clinical data or experience to inform their clinical recommendations or guide patient or surrogate decision making must be as precise as possible in discerning the benefits and burdens of each therapy or innovation. The increasing complexity and ambiguity of the spectrum of interventions used in clinical practice necessarily makes this process fraught with imprecision and uncertainty.

Justice

Justice pertains to fairness and equity in the treatment of others. It refers to an individual's access to an adequate level of health care and to the distribution of available health care resources, such as new or innovative therapies. Justice demands that individual patients are treated fairly, and decisions are not made based on subjective criteria such as race, age, sex, diagnosis, religious beliefs, or socioeconomic status (American Nurses Association, 2001). Questions of justice arise when the reasons for denying care is based on inherently discriminatory criteria such as ability to pay, social status, race, or age. Similarly, clinicians should be aware of the implications of research designs that exclude contextual, social, economic, cultural, or comorbid clinical issues on widespread adoption or translation to certain populations, particularly those underrepresented in research and those with limited access to health care services and treatments.

Ideally, ethical translation should ensure that innovations benefit all patients equitably, according to need or likelihood of benefit. Health care resources are always limited. Questions of resource allocation and the proper limits of treatment often arise when the use and consumption of resources is high. An appeal to fairness compels health care professionals to create equitable systems for the distribution of scarce health care resources. Insurance criteria, for example, may create unjustified barriers to providing necessary services based on inflexible interpretation of clinical or practice guidelines, or vulnerable populations may not have equal access to diagnostic or treatment regimens. Systems to prioritize access to those therapies and innovations with the highest level of evidence of benefit should be developed to maximize access to the largest number of people (Larkin et al., 2007). Although equal access by all is a laudable goal, it is currently not available in the United States. Hence, clinicians must be aware of these inequities and seek to neutralize them to the extent possible.

Health care professionals have dual obligations for allocating resources at the individual and societal levels. Clinicians struggle with how to balance the needs of our individual patients with the needs of the population. Considerations such as patient preferences, cost, time, and personnel become relevant as these issues are considered. Clearly, not all innovations will be sufficiently beneficial or cost-effective regardless of patient or clinician adoption. Likewise, questions regarding patient adherence to the prescribed medical regimen impact clinician willingness to recommend or initiate therapies with high levels of effectiveness but significant morbidity if not implemented properly raise questions of justice (Geppert & Arora, 2005).

Decisions for individuals must be balanced with cost-effectiveness and broader social and economic consequences. Currently, there is no systematic process in the United States to engage all the relevant stakeholders in a process for deciding how these conflicts will be resolved. Larkin et al. (2007) suggested a process of stakeholder engagement for translating science into practice. The taxonomy for engagement (The 8 P's) includes patients, public (community), press, physicians/providers, policymakers, private sector, payers, and public health representatives. Each of these stakeholders would work together to come to consensus about the criteria for access and distribution of translational science within communities. Such an approach is consistent with models for participatory community research.

Integrity

Attention to preserving integrity of patients, families, and clinicians reflects concerns about the impact of decisions on the character of the involved parties. Integrity, a state of wholeness, is necessary for each participant to remain faithful to their values (personal and professional) and to act in ways that are congruent with them. Questions of integrity arise when either person perceives that important values are in conflict or may be undermined through their actions. Patient/family values may be compromised, for example, when clinicians are unaware of the meaning or significance placed on values such as quality of life or suffering and do not recommend therapies that may have significance to their patients. In contrast, clinician integrity may be compromised when the interpretation of scientific evidence is contrary to their professional experience, and they feel pressured to recommend or prescribe certain therapies by patients, their families, other clinicians, or professional groups. Compromises of integrity may result in moral distress (Hamric & Blackhall, 2007).

■ TRANSLATIONAL ETHICS: QUESTIONS FOR DISCERNMENT

Clinicians involved in the translation of science into practice can benefit from having systematic process of ethical discernment and decision making. The following includes questions that may assist clinicians in this process.

- Is the level of evidence sufficient to justify recommending it to my patients?

- Are my patients enough like those in the study so that results are relevant and interpretable?

- Is the treatment feasible in my setting?

- Can I meet the standard of care if my options for screening and treatment are constrained by cost and access to treatment?

- What are the potential benefits and harms from the treatment for my patients?

- What are my patients' values and expectations about the treatment and the outcomes?

- Is recommending this innovation morally permissible?

- Does pursing this innovation violate other highly valued moral principles such as avoiding harm or self-determination?

- Are there competing personal or professional values that might affect my willingness to recommend or deliver this innovation?

- What kinds of objections might be raised about the proposed decision? How can you explain your decision in a way that addresses those objections?

■ APPLICATION OF ETHICAL FRAMEWORK INTO PRACTICE

The ethical issues of translation of evidence into practice are particularly poignant when applied to vulnerable populations:

> Mr. Smith, a 52-year-old African American, presents to the medical clinic as a walk-in patient stating, "I'm out of my medications." Mr. Smith has a past medical history of hypertension, hyperlipidemia, hepatitis C, chronic lower back pain, tobacco dependence, opiate dependence, which is currently in remission, and bipolar disorder.
>
> Mr. Smith missed his last two appointments and has not seen either his medical or psychiatric provider in the past 3 months nor has he received the result of his last blood test, which shows poorly controlled lipids, an elevated blood sugar, and rising liver function tests. Today, he is feeling on edge and has difficulty sitting in the crowded waiting room, which he attributes to his bipolar disorder.
>
> Today, Mr. Smith is seeing a new health care provider, as he does not have an appointment; this is his third provider this year. His blood pressure is 160/100. In reviewing the chart, the health care provider notes that the patient's [hepatitis C virus] HCV was never confirmed with a viral load (only a positive anti-HCV, which demonstrates exposure to the virus). Mr. Smith does have state-funded insurance and pharmacy assistance; he lives in a nearby men's shelter and is attending meetings regularly to sustain his abstinence. (Becker, 2010)

The ethical issues related to translation of evidence into practice in this case include respect for persons, balancing benefits and burdens, and justice.

Hepatitis C virus (HCV) is disproportionately represented in disadvantaged groups that raises questions of justice. In the United States, these include prisoners, people with mental health and substance abuse disorders, ethnic minorities, and the poor. The prevalence of HCV is highest among substance abusers and those with psychiatric conditions (Geppert & Arora, 2005). Evidence indicates that combination therapies are superior to single therapy and adherence to the treatment regimen effects outcomes (World Health Organization, 2003). Treatment is available, but costly at $10,000 to $24,168 (Geppert & Arora, 2005). Even when the disadvantaged patient does receive health insurance (usually through state or federal assistance), treatment may be withheld because of inability to meet stringent eligibility criteria in spite of multiple studies that demonstrate that treatment is effective in methadone users, IV drug users, and patients with major mental health issues that are comanaged by psychiatry.

Autonomy, a derivative of respect for persons, is threatened in this case because the diagnosis of HCV is not confirmed, and Mr. Smith has not been informed of the implications of his diagnostic data or the options for treatment. Access to confirmatory tests, effective treatments, and using current evidence to guide treatment decisions are needed to maximize benefits and reduce burdens.

Respect for persons requires that treatment decisions are made based on diagnosis, eligibility for therapy, patient preferences, feasibility, and willingness to implement the prescribed treatment. Prior to the implementation of a HCV algorithm, clinicians must determine the patient's diagnosis and eligibility for specific treatments. Clinicians involving persons such as

Mr. Smith may struggle with whether to offer an effective treatment that benefits or outweighs the risks or burdens, but the patient cannot pay for or because of concerns of nonadherence or other nonmedical factors such as race, gender, or diagnosis. Geppert and Arora (2005) argue that respect for persons and justice demands that "patients who are underprivileged and/or have stigmatizing conditions deserve access to effective HCV treatment." To categorically exclude them from receiving the therapy based on nonmedical criteria despite scientific evidence violates professional ethical norms (ANA, 2001), causes physical and psychosocial harms, and increases stigma and discrimination. Hence, based on fairness and equality, effective HCV treatment should be offered to all patients when benefits outweigh risks.

Justice also informs the analysis to determine whether risk factors such as substance abuse and psychiatric conditions negatively impact clinical outcomes in persons with HCV. These data are essential in weighing the benefits and burdens of the treatment and affect clinician recommendations. Without research designs that include similar subjects, the data is inconsistent and difficult to interpret and could lead to discriminatory decision making and violations of justice (Geppert & Arora, 2005).

■ CONCLUSION

Ethical and legal questions are inherent in translational science. Clinicians must consider the ethical and legal implications of their decisions and those of their patients and families. A systematic ethical framework can help to illuminate the aspects of clinical decision making and decisions regarding justified translation of evidence into clinical practice and the consequences—positive and negative of doing so.

■ REFERENCES

American Medical Association. (1993). Statement to Committee on Health, Committee on Ways and Means, 103d Cong., 1st sess., Ser. No. 103–23.

American Nurses Association (2001). *Code of ethics for nurses with interpretive statements.* Washington, DC: Author.

Beauchamp, T. L., & Childress, J. F., (Eds.). (2009). *Principles of biomedical ethics* (6th ed.). New York, NY: Oxford University Press.

Becker, K. (2010). Best care practices for homeless hepatitis C patients: Implementation of evidence-based adaptive clinical algorithm of care. Chatham University.

Field, M. J., & Lohr, K. N. (Eds.). (1990). *Clinical practice guidelines: Directions for a new program.* Washington, DC: National Academy Press.

Geppert, C. M., & Arora, S. (2005). Ethical issues in the treatment of hepatitis C. *Clinical Gastroenterology and Hepatology, 3*(10), 937–944.

Hamric, A. B., & Blackhall, L. J. (2007). Nurse-physician perspectives on the care of dying patients in intensive care units: Collaboration, moral distress, and ethical climate. *Critical Care Medicine, 35,* 422–429.

Hurwitz, B. (1994). Clinical guidelines: Proliferation and medicolegal significance. *Quality in Health Care, 3*(1), 37–44.

Larkin, G. L., Hamann, C. J., Monico, E. P., Degutis, L., Schuur, J., Kantor, W., & Graffeo, C. S. (2007). Knowledge translation at the macro level: Legal and ethical considerations. *Academic Emergency Medicine, 14*(11), 1042–1046.

McDonagh, R. J., & Hurwitz, B. (2003). Lying in the bed we've made: Reflection on some unintended consequences of clinical practice guidelines in the courts. *Journal of Obstetrics Gynaecology Canada, 25*(2), 139–143.

Rosoff, A. J. (2001). Evidence-based medicine and the law: The courts confront clinical practice guidelines. *Journal of Health Politics, Policy, and Law, 26*(2), 327–368.

Rushton, C. H. (2007). Respect in critical care: A foundational ethical principle. *AACN Advanced Critical Care, 18*(2), 149–156.

Rushton, C. H., Reina, M. L., & Reina, D. S. (2007). Building trustworthy relationships with critically ill patients and families. *AACN Advanced Critical Care, 18*(1), 19–30.

Sugarman, J., & McKenna, W. G. (2003). Ethical hurdles for translational research. *Radiation Research, 160*(1), 1–4.

Tanenbaum, S. (1994). Knowing and acting in medical practice: The epistmological politics of outcomes research. *Journal of Health Politics, Policy and Law, 19*, 27–44.

World Health Organization (2003). Hepatitis C. Retrieved from http://www.who.int/csr/disease/ hepatitis/whocdscsrlyo2003/en/index1.html

CHAPTER THIRTEEN

The Project Plan and the Work of Translation

Mary Terhaar

■ INTRODUCTION

When considering complex projects, building a house or landing a man on the moon may come to mind (Kennedy, 1962). These are high-stakes efforts that require precious resources and sustained commitment. Both invite scrutiny and both promise important gains for stakeholders if successful, and significant disappointment if not. Approaching any complex project will benefit from attention to detail, clear communication, effective cooperation between many individuals with highly specialized and frequently discrete knowledge and expertise, proper sequencing of work, precise timing of activities, and a detailed resource plan. Complex projects require quality controls to minimize or to mitigate untoward outcomes and thoughtful contingency planning to ensure achievement of critical activities and outcomes. Most importantly, complex projects require a clear statement of the purpose, aims, and the outcomes toward which all effort is directed. This is called the *project plan*.

Translation work aims to accomplish effective practice innovation in ways that significantly improve outcomes (Institute of Medicine [IOM], 2001, 2003; Mohide & Coker, 2005; Titler, 2002; Titler et al., 2003). Nurses engaged in the work of translation seek to reduce the cycle time from knowledge generation to its application in practice and achievement of the improved outcomes promised in original research findings (Foxcroft & Cole, 2008; Titler et al., 2003). Nurses engaged in this work can experience difficulty securing organizational support, achieving intervention fidelity, documenting outcomes, maintaining momentum for change, shifting organizational culture, and finding effective clinical leadership (Bradley et al., 2004). Project management and planning techniques can help mitigate each of these threats to the success of the project. Project management techniques can help to identify potential obstacles and orchestrate strategies to navigate around or over such challenges with minimal disruption to the plan or disturbance to important stakeholders.

Researchers use scientific process to ensure rigor and control across efforts to develop new knowledge. This process is incorporated in education from middle school onward. It is familiar, effective, and clearly articulated. PhD students, in traditional research-focused doctoral programs, follow a well-established and consistent approach designed to promote optimal compliance with scientific process. They prepare a proposal, defend it, and execute dissertation work using a time-tested approach that ensures fidelity with the scientific process and a consistent level of scholarship. The result is the development of new knowledge following a rigorous, well-vetted process. Universities are familiar with both the processes and the products of this approach because the faculty were themselves educated using that same approach. The product, that is called a disssertion, is traditionally presented in five chapters: the problem, the background, the methods, the findings, and the conclusions.

Project management is a process employed by many disciplines and enterprises engaged in high-stakes, complex work. The process is less well-known outside industry. Its purposes are to increase the probability of achieving target outcomes, fidelity to a plan, on-time completion of work, and overall success within budget (Project Management Institute [PMI], 2004a). Not intended for knowledge development, project management is a highly effective approach to knowledge translation and practice innovation, when combined with strategies for evidence based practice. Gawande (2010) proposed that health care today needs new leadership that looks more like a pit crew than a cowboy: leadership provided by engaged teams rather than by single physician leaders. Because of this need for new leadership, new patterns of behavior and new tools are required. Project management offers tools and strategies that can help these newly created pit crews with the work of translation and innovation. DNPs will be prepared to lead and facilitate these crews and these innovative translation projects. More importantly, the work products of their scholarship can be strengthened by following the framework of project management.

The purpose of this chapter is to introduce the phases of project management and present a set of tools and processes that can be used by teams and team leaders to enhance both the strength of success and the probability of its attainment by teams engaged in the work of translation. Project management has demonstrated value for teams charged with completing complex work. It is a strategy with great potential to facilitate translation science.

■ PROJECT MANAGEMENT

The PMI (2004a) defines a project as "a temporary endeavor undertaken to create a unique product, service, or result" (p. 5). Several thoughts here are worth emphasis with respect to translation. Projects are temporary. Projects are special activities, not the day to day work in which one routinely engages, which are referred to as operations. Projects, by contrast, have a particular focus and time frame related to one's primary work. Projects have a beginning and an end and generate a specific, valued outcome. They can help any enterprise to innovate and to adapt to changing market requirements and conditions. They can be used to help migrate knowledge into effective operations (Shenhar & Dvir, 2007).

Nurses and their colleagues from other health care disciplines are commonly required to engage in project activities because projects are well suited to accomplishing diverse strategic goals. Within any enterprise, many priorities compete for time and energy. Translation of specific evidence into practice is one strategy that cuts across many compelling priorities. Nurses and other health care professionals recognize that the common delay between knowledge generation and its effective application in practice is far too long: 7–11 years in fact (Foxcroft & Cole, 2008; Funk, Tornquist, & Champagne, 1995). As a result, nursing has invested significant intellectual capital in the evidence-based practice (EBP) process as a

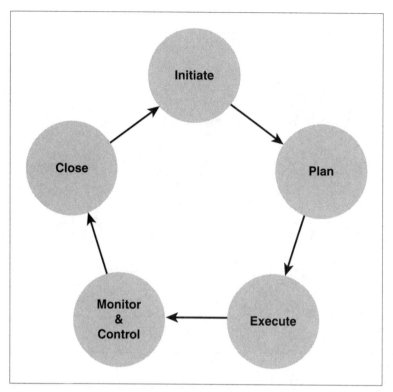

FIGURE 13.1   Phases of project management.

means to abbreviate that delay. Overlaying EBP processes with project management practices can help to secure the gains of EBP at an accelerated pace in ways that promote adaptability and sustainability within a particular context.

Translation projects, like other complex projects, progress through five phases: initiating, planning, executing, monitoring and controlling, and, finally, closing. Each focuses on a set of activities and benefits from use of a particular set of tools. Managing these phases and applying the respective tools can be of tremendous help to clinicians in translating evidence into practice (PMI, 2004a). Figure 13.1 presents the project management as a base for translation.

Phase 1: Initiating the Translation Project

The first phase of any project is initiation. During this phase, an idea is vetted to determine a fit between the outcome to be achieved and the mission, vision, values, and resources of the organization and work unit. During this phase, a few vital ideas are selected from the many good ideas generated by the team. The DNP student and the DNP can provide significant leadership during this phase.

The chief nursing officer (CNO) in any health care organization, serving any population in need, has a large set of initiatives in the "in box," all are seeking support. Many promise to improve care, reduce risk, control cost, or conserve precious human capital. From that universe of possibilities, the executive selects the critical few projects judged to have the highest probability of success and greatest congruence with the mission.

TABLE 13.1   **Cover Page and Approval Page**

Project Title

Project Leader

Advisor

Team Members

Site

Purpose

Background

Project Aims

Brief Summary of Project

Team Leader's Signature:

Approval Signature:

To position a project for favorable preliminary review, it is necessary to present a high-level summary that states the purpose of the project, the specific aims of the work, and the measurable outcomes to be achieved (clinical, operational, financial, or quality). A tool used for this purpose at the Johns Hopkins University School of Nursing is presented in Table 13.1.

In the case of translation projects within an EBP approach, the initiation phase also involves a rigorous evaluation of evidence that leads to a description of the best practices that address the specific clinical challenge at hand. The patient/problem, intervention, comparison, outcome (PICO) form, which was presented in the introduction to this text, is developed and guides the early work of gathering the evidence relevant to the identified problem. Next, the literature is reviewed and analyzed. Evidence is then aggregated and appraised. This evidence comprises the knowledge to be translated in response to a specific, well-defined clinical challenge in the context of the particular practice setting. It forms the foundation for the translation project. A template used at the Johns Hopkins University School of Nursing to outline the purpose and aims of a translation project is presented in Table 13.2.

Purpose
The purpose statement needs to be clear and compelling. It should capture the intent of the project, the interest of the team and stakeholders, and the support of those in the position to select the vital few projects that will be supported in a given cycle. The purpose should be specific and its scope appropriate to the problem or opportunity at the core of the project.

TABLE 13.2 **Summary of the Evidence**

#	1st Author	Year	Level of Research (or Nonresearch) Evidence	Sample Composition and Size	Results/ Recommen- dations	Limitations	RATING Strength / Quality

Aims

Critical outcomes to be accomplished during the translation project are determined and stated as project aims. These aims will guide all project work. They are to be clearly stated, outcome focused, and precise. Do not use compound statements because they make measurement difficult and determination of success elusive. Aims need to be sufficiently specific and inclusive to accomplish the project purpose and form the base for the evaluation plan.

Background

The background provides a high level summary of the evidence that supports the proposed innovation. It creates interest and establishes the project as a priority. This is best accomplished by citing strong evidence and connecting the project to the strategic intent and goals of the organization.

The Project Plan

Developing a project plan to represent the work is essential so the project can be fully understood and evaluated for potential effect on work units in the organization, key stakeholders, finances, and resources. A detailed summary of the project helps to establish the work of translation as important, well-considered, feasible, resource-conserving, and inclusive. The project plan helps create a reasonable expectation that the project will be successful, will produce important results that contribute to the success of the mission, will be completed on time and within budget, and will have a strong return on investment (PMI, 2004b).

The planning phase for any project is like the portion of the iceberg beneath the surface of the water because it is large and may go unrecognized. Lack of attention to planning is dangerous because it has the potential to end any endeavor: even an important one. Reasonable effort invested in a thoughtful project plan prevents allocation of time and resources to projects with low probability of success and minimal potential for gain.

Charge or Charter

The work of translation may be charged to a practice council, research committee, or other established group; or it may be conducted by a team that forms itself expressly for the purpose of conducting a single translation project. Regardless, the leadership team needs a charge that establishes the authority needed to complete the work. The charge needs to clearly identify the reason behind assembling the team, the problem to be solved, the time frame for the work, the members of the team, and the individual(s) named as the leader(s). The charge may be to improve quality, improve process, reduce rework, reduce cycle-time, decrease waste, or increase satisfaction. The clearer and more specific the charge, the greater the probability it will be attained. In translation projects, targets for time, resources, and outcomes are commonly included in the charge.

Leadership

An individual or a group of individuals may be assigned responsibility for the project. These team leaders are responsible to achieve the stated purpose as presented in the charge or charter. A coach can be provided to facilitate the work of leaders and team members. Because they are likely to be engaged in patient care at the same time they are asked to fill a leadership role, both may struggle to find the time required to manage a translation project of significant scope. Leaders may be consulted with respect to team formation or charged with actual assembly of the project team. Chapter 5 of this book summarizes evidence for effective leadership.

Team

The team of individuals who will play key roles in the project are selected and charged as the project team. This group will need to be comprised of individuals who together possess the necessary knowledge, skill, and authority to accomplish legitimate and sustainable change. A team that lacks any of the requisite knowledge, expertise, or skill can be expanded; can subcontract pieces of the work; or can be provided with education, coaching, or consultation to compensate for a deficit. The stronger and more inclusive the team, the higher the likelihood of success.

Support for the Team

Faculty members from schools of nursing, medicine, engineering, pharmacy, public health, or business may be able to provide support for projects and may prove to be good coaches for teams. They may be able to help with measurement plans, data analysis, and interpretation of findings. Faculty may also be able to help obtain Institutional Review Board (IRB) approval or extramural funding (see Exhibit 13.1).

Students from schools of nursing can also be helpful. Students value the opportunity to engage in meaningful work. They bring a strong set of skills that will prove helpful throughout the translation process. They are able to help with reviews of literature and evaluation of evidence. They can review charts, collect and enter data, and help with project management. Later, in the implementation phase, students can collect data, monitor processes, and maintain records and data.

The initiation phase focuses on establishing a good fit between the organization at a given time (including resources, commitments, and strategic intent) and the opportunities and requirements presented by a particular project. It involves two key factors: identifying opportunity or need and establishing readiness and preparation for action. Establishing readiness involves both situational and stakeholder analysis.

Situational Analysis

A situational analysis is a baseline evaluation that describes readiness of the organization for the work to come. This assessment identifies the strengths and weaknesses in the organization with

EXHIBIT 13.1

Translation and the Institutional Review Board, Sharon Dudley-Brown

The end result of translation is to apply evidence to practice, whether for the care of an individual patient, patient population, or system. Because evidence may not be immediately or directly applied to practice, a translation project may be helpful. Translation projects fall on the boundary between quality improvement (QI) and research where confusion remains (Beyea & Nicoll, 1998; Newhouse, 2007). As a result, it is important to make the distinction before beginning a translation project.

QI in health care is defined as a process by which individuals work together to improve systems and processes with the intention to improve outcomes (Committee on Assessing the System for Protecting Human Research Participants, 2002). It has also been defined as a data-driven systematic approach to improving care locally (Baily et al., 2006). "Quality improvement is not intended to generalize knowledge but improve care for a specific population, usually in limited application" (Newhouse et al., 2006, p. 212).

Research is defined by the U.S. Department of Health and Human Services (DHHS) as a systematic investigation (including development, testing, and/or evaluation) designed to develop or contribute to generalizable knowledge (DHHS, 2009). Newhouse et al. (2006) go on to state that research "includes any project that has the purpose of learning something that may apply to populations or administrative units beyond the primary site or setting of the research" (p. 212).

Differences between QI and research focus on the purpose and application. Again, research is conducted to generate new knowledge to be applied generally (DHHS, 2009), whereas QI is conducted to improve care for a specific health care facility/population (Beyea & Nicoll, 1998; Committee on Assessing the System for Protecting Human Research Participants, 2002). Although research generates knowledge to improve outcomes for people and populations, the subject in a research study may or may not benefit. In research, knowledge generation is the primary goal, not the care of the individual subject. In QI, the patient or population is expected to benefit directly from data because the goal is to improve health care delivery (Casarett et al., 2000).

Deciding whether a translation project falls under research or QI is important because Institutional Review Board (IRB) review and approval is required if a project involves human subjects. An IRB, or a human subjects review committee, reviews and approves conduct of human subjects research. Human subjects are defined as living individuals about whom an investigator conducting research obtains (a) data through intervention or interaction with the individual, or (b) identifiable private information (DHHS, 2009).

(Continued)

EXHIBIT 13.1

Translation and the Institutional Review Board *(Continued)*

The federal government requires each institution that receives federal funds to set up an IRB. These IRBs provide fair and impartial reviews of research proposals to protect human subjects from any unnecessary risks associated with participation in research. IRBs operate under a set of guidelines or principles that follow Code 45 of the code of federal regulations (CFR), Part 46 (Protection of Human Subjects). This is available at http://www.hhs.gov/ohrp/humansubjects/guidance/45cfr46.htm

When the jurisdiction of an IRB is determined by both the involvement of human subjects, as well as whether an activity involves research, a question that is sometimes not easy to answer. The DHHS have a frequently asked question page that can help one to sort out whether a project falls under research or QI. That website is http://www.hhs.gov/ohrp/qualityfaq.html. Most would agree that if there is any doubt whether an activity is research or QA, one should notify the IRB for assistance or review.

If the activity falls within the jurisdiction of the IRB, the level of IRB reporting and review must be identified. There are three levels of review, determined on the basis of the degree of risk inherent in the proposed activity, and those are exempt, expedited, and full.

To determine whether the federal regulations apply to a particular quality improvement activity, the following questions should be addressed in order: (a) Does the activity involve *research*? (45 CFR 46.102[d]); (b) Does the research activity involve human subjects? (45 CFR 46.102[f]); (c) Does the human subjects research qualify for an exemption? (45 CFR 46.101[b]); and (d) Is the nonexempt human subjects research conducted or supported by DHHS or otherwise covered by an applicable Federal Wide Assurance (FWA) approved by the Office for Human Research Protections (OHRP; DHHS, 2009)? There are decision charts to assist in this as well, and are available at http://www.hhs.gov/ohrp/humansubjects/guidance/decisioncharts.htm

Some institutions, including the Johns Hopkins Medicine (university and health system), have worksheets to guide the decision making on whether an activity is human subjects research and regulated by the DHHS, and, thus, require an IRB application. These worksheets, although optional, can be submitted for review and assist in determination of research or QI. Johns Hopkins also has a website devoted to Organization Policy on Quality Improvement/Quality Assurance Activity (Policy No. 102.2[a]; Johns Hopkins Medicine [JHM], 2007).

Therefore, as part of developing a plan for translation, the consideration of whether the translation activity is research or quality improvement is an important one.

respect to the project, the opportunities inherent in the work of the project, and any potential threats to project success. It is best conducted in an open dialog with key stakeholders and customers. The assessment frequently identifies strengths, weaknesses, opportunities, and threats (SWOT).

Strengths are key functions the organization does well. Experienced clinical leaders, strong financial position, committed customers, dedicated clinicians, an established program of research, and an engaged executive are examples of organizational strengths. Each of these attributes positions an organization or work unit for success. A unit with stable staff, strong leadership, and a good physical plant is favorably positioned to engage in innovation. These are its strengths.

Weaknesses are particular areas where the organization identifies need or deficiency. High staff turnover, vacancies in critical roles, knowledge or skill deficits, undesirable payer mix, outdated processes, and old technology are examples of organizational or work unit weaknesses. These can compromise any organization's position in the market and ability to innovate. A unit where staff turnover is high, commitment is low, and staff members are inexperienced will need to address these weaknesses in any plan for innovation.

Opportunities are factors that position an organization for success. Some are external, such as a change in the demographic in the community that has potential to increase business. Some are internal, such as a strong department that is ready and eager to take on a challenge. Connecting opportunity to strategic intent supports innovation. Therefore, a pediatric primary care group whose pediatric nurse practitioner (PNP) is earning his or her doctor of nursing practice (DNP) degree has an opportunity to benefit from hosting that PNP's doctoral project because that DNP student will provide the scholarship to drive meaningful performance improvement.

Threats are factors that can prevent the success of a project. Competition, unforeseen demands on staff and resources, and new technology or knowledge can threaten a project. To the extent that external conditions can be evaluated with respect to a project, strategies to reduce their effect can be developed. For example, innovative education for breastfeeding can be threatened when reimbursement is reduced to hold down health care costs and when lactation support is on the list of programs to be cut.

Based on the SWOT analysis, the project team develops strategies to exploit strengths, compensate for weaknesses, exploit opportunities, mitigate threats, and communicate essential information with those affected by the work of the project. A tool that can be used during the situational assessment that identifies strengths, weaknesses, opportunities, and threats is presented in Figure 13.2.

Stakeholders

Stakeholders are those "individuals or organizations actively involved in the project or those whose interests may be affected by the project execution or project outcome" (PMI, 2004b, p. 24). Engaging stakeholders effectively is critical to the success of any project. To do so, it is necessary to establish an understanding of their expectations and requirements so these can be taken into account when planning and executing the project.

A stakeholder assessment is conducted to identify the extent to which individuals in the organization are affected by the work of the project. It can be used to identify the reasons they are interested or affected and the ways they may become engaged in the work. Take the

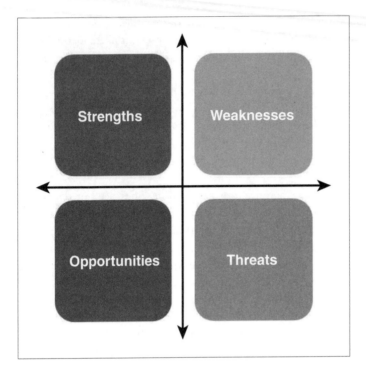

FIGURE 13.2 Situational assessment.

time to map out key individuals, their level of investment, their perspective with respect to the project work and aims, and their importance with respect to the success of the project. Conducting such an assessment can help to surface expectations, identify potential barriers, and discover individuals and conditions that support the project aims. It will also help to plan inclusion strategies, responsibilities, and communication throughout the lifecycle of the project. The template for a stakeholder assessment is presented in Table 13.3 and a template to be used to develop a stakeholder map and identify helpful engagement strategies is presented in Figure 13.3.

TABLE 13.3 **Stakeholder Analysis**

Individual or Team	**Stake or Mandate**	**Potential Involvement**	**Involvement**

Note. C = Critical; M = Marginal.

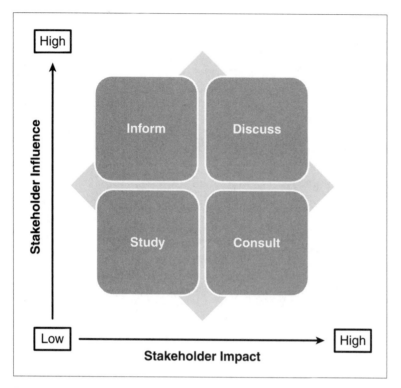

FIGURE 13.3   Stakeholder map.

Approval

In order for Phase 1 (initiation) to be complete, due diligence is required. A project proposal that presents clear and specific aims is developed and formal approval obtained. Such approval may be given directly by the CNO, by the administration, or by a governance body, practice committee, or research committee charged with oversight of translation. Like the original charge or charter, the approval is most effective when it is clear, specific, and detailed.

Phase 2: Project Planning

The purpose of the project plan is to provide deep detail with respect to the activities that will be completed to achieve the purpose and aims of the project. This critical information is communicated in the form of a work breakdown structure that is used as the base for all time management, resource management, communication, coordination, and evaluation work.

Managing the Work

The work breakdown structure (WBS) is a concept map for the project. The document itself looks simple, but creating this representation of all project work takes considerable thought and attention to detail. Begin with the end in mind (Covey, 1989). State that end clearly as the overall purpose of the project. Then, determine what is necessary to accomplish that end and write those as project aims. In addition, drill deeper to describe all actions required to accomplish those project aims and write those as activities. Continue to drill deeper until the

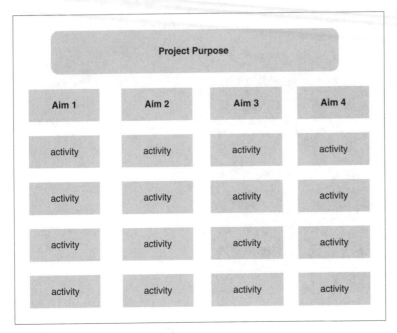

FIGURE 13.4   Work breakdown structure.

plan is clear and complete. That will form the basis for your WBS. Figure 13.4 contains a schematic for the WBS. This template allows a visual representation of the work. For large or complex projects, a list may be more helpful than a visual model. Figure 13.5 contains a segment of WBS used to manage performance improvement activities undertaken by the faculty in the DNP program at the Johns Hopkins University School of Nursing.

Work Breakdown Structure Development Process

Some people find it helpful to create the WBS by writing "to do" items on Post-it notes and then placing them on the wall. This approach requires that team members help to state all the activities required to achieve an aim. Members then brainstorm the ways the aims can be accomplished and post those activities or actions beneath each related aim. Brainstorming continues with a focus on actions and activities required to achieve the aims, and those threads are posted in the subsequent text. This process is repeated until the group has described all activities necessary to achieve the project aims. It is particularly helpful when the team is comprised of members with different knowledge bases and expertise. It helps to bring the specialty knowledge to the surface and create a shared understanding of a process or processes. In the end, content is recorded and shared by members who work on crafting the final draft of the WBS that is free of redundancies, inconsistencies, or omissions. A common vocabulary can be developed along with a sense of identity and affiliation with other team members and the aims to be achieved.

In the end, the WBS is comparable with the methods section of a dissertation or research paper. It should contain sufficient detail to allow any reader to replicate the work and, in so doing, recreate the outcomes. Creating the WBS is a challenge that requires those engaged in its development to describe a process or processes in minute detail. Benner (1984) reports

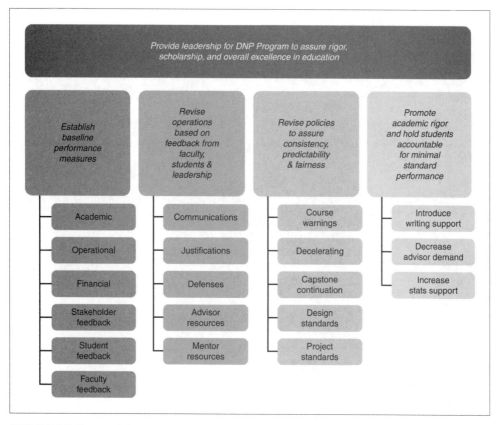

FIGURE 13.5   Work breakdown structure for doctor of nursing practice program performance improvement activities.

that even experts have a difficult time breaking down what they do to basic components. Ask the expert nurse how they recognized that a specific patient was in trouble and that nurse will often share some high-level, integrated thoughts, which could not lead a novice through the same clinical challenge and would not lead to the same resolution of the problem. Creating the WBS is like asking the expert to break down expert thinking into basic steps. It can be tedious work for the expert and, yet, failure to complete this work is certainly planning for project failure. There are many ways to represent the work, but the detail must be included for the project to be successful. The challenge to the team leader is to hold experts captive in discussions about details and dialog that takes time away from direct care.

It may be easier to see the value of the WBS using content less familiar to the clinical expert. Consider changing a tire. How does one go about the work? What resources are needed? How does one avoid the risk? What can be learned from experience? What can be learned from the users' manual? Figure 13.6 presents a WBS for changing a flat tire. As translation work, this is a poor example because the sources are anecdotal or industry-sponsored driver's manuals. On the other hand, as detailed work developed to help the user, it is illustrative. Because the aims drive the work, explicitly including safety in the aim requires the addition of steps that might otherwise not have been recognized as important.

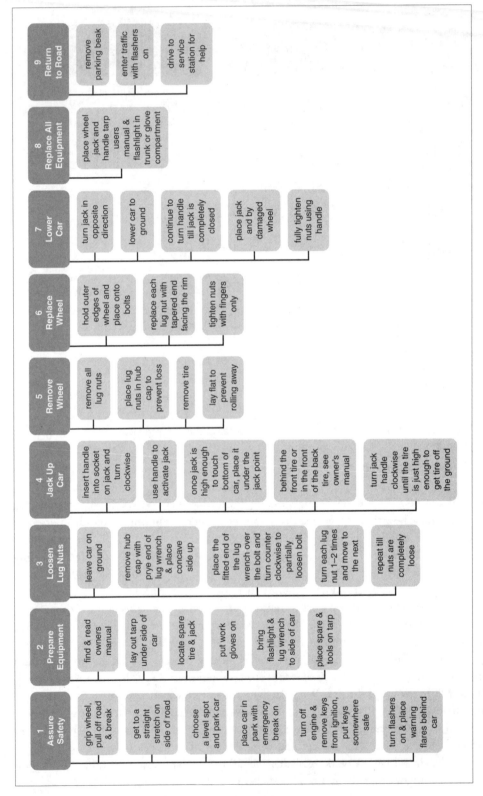

FIGURE 13.6   Work breakdown structure for changing a flat tire.

Project Approval and Support

For the purpose of considering project approval, it is useful to return to the contrast drawn earlier between the PhD and the DNP. The PhD student conducts research called a dissertation. Research generates new knowledge. It is rigorous, follows a prescribed process, and is reviewed for quality, rigor, and scholarship. It is also evaluated for its effect on participants known as human subjects. The DNP student conducts a translation project or quality improvement project. Translation applies findings from quality research endeavors to practice, and the authors use a prescribed process known as *project management* to facilitate disciplined implementation and evaluation of the knowledge application.

Entities engaged in the care of patients have in place IRBs responsible for the oversight of all activities that involve research on human subjects with the purpose of generating new, systematically collected knowledge that can be generalized to populations other than the subjects engaged in the study. Depending on the nature of the translation project, review by the IRB may be indicated or required. Because nurses have a privileged relationship with patients, characterized by a high level of trust and a high degree of dependency, a conversation with the IRB is wise at the beginning of any translation project. In many cases, the translation project plan is presented to the IRB for review just like a research project. This assures that the rights of all participants are protected, data are kept confidential, participants face no unnecessary harm or risk, procedures for recruiting subjects are appropriate, and methods and documents to be used in obtaining consent are clear, complete, and appropriate for the population of concern. Further detail is presented in Exhibit 13.1.

Managing Time

It is common to create at least a mental timeline for a project, but going through the effort to actually create a detailed representation of the activities to be conducted over time forces a more thorough and useful plan. This in turn makes execution more manageable and helps to keep all team members both informed and accountable for progress.

Develop Gantt charts to keep each project on track. Gantt charts are visual representations of a project over time that can be used to schedule, coordinate, and allocate the resources needed to complete a project. Gantt charts show the start, end, and specific target dates called "milestones" specific to each project. These tools can easily be customized to each project. They communicate a great deal of information succinctly and in the context of the overall project work.

To develop a Gantt chart, engage the team in a discussion of the items on the WBS. Stipulate the time required for each activity. Establish the sequence of activities. Identify antecedents when relevant. Identify activities where timing of the execution is flexible and those where it is not.

To build the Gantt chart, create a table. Along the vertical axis on the left hand side, enter one activity from the WBS into each cell (for particularly complex projects you may choose to create a separate Gantt chart for each aim). Then enter increments of time that are appropriate for your project in the top row of cells across the horizontal axis of the chart. Mark the deadline or target date for each activity to be completed. Then as the work progresses, you can track your progress to the targets you have set. A sample Gantt chart is presented in Table 13.4.

TABLE 13.4   **Gantt Chart for Managing Work Over Time**

Aim:

Activity	1	2	3	4	5	6	7	8	9	10

Aim:

Activity	1	2	3	4	5	6	7	8	9	10

Shared Responsibility

The work of translation often requires collaboration among many individuals, from various disciplines and work units. Coordinating the activities and accountabilities of such a team requires fine tuning and clear communication. Responsibility charts (R charts) help in situations like these, when many people are legitimately and necessarily involved in the work. In such a situation, it becomes important that each person understands his or her responsibilities, that those in positions of authority approve work appropriately, and that those who are affected by the work are provided with information they require to perform their own work. Use the stakeholder analysis and the WBS to facilitate a discussion of responsibilities and to generate a responsibility chart like the one presented in Table 13.5.

Planning Evaluation

The aims and the WBS provide the infrastructure for the evaluation plan. Each aim is assigned a metric selected for its sensitivity, specificity, and reliability that will be evaluated to determine whether the aim has been achieved. For example, a *fast track* may be implemented in the emergency department to reduce waiting time. Metrics for this project may include time waiting for intake, time waiting to see the physician, number of people in the waiting room, and patient satisfaction. For the purpose of planning evaluation, the team will identify the measures to be used, determine the source of the data, and plan the statistics to be used to determine the outcome. A template for the evaluation plan is presented in Table 13.6. A full discussion of the evaluation process is presented in Chapter 14. It is important to note that evaluation must be planned in advance along with all the other work of the project. This is necessary to assure that the necessary data are collected throughout the project to evaluate with a high level of confidence the effectiveness of the innovation derived of the evidence.

TABLE 13.5   **Responsibility Chart for Managing the Integrated Work of Diverse Individuals**

Aim:

Activity	Stakeholder 1	Stakeholder 2	Stakeholder 3	Stakeholder 4	Stakeholder 5	Stakeholder 6	Stakeholder 7	Stakeholder 8	Stakeholder 9	Stakeholder 10

Note. A = needs to provide Approval; R = Responsible; r = coresponsible; C = Consultant; I = needs to be Informed.

Strategic Communication

All stakeholders require information about the progress of the project. They need to receive updates on completion of work and attainment of the project aims. Working from the stakeholder analysis and the stakeholder map, and in collaboration with the stakeholders identified as having legitimate need for information, develop a plan for communication. Identify standing meetings and forums where information can be conveniently and regularly shared. Identify vehicles for conveying information that are used by the group and helpful to the stakeholders. Plan to use these forums and vehicles to keep all stakeholders informed. Identify the plan and seek improvement and approval by the parties involved. Then stick to the plan.

TABLE 13.6   **Evaluation Plan**

Measure	Data Source	Benchmark or Norm	Schedule	T1	T2
Aim 1:					

TABLE 13.7   **Quality Management Plan**

Deliverable	Relevant Quality Criteria	Recovery Procedure (If item does not meet standard)	Person(s) Responsible

Quality
- Learn how stakeholders describe and measure quality.
- What quality improvement activities are under way on the unit?
- What are the quality goals for the group?
- Understand baseline measures of quality before the project begins.
- Work to identify the level of quality below which performance must not fall.
- Engage others in monitoring the quality and the outcome of the project.
- Develop plans to stop the project or address problems if there is a negative effect on quality.
- Be certain to understand how a problem is to be reported and addressed should it occur.
- Understand the likelihood that this project might compromise quality even though the goal is to improve it.
- Plan ways to document and communicate quality throughout the life cycle of the project.
- Use graphs, reports, and dashboards, share information, recruit staff when interpreting findings, and be accountable for quality.

A template to develop the quality plan is presented in Table 13.7.

Minimizing Risk

As always, any project that involves human subjects requires that any potential risk to subjects be identified. As caregivers, nurses advocate that patients be fully informed of any risks inherent in a new treatment or approach to care. The IRB will require full disclosure of risk and a plan to manage any identified risk.

In translation projects, the staff also need to be assured that they too are protected against risk. For example, if the translation project seeks to increase caregiver knowledge based on evidence, then baseline knowledge will need to be assessed along with knowledge following the intervention. Caregivers deserve assurance that knowledge deficit at baseline will not bring discipline or retaliation. The goal of quality improvement is not to eliminate staff members who would benefit from education but to raise the level of knowledge across the staff.

To protect both groups, a risk management plan is prepared. Its purpose is to predict any potential risks, to identify the means to identify those who may face risk, and to take appropriate action to mitigate that risk. A template for such a plan is presented in Table 13.8.

TABLE 13.8   **Risk Management Plan**

	Response to Reduce, Avoid, or Manage Risk	**Indicator & Threshold**	**Probability L/M/H**	**Effect L/M/H**	**Status**
Risk 1 *if*					
1.1	*then*				
1.2	*then*				
1.3	*then*				
1.4	*then*				
1.5	*then*				
Risk 2 *if*					
2.1	*then*				
2.2	*then*				
2.3	*then*				
2.4	*then*				
2.5	*then*				

Organizational Learning

Health care, like any enterprise, depends on two primary streams of work. The first is the day-to-day operations necessary to accomplish the mission. This is the work of operations and is the focus of traditional management. The second is the work of innovation and growth. This is the work of teams and projects, the work of organizational learning. Both are critical to

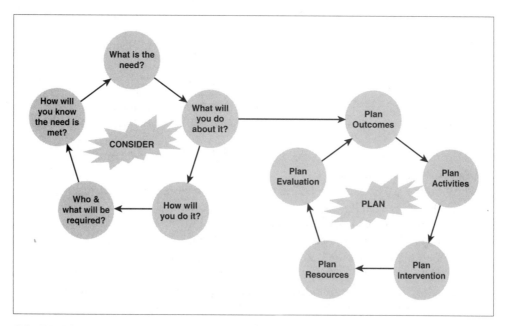

FIGURE 13.7   Processes for translation and organizational learning.

success. Both are the work of leaders (Shenhar & Dvir, 2007). Consequently, leadership must fully exploit all learning and development achieved in the conduct of projects it supports. At every phase of the project, leaders need to ask: "What has been learned?" and "How can that be applied across the organization?" Through engaged and inquisitive leadership, enterprises can achieve their potential as learning organizations whose practices are consistently disciplined by evidence, where the time between knowledge generation and its application is as brief as possible, and business is strong as a result.

A well-managed project is like a story well told. With a good book, the beginning captures the interest of the reader and makes them want to turn the page. The chapters are compelling, in and of themselves, and all connect to the final effect. In the end, the reader judges that a book was worth the time because they know more, feel something new, or are motivated to change.

A good project plan is much like a good book. The proposal generates interest in the project that converts to commitment. The plan itself guides the work. In the end, the project is favorably judged when the aims are achieved.

■ CONCLUSION

The work of translation is well served by thoughtful, inclusive planning that makes good use of project management tools and strategies. Clinicians can begin to plan by asking "What is the need?" and then plan the desired outcomes using the literature. They can ask "What ought to be done?" and then plan the intervention. They can ask "How would the thing best be done?" and then plan the interventions, the controls, and the monitoring required to ensure safety. They can ask "Who and what will be required?" and then plan for those resources. They can ask "How will it be determined that the need is met?" and then plan for a rigorous evaluation.

The result will be that evidence is translated into practice by clinicians who are best able to judge its efficacy, monitor its outcomes, and refine practice across health care.

■ REFERENCES

Baily, M. A., Bottrell, M., Lynn, J., & Jennings, B. (2006). *The ethics of using QI methods to improve health care quality and safety: A Hastings Center special report.* Garrison, NY: The Hastings Center.

Benner, P. (1984). *From novice to expert: Excellence and power in clinical nursing practice.* Menlo Park, CA: Addison-Wesley.

Beyea, S. C., & Nicoll, L. H. (1998). Is it research or quality improvement? *AORN, 68*(1), 117-119.

Bradley, E. H., Webster, T. R., Baker, D., Schlesinger, M., Inouye, S. K., Barth, M. C., . . . Koren, M. J. (2004). Translating research into practice: Speeding the adoption of innovative health care programs. *Issue Brief (Commonwealth Fund),* (724), 1–12. Retrieved from http://www.commonwealthfund.org/usr_doc/Bradley_translating_research_724_ib.pdf

Casarett, D., Karlawish, J. H. T., & Sugarman, J. (2000). Determining when quality improvement initiatives should be considered research: Proposed criteria and potential implications. *Journal of the American Medical Association, 283*(17), 2275-2280.

Committee on Assessing the System for Protecting Human Research Participants, Institute of Medicine (2002). Responsible research: A systems approach to protecting research participants. Federman, D. D., Hanna, K. E., & Rodriguez, L. L. (Eds). Washington: National Academies Press.

Covey, S. R. (1989). *The seven habits of highly effective people.* Salt Lake City, UT: Franklin Covey Company.

Department of Health and Human Services (DHHS). (2009). Office of Human Research Protections (OHRP). Available at: http://www.hhs.gov/ohrp. Downloaded 7/20/11.

Foxcroft, D. R., & Cole, N. (2008). Organisational infrastructures to promote evidence based nursing practice. *The Cochrane Database of Systematic Reviews,* (4), CD002212. doi: 10.1002/14651858.CD002212

Funk, S. G., Tornquist, E. M., & Champagne, M. T. (1995). Barriers and facilitators of research utilization: An integrative review. *Nursing Clinics of North America, 30*(3), 395–407.

Gawande, A. (2010). *Health care needs a new kind of hero.* Interview by Gardiner Morse. *Harvard Business Review, 88*(4), 60–61.

Institute of Medicine. (2001). *Crossing the quality chasm: A new health system for the 21st century.* Washington, DC: National Academies Press.

Institute of Medicine. (2003). *Priority areas for national action: Transforming health care quality.* Washington, DC: National Academies Press.

Johns Hopkins Medicine (JHM). (2007). Organization Policy on Quality Improvement/ Quality Assurance Activity (Policy No. 102.2(a)). Available at: http://www.hopkinsmedicine. org/institutional_review_board/guidelines_policies/organization_policies/102_2a.html. Downloaded 7/20/11.

Kennedy, J. F. (1962). *We choose to go to the moon.* A speech delivered at the Rice University. Houston, TX. Retrieved from http://www.historyplace.com/speeches/jfk-space.htm

Mohide, E. A., & Coker, E. (2005). Toward clinical scholarship: Promoting evidence-based practice in the clinical setting. *Journal of Professional Nursing, 21*(6), 372–379.

Newhouse, R. P. (2007). Diffusing confusion among evidence-based practice, quality improvement and research. *The Journal of Nursing Administration, 37*(10), 432-435.

Newhouse, R. P., Pettit, J. C., Poe, S., & Rocco, L. (2006). The slippery slope: Differentiating between quality improvement and research. *The Journal of Nursing Administration, 36*(4), 211-219.

Project Management Institute. (2004a). *Project management body of knowledge.* Newtown Square, PA: ANSI Publication.

Project Management Institute. (2004b). *A guide to the project management body of knowledge (PM-BOK Guide;* 3rd ed.). Newtown Square, PA: ANSI Publication.

Shenhar, A. J., & Dvir, D. (2007). *Reinventing project management: The diamond approach to successful growth and innovation.* Boston, MA: Harvard Business School Press.

Titler, M. G. (2002). Use of research in practice. In G. LoBiondo-Wood & J. Haber (Eds.), *Nursing research methods: Critical appraisal and utilization* (5th ed., pp. 411–444). St. Louis, MO: Mosby.

Titler, M. G., Herr, K., Ardery, G., Brooks, J., Buckwalter, K. C., Clarke, W. R., . . . Xie, X. J. (2003). TRIP intervention saves healthcare dollars and improves quality of care. In *Translating research into practice: What's working? What's missing? What's next?* Washington, DC: Agency for Healthcare Research and Quality. Sponsored by the Agency for Healthcare Research and Quality.

CHAPTER FOURTEEN

Evaluation of Translation

Sharon Dudley-Brown

Translation is not complete until the impact and extent of innovation use are examined and understood.

—Donaldson, Rutledge, & Ashley, 2004, p. S43

■ INTRODUCTION

Evaluation has been defined as systematic investigation of the merit, worth, or significance of an object (Scriven, 1998; Shadish, Cook, & Leviton, 1991). Evaluation needs to begin when the project begins. Evaluation of a translation project should include evaluation of the outcomes and project goals, as well as the structure and process of the initiative. Evaluation should relate back to the identification and assessment of the barriers, strengths, and limitations of the translation plan. The evaluation should provide information for dialogue and planning related to applicability and sustainability and should highlight future needs. This chapter will describe the critical components of evaluation of translation and will include models to assist in evaluation.

■ SHORTCOMINGS OF EVALUATION OF QUALITY IMPROVEMENT PROGRAMS

Øvretveit and Gustafson (2002) report on the lack of evidence on the effectiveness of quality improvement (QI) programs. They cite five most common shortcomings of research on QI programs (p. 273). These include (a) implementation assessment failure, (b) outcome assessment failure, (c) outcome attribution failure, (d) explanation failure, and (e) measurement variability. They follow with eight suggestions for evaluation, which are helpful when exploring the evidence on evaluation:

1. Assessment or measurement of the level of implementation of the intervention, which includes such questions as "How broad?", "How deep?", and "How long?"
2. Validation of *implementation assessment*, where they suggest obtaining responses from a cross-section of personnel involved to validate the project's implementation
3. Wider outcome assessment, which includes how to attribute the outcomes to the intervention and links to the overall objectives

4. The need for longitudinal studies and prospective evaluation of programs over time
5. More attention to economics and sustainability costs
6. Use of theory-driven evaluation, as described succeedingly by Walshe (2007)
7. Use of common definitions and measures across programs
8. The need for the development of tools to predict and explain program effectiveness

■ THEORY-DRIVEN EVALUATION

Walshe (2007) proposes the need for theory-driven evaluation in QI. He proposes that the theoretical basis for the intervention (why and how it works) is more important than its empirical performance (whether it works). Citing that QI initiatives are complex social interventions, their evaluation must look at understanding the interconnections between context (the situation, setting, or organization), content (the nature or characteristics of the intervention), application (the process through which the intervention is delivered), and outcomes (the results of the intervention).

Theory-driven evaluation, according to Walshe (2007), attempts to map out the program theory behind an intervention, and then designs an evaluation to test the theory. The aim in QI is not to find out "whether it works," but rather, to establish when, how, and why the intervention works, or to "unpick the complex relationship between context, content, application, and outcomes, and to develop a necessary contingent and situational understanding of effectiveness" (p. 58). One should seek theoretical, rather than empirical, generalizability because of situational differences in context, content, application, and outcomes.

■ REVISITING TRANSLATION FRAMEWORKS

Translation should be evaluated against the criteria used to develop the translation framework, as well as the translation plan. For example, using the Promoting Action on Research Implementation in Health Services (PARIHS) framework (Kitson et al., 1996; Kitson, 2002), evaluation, a part of context, relates to how the organization measures its performance, and how (or whether) feedback is provided to people within the organization, as well as the quality of measurement and feedback. In fact, Donaldson, Rutledge, and Ashley (2004) compared four translation frameworks (Havelock, 1986; Lewin, 1951; Rogers, 2003; and the PARIHS framework, Kitson et al., 1996; Kitson, 2002) in measuring evidence uptake by individuals and organizations. Each framework suggests that translation is not complete until the extent and impact of use is examined. In addition, evaluation should use process measures that integrate clinician knowledge, actual performance of the practice, and patient/clinician outcomes. Donaldson et al. argue that the PARIHS framework (Kitson et al., 1996; Kitson, 2002) also includes changes in patterns of care and changes in policies, procedures, or protocols. The impact of change must be validated by the integration of monitoring and evaluation of specific target outcomes of adoption (Donaldson et al., 2004).

As Planas (2008) states, there is a need to look at both the effectiveness and adoptability of evidence-based interventions in practice settings (p. 1854). Exploring the research continuum, from basic research (bench) to clinical investigations with patients (bedside) to health care decision making (practice), between each phase translation must occur (Sung et al., 2003). Type 1 translation involves the transfer of knowledge from lab or bench to clinical trials, whereas Type 2 translation translates evidence-based recommendations into everyday practice and health care decision making and by identifying the gap between recommended and actual care (Sussman, Valente, Rorhrbach, Skara, & Pentz, 2006). Sussman et al. (2006) define *translation* as an extended process of how research knowledge that is directly or indirectly relevant to health behavior eventually serves the public. Planas (2008) suggests using the RE-AIM model to improve Type 2 translation efforts.

The RE-AIM model, a planning and evaluation framework, was originally developed to evaluate the public health or population-based impact of an intervention (Glasgow, Vogt, & Boles, 1999). The components include reach, efficacy, adoption, implementation, and maintenance. Reach, an individual level measure, includes participation rate and representativeness of participants. Efficacy, also at the individual level of measure, includes positive and negative outcomes, as well as biological, behavioral, humanistic, and economic outcomes. In addition, this includes evaluating the processes of care associated with the outcomes. Adoption, measured at the organization level, refers to the representativeness of the setting and the participation rate. Implementation, also at the level of the organization, is the extent to which the intervention is delivered as intended (fidelity of the intervention) and includes both integrity and differentiation. Implementation interacts with efficacy to determine effectiveness. Maintenance, measured at the individual and organization level, is the exploration of the long-term effect of the intervention and extent of continuation (Glasgow et al., 1999; Planas, 2008). In terms of evaluation, Glasgow et al. (1999) suggests that all of the dimensions are incorporated into an evaluation.

Another model for translating research to practice is the PRISM model—the practical, robust, implementation, and sustainability model (Feldstein & Glasgow, 2008). This model evaluates how the program or intervention interacts with recipients to influence program adoption, implementation, maintenance, reach, and effectiveness. Developed from the safety sector in health care, the model contains components of the RE-AIM model, the PARIHS framework, and Rogers' Diffusion of Innovations, as well as the Chronic Care Model. Specifically, the model explores the interaction between the intervention and the recipients; from a patient and organizational perspective; the influence of the external environment; the implementation and sustainability infrastructure; and how these feed into the adoption, implementation, and maintenance of the program. In terms of evaluation, it includes much of the RE-AIM components, and also characteristics of patients and organizations in exploring the intervention and the recipients.

■ EVALUATION OF TRANSLATION

The evaluation of a translation project should begin when the plan for the project is developed (see Chapter 13 on creating a plan for translation). Key components of the evaluation include five major components. First is an evaluation of the overall project goals and specific aims. Simply, it was the overall goal met and why or why not. If there were specific aims, each should be addressed separately.

Second is an evaluation of the outcomes (see Chapter 4 on outcomes). Outcomes should include both patient and provider and system/institution outcomes identified in the planning phase. Outcomes can be clinical indicators, clinician or patient behavior, and can be quantitative or qualitative in nature. As Planas (2008) describes, typical outcomes in health care include the biological (blood pressure), behavioral (adherence), humanistic (quality of life), and economic outcomes. Kleinpell & Fulmer (2001) groups outcomes as to whether they are care-related, patient-related, or performance-related. Another way to classify outcomes is by short-term, intermediate, or long-term outcomes. Any change in outcomes should be matched to the intervention. Essentially, outcomes are compared to baseline data to draw conclusions about the effectiveness of the innovation or intervention (Rich, 2009). An evaluation of outcomes usually involves statistical analysis of the quantitative data collected in the project (see Chapter 4). The most common statistical test used in QI or quality assurance (QA) projects is the *t* test, which measures difference between two groups when data are at interval or ratio level (see Table 14.1). However, an important consideration with *t* tests are whether the data is paired or independent. Paired *t* tests are stronger and, thus, require smaller sample sizes to meet significance. However, paired data must be available to use this test. In a QI project, typically, it is before and after the data that are used. However, to use a paired *t* test, the before-and-after data must be from the same subject. Although this is not always possible, the use of paired data is preferred.

However, many would argue that the data need to be collected in a time series, rather than just before and after, to be sure that any improvement in the outcome is caused by the intervention/project (Carey, 2003). Thus, various authors have proposed expanding the design of QA/QI projects beyond the usual before-and-after design (Shojania & Grimshaw, 2005).

Shojania and Grimshaw (2005) describe the weak designs used in the evaluation of QI projects—not only the use of the simple before-and-after design, but also using it at single sites. They do state that when resources prevent a randomized controlled trial (RCT), institutions should avoid the simple before-and-after design, and suggest instead, the use of a time-series design or a controlled before-and-after design. In a time-series design, or interrupted time-series design, data are collected at multiple periods. This can strengthen the notion that the outcome is attributable to the intervention. A controlled before-and-after design can be used when the use of multiple time points is not feasible and essentially compares outcomes between two institutions or settings—one that implemented the intervention and one that did not.

Third is an evaluation of the structure and process of the initiative. The evaluation should provide validation of the implementation and fidelity to the intervention. Whether outcomes were met or not, identification of structure and process variables involved may be significant. Because many QI initiatives are effective in some settings but not in others, the influence of structure and process is significant. In addition, one must know that any

TABLE 14.1 **Guide to Bivariate Statistical Tests for Two Groups**

Level of Measurement of Dependent Variable	Two-Group Comparison (Independent Variable)	
	Independent groups	*Dependent groups*
Nominal (categorical)	X^2	McNemar test
Ordinal (rank)	Mann–Whitney test	Wilcoxon signed rank test
Interval or ratio (continuous)	Independent group *t* test	Paired *t* test

change in before-and-after (outcome) data (improvement) was because of the fact that the intervention/project is critical, and relates to the stability and predictability of the process (Carey, 2003). Although an intervention can be thought to be effective, it may not be effective in translation because of structural (personnel, organization) or process (exposure, feasibility, timing, clinic flow) issues. Elucidation of these is important for future translation and sustainability of change.

Carey (2003) argues that process measures complement outcome measures and should be used together. Outcomes can be negative even when correct processes occur, and vice versa. He states that process measures are early indicators of outcomes (p. 97) and are selected by moving upstream and asking what might affect a change in a desired outcome, although a clear connection between indicators is necessary.

Hulscher, Laurant, & Grol (2003) explores the purpose and value of process evaluation in QI. They describe three key aspects of process evaluation: (a) to describe the QI intervention itself, (b) to explore the actual exposure to the intervention, and (c) to describe the experience of those who were exposed (the participants). They propose a framework for describing the key features of a QI intervention, in which attention is paid to the features of the target group, the implementers or change agents, the frequency of the intervention activities, and the information imparted. They propose that by using the framework, all three key aspects of process evaluation will be addressed.

Fourth, the evaluation should relate back to the identification and assessment of the barriers, strengths, and limitations of the translation plan. Were the barriers found the ones that were identified a priori? If not, why or why not? In addition, describing any discrepancies from the strengths, weaknesses, opportunities, and threats (SWOT) analysis conducted in the planning phase would be helpful for future translation projects in the organization. Evidence of clinical adoption and sustainability should be included—for example, the changes in patterns of care provided, changes in organization, or changes in policies, procedures and protocols, and evidence of benchmarking.

Fifth, and last, the evaluation should provide information for dialogue and planning related to sustainability and should highlight future needs. Barriers and needs for sustainability need to be identified for continued and ongoing endurance and extension of the intervention. Sustainability requires energy and resources. The RE-AIM planning tool can be used to identify key issues in evaluating the potential sustainability of an innovation (Brach, Lenfestey, Roussel, Amoozegar, & Sorensen, 2008). Planning for ongoing evaluation is important; as with any new evidence, there will need to be a new plan for translation.

■ PROGRAM EVALUATION

In 1999, the Centers for Disease Control and Prevention (CDC) proposed a framework for program evaluation in public health practice (CDC, 1999). The framework for program evaluation involves a series of six steps that should be taken in each evaluation. These steps include the following: Step 1, engage stakeholders; Step 2, describe the program; Step 3, focus the evaluation design; Step 4, gather credible evidence; Step 5, justify conclusions; and Step 6, ensure use and share lessons learned. The second element of the framework is a set of 30 standards for assessing the quality of evaluation activities that are organized to the following four groups: (a) utility, (b) feasibility, (c) ethics, and (d) accuracy. The standard of utility is defined as serving the information needs of the intended users. As for feasibility, the evaluation should be realistic, prudent, diplomatic, and frugal. The standard of ethics suggests that the evaluation be legal, ethical, and with regard for the welfare of those involved and those affected. The last standard, accuracy, is defined as to reveal and convey technically accurate information.

This framework was expanded in the *Introduction to Program Evaluation for Comprehensive Tobacco Control Programs*, which delineates the principles used for research versus program evaluation (MacDonald et al., 2001). For example, comparing the concept of planning between research and program evaluation, research uses the scientific method; specifically, state the hypothesis, collect the data, analyze the data, and draw the conclusions. This is in contrast to that of program evaluation, which uses the aforementioned 6-step framework for program evaluation. Contrasting the concept of standards, they are again distinguished by the use of validity (internal and external) in research, and the use of the aforementioned program evaluation standards for program evaluation. In the concept of questions, research principles include facts (descriptions, associations, and effects), whereas program evaluation includes values (merit, worth, and significance). These can all be useful in the evaluation process.

A more recent publication, building on the aforementioned two topics, provides information on selecting indicators and linking them to outcomes (Starr et al., 2005). They use the definition of an outcome indicator by the United Way of America, which states that an outcome indicator is a specific, observable, and measurable characteristic or change that will represent achievement of the outcome (United Way of America, 1996). In contrast, outcomes are the outputs or direct products of implementation activities. Outcome components are categorized as short term, intermediate, or long term.

In terms of evaluation, Starr et al. (2005) describe steps in program evaluation as the following: Step 1, select the goal; Step 2, select long-term outcomes; Step 3, select short-term and intermediate outcomes; Step 4, select indicators of progress toward outcomes; Step 5, select or design activities to achieve selected outcomes; Step 6, implement selected intervention activities; and Step 7, evaluate progress toward achieving selected outcomes.

However, the authors (Starr et al., 2005) go on to state that measuring outcomes only is insufficient for evaluation, and that what is equally important is process evaluation, which measures program implementation. Recently, the CDC published a guide to process evaluation (CDC, 2008), which delineates the differences between process evaluation from outcome evaluation. Outcome evaluation allows for documentation of outcomes and linkages between an intervention and an effect. Process evaluation focuses on inputs, activities, and outputs, allowing for a description of the project's activities and to link progress to the outcomes. The authors describe process evaluation as "the systematic collection of information on a program's inputs, activities, and outputs as well as the program's context and other key characteristics" (CDC, 2008, p. 4). "Process evaluation involves the collection of information to describe what a program includes and how it functions over time" (CDC, 2008, p. 4). It helps to focus time and resources. Process evaluation can be conducted once during a project or continuously.

The CDC (2008) describes four main purposes of process evaluation: (a) program monitoring, (b) program improvement, (c) development of effective program models, and (d) program accountability. First, in program monitoring, one can track, document, and summarize the inputs, activities, and outputs of programs. In program improvement, one can compare the inputs, activities, and outputs to standards or criteria, or recommended practice. In addition, one can measure the fidelity of the implementation with that of the planned program. In developing effective program models, one can assess how process is linked to outcomes to identify the most effective program components. In program accountability, one can demonstrate the use and allocation of resources.

The materials developed by the CDC on program evaluation, outcome indicators, and process evaluation are all helpful in the evaluation of translation projects. Although not formally described as such, these include both formative and summative types of evaluations. Scriven (1967) described formative evaluation as being done throughout program development and implementation to improve or make changes while the program is proceeding in implementation. Formative evaluations focus on ways of improving the effectiveness of a program, a policy, an organization, a product, or a staff unit. Such evaluations have a formal design, and the data is collected, analyzed, or both, at least in part, by an evaluator. Scriven (1967) defines summative evaluation as assessment of effects and outcomes, which is completed at the end of a program and serves as a decision-making tool about program continuation or change. According to Puddy et al. (2008), the evaluation paradigm of summative and formative assessment has the potential to contribute to current conceptualizations of program evaluation.

■ EVALUATION OF TRANSLATION: A PRACTICAL GUIDE

In reality, and despite proper planning, the evaluation of translation and of the translation project may reveal both process and outcome shortfalls. These are helpful in deciding sustainability of the project and in a continuous loop of planning for the next project implementation. It often seems that the initial preplanned-for barriers to implementation are, in the end, not major barriers, whereas the major hurdles of a project end up to be those that were unanticipated, as so it is with Biondi's law. Biondi's law states that if your project does not work, look for the part that you did not think was important.

To assist in minimizing these issues, one should use a translation framework to assist in guiding any translation project. Beginning with the planning phase of the project, one should consider both evaluation questions as well as evaluation methods that will be used. In terms of questions for evaluation, the following should be considered: (a) How will the project's success be measured? (b) How will success in achieving aims be measured? (c) How will outcomes and indicators (your data) be measured? (d) Are indicators and outcomes able to be achieved with intervention proposed? (e) How will the project improve quality? (f) Can you identify areas that will need improvement? (g) Are timelines being met? (h) How will resources be allocated and evaluated? (i) How will impact be assessed? (j) How will sustainability and dissemination occur?

Time involved in completion of a project (whether it be a research or evidence-based practice project) tends be underestimated. As Drazen's law of restitution states, the time it takes to rectify a situation is inversely proportional to the time it took to do the damage. Thus, when considering translation into practice, and the evaluation process, if the translation plan and project does not meet its goals, more time may be needed to return to a state of equilibrium. To minimize this problem of restitution, ongoing evaluation is important. In addition, time for project completion should be factored into the evaluation process. For example, a project may be deemed to be ineffective in changing outcomes, but perhaps with a change in (lengthening of) time frame, the outcomes could be successfully improved.

Finally, the evaluation process needs to be considered in light of the entire translation process, as a feedback loop. Project planning and implementation typically concludes with evaluation. However, that evaluation should directly feed into another project and implementation of translation. Perhaps the results of one cycle may be that research is needed to test whether an intervention is effective, or perhaps another translation project may be needed in redefining the details for applicability in a specific setting. Thus, evaluation is one piece necessary for the successful implementation of the translation of evidence into practice.

■ CONCLUSION

In conclusion, the evaluation of translation needs to be a part of the planning process and should be consistent with the framework chosen for translation. Evaluation is an important component and can, and should, provide continuous feedback on the translation of evidence.

■ REFERENCES

Brach, C., Lenfestey, N., Roussel, A., Amoozegar, J., & Sorensen, A. (2008). *Will it work here? A decisionmaker's guide to adopting innovations.* Prepared by RTI International under Contract No. 233-02-0090. (AHRQ Publication No. 08-0051). Rockville, MD: Agency for Healthcare Research and Quality.

Carey, R. G. (2003). *Improving health care with control charts: Basic and advanced SPC methods and case studies.* Milwaukee, WI: ASQ Quality Press.

Centers for Disease Control and Prevention (1999). Framework for program evaluation in public health. *Morbidity and Mortality Weekly Report, 48*(RR-11), 1–40.

Centers for Disease Control and Prevention (2008). *Introduction to process evaluation in tobacco use prevention and control.* Atlanta, GA: US Department of Health and Human Services, Author, National Center for Chronic Disease Prevention and Health Promotion, Office on Smoking and Health. Retrieved from http://www.cdc.gov/tobacco/publications/index.htm

Donaldson, N. E., Rutledge, D. N., & Ashley, J. (2004). Outcomes of adoption: Measuring evidence uptake by individuals and organizations. *Worldviews on Evidence-Based Nursing, 1*(Suppl. 1), S41–S51.

Feldstein, A. C., & Glasgow, R. E. (2008). A practical, robust implementation and sustainability model (PRISM) for integrating research findings into practice. *The Joint Commission Journal on Quality and Patient Safety, 34*(4), 228–243.

Glasgow, R. E., Vogt, T. M., & Boles, S. M. (1999). Evaluating the public health impact of health promotion interventions: The RE-AIM framework. *American Journal of Public Health, 89*(9), 1322–1327.

Havelock, R. G. (1986). Linkage: Key to understanding the knowledge system. In G.M. Beal, W. Dissanayake, & S. Konoshima (Eds.), *Knowledge generation, exchange, and utilization* (Ch. 9). Boulder, CO: Westview Press.

Hulscher, M. E., Laurant, M. G., & Grol, R. P. (2003). Process evaluation on quality improvement interventions. *Quality & Safety in Health Care, 12*(1), 40–46.

Kitson, A. (2002). Recognizing relationships: Reflections on evidence-based practice. *Nursing Inquiry, 9*(3), 179-186.

Kitson, A., Ahmed, L. B., Harvey, G., Seers, K., & Thompson, D. R. (1996). From research to practice: One organizational model for promoting research-based practice. *Journal of Advanced Nursing, 23*(3), 430-440.

Kleinpell, R. M., & Fulmer, T. T. (2001). *Outcome assessment in advanced practice nursing.* Springer.

Lewin, K. (1951). *Field theory in social science.* New York: Harper & Row.

MacDonald, G., Starr, G., Schooley, M., Yee, S. L., Klimowski, K., & Turner, K. (2001). *Introduction to program evaluation for comprehensive tobacco control programs.* Atlanta, GA: Centers for Disease Control and Prevention.

Øvretveit, J., & Gustafson, D. (2002). Evaluation of quality improvement programmes. *Quality and Safety in Health Care, 11*(3), 270–275.

Planas, L. G. (2008). Intervention design, implementation, and evaluation. *American Journal of Health-System Pharmacy, 65*(19), 1854–1863.

Puddy, R.W., Boles, R. E., Dreyer, M. L., Maikranz, J., Roberts, M. C., & Vernberg, E. M. (2008). Demonstrating support for the formative and summative assessment paradigm in a school-based intensive mental health program. *Journal of Child & Family Studies, 17*(2), 253–263.

Rich, K.A. (2009). Evaluating outcomes of innovations. In N.A. Schmidt & J.M. Brown (Eds.) *Evidence-based practice for nurses: Appraisal and application of research* (pp. 385–398). Sudbury, MA: Jones and Bartlett.

Rogers, E.M. (2003). *Diffusion of innovations,* (5th ed.) New York: Free Press.

Scriven, M. (1967). The methodology of evaluation. In R. W. Tyler, R. M. Gagne, & M. Scriven (Eds.), *Perspectives of curriculum evaluation* (pp. 39–83). Chicago, IL: Rand McNally.

Scriven, M. (1998). Minimalist theory of evaluation: The least theory that practice requires. *American Journal of Evaluation, 19*(1), 57–70.

Shadish, W. R., Jr., Cook, T. D., & Leviton, L. C. (1991). *Foundations of program evaluation: Theories of practice.* Newbury Park, CA: Sage Publications.

Shojania, K. G., & Grimshaw, J. M. (2005). Evidence-based quality improvement: The state of the science. *Health Affairs, 24*(1), 138–150.

Starr, G., Rogers, T., Schooley, M., Porter, S., Wiesen, E., & Jamison, N. (2005). *Key outcome indicators for evaluating comprehensive tobacco control programs.* Atlanta, GA: Centers for Disease Control and Prevention.

Sung, N. S., Crowley, W. F., Jr., Genel, M., Salber, P., Sandy, L., Sherwood, L.M., . . . Rimoin, D. (2003). Central challenges facing the national clinical research enterprise. *Journal of the American Medical Association, 289*(10), 1278–1287.

Sussman, S., Valente, T. W., Rorhrbach, L. A., Skara, S., & Pentz, M. A. (2006). Translation in the health professions: Converting science into action. *Evaluation & the Health Professions, 29*(1), 7–32.

United Way of America. (1996). *Measuring program outcomes: A practical approach.* Alexandria, VA.

Walshe, K. (2007). Understanding what works—and why—in quality improvement: The need for theory-driven evaluation. *International Journal for Quality in Health Care, 19*(2), 57–59.

CHAPTER FIFTEEN

Dissemination of Translation

Sharon Dudley-Brown

The overall purpose of dissemination is the utilization of knowledge.
—Cronenwett, 1995; Ordonez & Serrat, 2009

■ INTRODUCTION

Dissemination is an important component of translation of evidence, because if the translation is not disseminated, then no change in care will occur, and innovations will not be adopted. Dissemination is the communication of clinical, research, and theoretical findings for the purpose of transitioning new knowledge to the point of care (Brown & Schmidt, 2009). This chapter will describe the methods and issues in dissemination of translation of evidence.

■ RESEARCH DISSEMINATION

Funk, Tornquist, and Champagne (1989) had a model of research dissemination that outlined the three factors that were important and necessary for research to be disseminated.

- First are the qualities of the research. This includes the topic, relevance, applicability, availability of research, scientific merit, significance, level of control practitioners have over their own practice, and the gap between research and practice.
- Second are the characteristics of the communication. This includes the use of non-technical language, clarification on limits of generalizability, strategies for implementation, demonstration of new techniques, broad dissemination, and discussion between researchers and clinicians.
- Third is the facilitation of utilization. This factor includes the reinforcement of new knowledge, ongoing dialogue between researchers and clinicians, updates on research in the area, sharing of experiences, and giving support during implementation experiences. Attention to these categories can increase dissemination in any area.

Levels of Dissemination

Dissemination occurs at multiple levels. Once the translation project is complete, the first area for dissemination is internally at the site of the adoption or innovation. This is usually institutionally based and can include clinical staff as well as administrative staff. The translation can also be disseminated to upper management. Presentation at clinical or grand rounds can be accomplished through small or large group presentations. The focus of each of these may be different in order to meet the needs of the audience. After the translation is disseminated at the site, it should be disseminated at the institutional level. This can be accomplished by hospital or organization professional committee meetings or journal clubs. Third, one must consider how and in what venue to disseminate the translation externally—beyond the institution or both nationally and internationally. In addition, external dissemination to influence policy may occur through the use of the media or through government advocacy. Dissemination is most successful if multiple methods are used over time (Brown & Schmidt, 2009).

Highlighting challenges in the dissemination of evidence internally, Oermann, Roop, Nordstrom, Galvin, and Floyd (2007) described an intervention for disseminating Cochrane reviews to nurses. The authors sought to determine if short summaries of a systematic review that presented the findings without requiring a background in research and statistics were effective in increasing nurses' awareness of research results and understanding of the evidence. Subjects included staff and advanced practice nurses in seven hospitals, and subjects received either the intervention or served as a control. Although the number of nurses who completed the posttest was small, results support the feasibility of disseminating the findings of systematic reviews to bedside nurses and advanced practice nurses. Nurses reported increased awareness of the research evidence, which was most apparent in the staff nurses.

Indeed, because dissemination and diffusion of evidence internally, within an organization, is influenced by the organization's contextual factors, external dissemination is influenced by larger organizational and social systems and values.

Strategies for Improving Dissemination

In a recent brief by the Commonwealth Fund on the dissemination of evidence-based practices in health care, Yuan et al. (2010) cite key strategies to improve the dissemination of best practices in quality improvement (QI). These include (a) highlighting the evidence base and the relative simplicity of recommended practices; (b) aligning the campaigns with strategic goals of adopting organizations; (c) increasing the recruitment by integrating opinion leaders into the enrollment process; (d) forming a coalition of credible campaign sponsors; (e) generating a threshold of participating organizations that maximizes network exchanges; (f) developing practical implementation tools and guides for key stakeholder groups; (g) creating networks to foster learning opportunities; and (h) incorporating monitoring and evaluation of milestones and goals (Yuan et al., 2010, p. 1).

Kreuter and Bernhardt (2009) describe the challenge in dissemination of evidence as a marketing and distribution problem. They describe a lack of infrastructure to move public health programs from research to practice, and propose recommendations for building that needed infrastructure within the public health system.

The Three P's of Dissemination

There are three main methods of dissemination, also known as the *three P's*: posters, presentations, and papers (manuscripts). All three require an abstract for acceptance. A good abstract targets the audience and aim (whether it be a poster or presentation at a conference, or a manuscript), and provides key information in a clear manner. Formatting is important and depends on the use of the abstract, but following recommended fonts and word limit is crucial to acceptability. An abstract should be written in the past tense, and the American Psychological Association (APA) publication manual has clear and useful guidelines for both a research and nonresearch abstract (APA, 2010). The APA suggests that an abstract be accurate, self-contained, concise and specific, nonevaluative, and coherent and readable. They suggest an abstract be less than 120 words, but this length is more likely dictated by the conference organizing committee or journal.

Poster

A poster is a versatile medium, and is used to disseminate research or nonresearch at a conference or other venue, such as in the community. The primary purpose of a poster presentation is to facilitate scholarly dialogue among colleagues (Betz, Smith, Melnyk, & Rickey, 2005). One advantage is that work presented on a poster can (usually) still be in progress. Posters also need to be prepared to guidelines provided by the organizer. The message needs to be scholarly, straightforward, and clear. Incomplete sentences can be used, and bulleting of items is recommended. Posters should be more detailed than a speech, less detailed than a presentation, but more interactive than either (Schaffner, 2008). The use of charts and graphs provide visual stimulation as well as complement the data presented in verbal form. The reader's eye (in the United States) moves from top to bottom, left to right, and, therefore, the individual sections of the poster needs to be structured in this way. It has been suggested that the font of the title be more than 96 points and the font of the text be more than 24–36 points. A suggested guide is to make the text large enough to read from 3 to 6 ft away, or be able to read the material easily standing, when the poster is laid on the ground. A prominent title can also help lure people to the poster. There are numerous resources with suggested guidelines and methods for poster designs and construction available via the Internet (Table 15.1). Using a search engine to search "poster presentation guidelines" will undoubtedly provide numerous options. The website www.posterpresentations.com provides (free) PowerPoint templates for varying sizes of posters, with templates, and (for a fee) will print and ship the poster to you or to your meeting site.

Content will vary whether the authors are presenting a research project, an evidence-based practice project, or presenting a clinical case or review. For a research poster, categories might include background, research aims/hypothesis, review of the literature, design/methods, sample and setting, data analysis, results, limitations, discussion, and conclusion/implications. For a poster on an evidence-based practice project, topics might include background/significance, clinical question, search methods, appraisal of the evidence, method of grading the evidence, synthesis of findings, translation of evidence/intervention, findings, evaluation, and discussion (Table 15.2).

Once the poster is made, the author has to fulfill the obligations of a presenter because poster viewing and presentations involve communication and networking among colleagues. The author should be prepared to learn from the viewers, and should consider a poster as a

TABLE 15.1   **Helpful Websites for Posters and Oral Presentations**

http://www.ncsu.edu/project/posters/NewSite/
  This site creates effective poster presentations, has a quick reference guide, and has start-to-finish instructions.

http://www.bio.miami.edu/ktosney/file/PosterHome.html
  This site has examples of both good and bad posters.

http://lorien.ncl.ac.uk/ming/dept/tips/present/posters.htm
  This site provides information on the "how to's" of a scientific poster presentation.

http://library.buffalo.edu/asl/guides/bio/posters.html
  This library site has guidelines for creating academic posters.

http://gradschool.unc.edu/student/postertips.html
  This site covers everything you need to know about creating a professional poster.

http://pages.cs.wisc.edu/~markhill/conference-talk.html
  This site provides an advice on giving an effective oral presentation.

http://www.nwlink.com/~donclark/leader/leadpres.html
  This site on leadership contains useful information on presentations.

way to market his or her work. For example, the authors need to be available by their poster at stated time frames. The author or representative should bring handouts, abstract, and business cards. After the poster session, Smith and Mateo (2009) suggest the author(s) evaluate their poster. In addition, author(s) should jot down the feedback received from viewers, whether related to that project or ideas for future projects.

Presentation

Oral presentations can be invited or juried. If juried, the abstract is necessary and is crucial for acceptance. Conference sponsors usually solicit presenters by announcing a call

TABLE 15.2   **Poster Content**

Research Poster	Evidence-Based Practice Project Poster
Background	Background/significance
Research aims/hypotheses	Clinical question
Review of literature	Search methods
Methods/design	Appraisal of evidence
Sample and setting	Method of grading evidence
Data analysis	Synthesis of findings
Results	Translation of evidence/intervention
Limitations	Findings
Discussion	Evaluation
Conclusions/implications	Discussion

for abstracts. Typically, an invited speaker does not need to prepare an abstract. An oral presentation is better than a poster for dissemination of philosophical and theoretical topics. Oral presentations must be of completed work, and thus the abstract is completed in the past tense.

Once an abstract is accepted for an oral presentation, the author(s) need to ascertain the target audience, the room setting (size and seating arrangement) and the time allotted (both for the presentation as well as questions), and whether the presentation (frequently in PowerPoint) needs to be submitted in advance.

In preparation, the content of the presentation needs to be dictated by what was submitted in the abstract. Developing an outline from the abstract is one method to begin preparation. Because the purpose of the slides is to enhance the presentation of the content (Smith & Mateo, 2009), the author(s) must decide the number and type of slides (words, pictures/graphs, or both), depending on the content and audience. The recommendation is a maximum of one slide per minute of talk. This also requires that the presenter understand the exact time he or she has to present and for entertaining any questions or for discussion. Considerations for developing slides include the following: (a) use contrasting colors (such as navy blue background and yellow lettering); (b) keep a consistent template and font throughout; (c) choose a simple font (Arial, sans serif, or Times New Roman); (d) keep the number of words per slide to a minimum; (e) left-justify the text; and when using graphs, orient the audience (Betz et al., 2005; Smith & Mateo, 2009). As with posters, there are numerous resources on the Internet to assist not only in preparing the slides, but also with tips on presenting.

Once the presentation is completed, follow conference guidelines for submission, if requested. Because most presentations are done on computer software (as opposed to actual slides), make and bring another copy of the presentation to the conference (e.g., on a flash drive), as well as a printed copy of the slides, for use in the event of a technological malfunction.

Public speaking is a skill, and thus requires learning and practice (Englehart, 2004). Rehearsing the presentation is a must, especially for those new to oral presentations. Presenting to colleagues at work is an excellent way to not only rehearse but also obtain any suggestions and feedback on the content, and to enhance clarity. A common pitfall in oral presentations is staying to the allotted time. The sole responsibility of staying on time is with the presenter.

Publication

Papers or manuscripts for publication can be on research, evidence-based practice projects, or on case studies or clinical reviews. Manuscripts are almost always required to be of completed work. All posters and presentations should also be considered for a manuscript submission. Whereas posters and presentations are only for the people in attendance, a manuscript is considered a permanent contribution and method of dissemination to the profession. Publication options include professional journals, electronic journals, the Internet (including listservs, Twitter, and blogs), newsletters, and newspapers.

In developing a manuscript for a professional journal, the journal for publication needs to be considered early on. Peer-reviewed journals publish more rigorously reviewed manuscripts than non-peer-reviewed journals. Both the target audience and the target journal need to be defined. Authorship should also be decided and agreed upon in advance. The author(s) need to review the author guidelines from the specific journal and comply with suggested length, reference style, and other specific manuscript details. Most of this information is now available online. Many journals will accept and respond to queries from authors, usually submitted electronically through the journal/editor website, or via e-mail. In a query to the editor, the author(s) must succinctly explain their plans for the structure and content of the manuscript. This can save authors considerable time and effort.

Just as there are guidelines for the publication of randomized controlled trials (RCTs; consolidated standards of reporting trials [CONSORT]) and preferred reporting items for systematic reviews and meta-analyses (PRISMA), there are also guidelines for the publication of QI projects in health care (Altman et al., 2001; Liberati et al., 2009). Standards for Quality Improvement Reporting Excellence (SQUIRE) guidelines have been developed for authors describing the development and testing of interventions to improve the quality and safety of health care (Davidoff et al., 2008). Journals, such as *The Journal of Nursing Care Quality* and *The Joint Commission Journal on Quality and Patient Safety*, have adopted these guidelines for reporting QI projects to ensure that the project is sufficiently reported so readers can understand the problem, intervention, setting, and outcomes (Oermann, 2009). The SQUIRE guidelines assist in the reporting of QI projects, including details of the intervention and circumstances leading to the need for the change, and the setting and local conditions that could influence the outcomes. In addition, as Oermann (2009) points out, these guidelines can be used to educate nurses and other health care professionals on the QI process and as a framework for the project plan (p. 94). Categories include the following sections (and subsections): (a) title and abstract (title, abstract); (b) introduction (background knowledge, local problem, intended improvement, study question); (c) methods (ethical issues, setting, planning the intervention, planning the study of the intervention, methods of evaluation, and analysis); (d) results (outcomes); (e) discussion (summary, relation to other evidence, limitations, interpretation, and conclusions); and (f) other information (funding; Davidoff et al., 2008; Table 15.3).

Developing the manuscript content, proofreading, and responding to suggestions all take time, perseverance, and a positive attitude (Betz et al., 2005). To increase the chances that a manuscript will be accepted, the following guidelines are recommended: select the appropriate audience, select the appropriate journal, query the editor, include implications for practice and significance of your project, conform to submission requirements, adhere to copyright laws, use recent references, maintain organization, use tables and graphs, determine authorship in advance, acknowledge appropriately, and conform to ethical practice (Smith & Matteo, 2009).

■ ETHICAL CONCERNS

Ethical issues in publication have recently come to the forefront. Siedlecki, Montague, and Schultz (2008) describe common ethical pitfalls that authors may encounter during the preparation and submission of a manuscript, and how to avoid them. These include plagiarism, failure to cite sources correctly, dual publications, and authorship decisions. Plagiarism can be intentional or unintentional, but involves stealing (knowingly or unknowingly) another person's work or ideas and using them as your own. It also includes self-plagiarism that occurs when an author borrows extensively from one of his or her prior works, and does not

TABLE 15.3 **SQUIRE Guidelines for Reporting QI Studies**

Section of Paper	Description
Title and Abstract	Did you provide clear and accurate information for finding, indexing, and scanning your article?
1. Title	a. Indicate article is on improvement of quality b. State aim or intervention c. Indicate study method
2. Abstract	Summarize key information using journal abstract format
Introduction	Why did you start?
3. Background knowledge	Provide a brief summary of the current knowledge of problem being addressed in the project: include characteristics of setting
4. Local problem	Describe the specific local problem addressed in the project
5. Intended improvement	a. Describe changes/improvements in processes and outcomes of proposed intervention b. Specify who and what led to decision to make changes, include why project is done now (timing)
6. Study question	State primary and other questions that QI study was intended to answer
Methods	What did you do?
7. Ethical issues	Indicate ethical concerns of implementing the improvement and study and how they are addressed
8. Setting	Specify elements and characteristics of setting most likely to influence change/improvement
9. Planning the intervention	a. Describe intervention in enough detail for others to reproduce it b. Indicate factors that contributed to decision about specific intervention to implement c. Describe plans for how intervention was to be implemented: what was done, how tests of change would be used to modify intervention, and by whom
10. Planning the study of the intervention	a. Outline plans for assessing how well the intervention was implemented b. Describe mechanisms by which intervention components were expected to cause changes, and plans for testing if they were effective c. Identify study design for measuring the effects of intervention d. Discuss plans for implementing essential aspects of study design e. Describe the aspects of study design that addressed internal validity (integrity of data) and external validity (generalizability)

(continued)

TABLE 15.3   SQUIRE Guidelines for Reporting QI Studies (*Continued*)

Section of Paper	Description
11. Methods of evaluation	a. Describe instruments and procedures to assess effectiveness of implementation, contributions of intervention components and context factors to effectiveness of intervention, and outcomes b. Report validity and reliability of assessment instruments c. Explain methods to ensure data quality and adequacy
12. Analysis	a. Provide details of qualitative and quantitative (statistical) methods b. Align unit of analysis with level at which intervention was implemented, if applicable c. Specify degree of variability expected in implementation, change expected in primary outcome (effect size), and ability of study design (including size) to detect those effects d. Describe analytic methods to demonstrate effects of time as variable
Results	

13. Outcomes	What did you find?
	a. Nature of setting and improvement intervention:
	  i. Indicate relevant elements of setting and structures and patterns of care that provided context for the intervention
	  ii. Explain actual course of intervention
	  iii. Document success in implementing intervention components
	  iv. Describe how and why initial plan evolved and lessons learned
	b. Changes in processes of care and patient outcomes associated with intervention:
	  i. Present data on changes observed in care delivery process
	  ii. Present data on changes observed in patient outcomes
	  iii. Consider benefits, harms, unexpected results, problems, and failures
	  iv. Present evidence on strength of association between observed changes/improvements and intervention components/context factors
	  v. Include summary of missing data for intervention and outcomes

Discussion	
14. Summary	What do the findings mean? a. Summarize the most important successes and difficulties in implementing intervention and main changes observed b. Highlight study's strengths
15. Relation to other evidence	Compare and contrast study results with relevant findings of others

16. Limitations
   a. Consider possible sources of confounding, bias, or imprecision in design, measurement, and analysis that might affect study outcomes
   b. Explore factors that could affect generalizability
   c. Address likelihood that observed gains may weaken over time, and describe plans for sustainability
   d. Review efforts to minimize study limitations
   e. Assess effect of limitations on interpretation and application of results

17. Interpretation
   a. Explore possible reasons for differences between observed and expected outcomes
   b. Draw inferences consistent with strength of data about causal mechanisms and size of observed change
   c. Suggest steps that might be modified to improve future performance
   d. Review issues of cost of intervention (opportunity and financial)

18. Conclusions
   a. Consider practical usefulness of intervention
   b. Suggest implications for health care and other QI studies

Other information

19. Funding
   Were there other factors relevant to the conduct and interpretation of the study?
   List funding sources, if any, and role of funding organization in design, implementation, interpretation, and publication

Note. QI = quality improvement. Adapted from Davidoff, F., Batalden, P., Stevens, D., Ogrinc, G., Mooney, S., & SQUIRE Development Group. (2008). Publication guidelines for improvement studies in health care: Evolution of the SQUIRE project. *Annals of Internal Medicine, 149*(9), 670–676. Oermann, M. H. (2009). SQUIRE guidelines for reporting improvement studies in healthcare: Implications for nursing publications. *Journal of Nursing Care Quality, 24*(2), 91–95.

properly acknowledge the source through a citation. Although citation errors are common in the health care literature, they connote sloppiness by the author, and may greatly hinder the reader's ability to locate a source. The use of citation management software programs, such as EndNote, can help eliminate this problem. Dual publication, or salami publishing, is the publication of multiple manuscripts for one project or study (Baggs, 2008; Siedlecki et al., 2008). Authorship problems can arise when several individuals submit an article as a group. Everyone who made a "substantial contribution" to the project should be listed as an author, and conversely, all individuals listed as authors should be involved in writing and reviewing the manuscript (Baggs, 2008; Broome, 2008; Graf et al., 2007; Siedlecki et al., 2008). Clear guidelines on authorship can be found on the website of the International Committee of Medical Journal Editors at http://www.icmje.com

Another component to ethical issues in dissemination is the ethical issues surrounding the dissemination of sensitive data and information. For example, if the translation of evidence identifies an improvement in outcomes, safety, or cost, the preimplementation data may be viewed as a poor outcome by some. A good rule of thumb is to be sure administrators are aware of outcomes preimplementation and postimplementation of a translation project, prior to any dissemination. Another suggestion is to disseminate the information at the institutional level first prior to any dissemination outside of the institution.

■ SUMMARY

In sum, dissemination is the final phase of translation, and an imperative for moving evidence into practice. Preparation for dissemination for any venue and by any method will enhance the success of any dissemination and translation initiative (Betz et al., 2005).

■ REFERENCES

Altman, D. G., Shulz, K. F., Moher, D., Egger, M., Davidoff, F., Elbourne, D., et al. for the CONSORT Group. (2001). The revised CONSORT statement for reporting randomized trials: Explanation and elaboration. *Annals of Internal Medicine, 134,* 663–694.

American Psychological Association. (2011). *Publication manual of the American Psychological Association* (6th ed.). Washington, DC: Author.

Baggs, J. G. (2008). Issues and rules for authors concerning authorship versus acknowledgements, dual publication, self plagiarism, and salami publishing. *Research in Nursing and Health, 31*(4), 295–297.

Betz, C. L., Smith, K., Melnyk, B. M., & Rickey, T. (2005). Disseminating evidence. In B. M. Melnyk & E. Fineout-Overholt (Eds.), *Evidence-based practice in nursing and healthcare: A guide to best practice* (pp. 361–403). Philadelphia, PA: Lippincott, Williams & Wilkins.

Broome, M. E. (2008). The "truth, the whole truth and nothing but the truth." *Nursing Outlook, 56*(6), 281–282.

Brown, J. M., & Schmidt, N. A. (2009). Sharing the insights with others. In N. A. Schmidt & J. M. Brown (Eds.), *Evidence-based practice for nurses: Appraisal and application of research* (pp. 399–417). Sudbury, MA: Jones and Bartlett.

Cronenwett, L. R. (1995). Effective methods for disseminating research findings to nurses in practice. *Nursing Clinics of North America, 30*(3), 429–438.

Davidoff, F., Batalden, P., Stevens, D., Ogrinc, G., Mooney, S., & SQUIRE Development Group. (2008). Publication guidelines for improvement studies in health care: Evolution of the SQUIRE project. *Annals of Internal Medicine, 149*(9), 670–676.

Englehart, N. (2004). Giving effective presentations. *Canadian Operating Room Nursing Journal, 22*(1), 22–24.

Funk, S. G., Tornquist, E. M. & Champagne, M. T. (1989). A model for improving the dissemination of nursing research. *Western Journal of Nursing Research, 11*(3), 361–367.

Graf, C., Wagner, E., Bowman, A., Flack, S., Scott-Lichter, D., & Robinson, A. (2007). Best practice guidelines on publication ethics: A publisher's perspective. *International Journal of Clinical Practice, 61*(suppl 152): 1–26.

Kreuter, M. W., & Bernhardt, J. M. (2009). Reframing the dissemination challenge: A marketing and distribution perspective. *American Journal of Public Health, 99*(12), 2123–2127.

Liberati, A., Altman, D. G., Tetzlaf, J., Mulrow, C., Gotzsche, P. C., Ioannidis, J. P. A., et al. (2009). The PRISMA statement for reporting systematic reviews and meta-analysis of studies that evaluate health care interventions: Explanation and elaboration. *Journal of Clinical Epidemiology 62*, e1–e34.

Oermann, M. H. (2009). SQUIRE guidelines for reporting improvement studies in healthcare: Implications for nursing publications. *Journal of Nursing Care Quality, 24*(2), 91–95.

Oermann, M. H., Roop, J. C., Nordstrom, C. K., Galvin, E. A., & Floyd, J. A. (2007). Effectiveness of an intervention for disseminating Cochrane reviews to nurses. *Medsurg Nursing, 16*(6), 373–377.

Ordonez, M., & Serrat, O. (2009). Disseminating knowledge products. *Asian Development Bank: Knowledge Solutions, 43*, 1–6.

Schaffner, M. (2008, May). *Preparing a research poster.* Paper presented at the 35th annual course of the Society of Gastroenterology Nurses and Associates, Salt Lake, UT.

Siedlecki, S. L., Montague, M., & Schultz, J. (2008). Writing for publication: Avoiding common ethical pitfalls. *Journal of Wound, Ostomy, and Continence Nursing, 35*(2), 147–150.

Smith, S. P., & Matteo, M. A. (2009). Reporting results through publication. In M. A. Mateo & K. T. Kirchhoff (Eds.), *Research for advanced practice nurses: From evidence to practice* (pp. 441–455). New York, NY: Springer Publishing.

Yuan, C. T., Nembhard, I. M., Stern, A. F., Brush, J. E., Krumholz, H. M. & Bradley, E. H. (2010). Blueprint for the dissemination of evidence-based practices in health care. *The Commonwealth Fund, Issue Brief, 1399*(86), 1–14.

Index

Note. *b* refers to a box; *e* refers to exhibit; *f* refers to a figure; *t* refers to a table.

NATIONAL
GEOGRAPHIC

Tropical
Rain Forests

PLANTS IN THEIR HABITATS

Tracey Reeder

PICTURE CREDITS

Cover: Brualio Carrillo National Park, Costa Rica © Gail Shumway/
Taxi/Getty Images.

Page 1 © Gary Braasch/Stone/Getty Images; page 4, Digital
Vision; page 5 (top) © B. Bird/Zefa/Corbis/Tranz; page 5 (bottom
left), Corbis; page 5 (bottom right), Photodisc; page 6 © Paul A.
Souders/Corbis/Tranz; page 7 © Ralph Clevenger/Corbis/Tranz;
page 8 © Gary Braasch/Corbis/Tranz; page 9 © Peter Campbell;
page 10 © Frank Krahmer/Zefa/Corbis/Tranz; pages 11–12
© Peter Campbell; page 13 © Wolfgang Kaehler/Corbis/Tranz;
page 14 © Kuljit Kaur; page 15 (top) © Carl and Ann Purcell/
Corbis/Tranz; page 15 (bottom) © Wayne Lawler/Ecoscene/Corbis/
Tranz; page 16 (top) © Joel W. Rogers/Corbis/Tranz; page 16
(bottom left) © Macmillan Education Australia; page 16 (bottom
right) © Chris Mattison/Frank Lane Picture Agency/Corbis/Tranz;
page 17 (top) © Terry Whittaker/Frank Lane Picture Agency/
Tranz; page 17 (bottom) © Michael and Patricia Fogden/Corbis/
Tranz; page 18 © Buddy Mays/Corbis/Tranz; page 21 © Peter
Campbell; page 23 (top), Photodisc; page 23 (bottom) © John
and Lisa Merrill/Corbis/Tranz; page 24 (bottom) © Photolibrary;
page 24 (Brazil nut), Alamy; page 25 (left) © Bob Krist/Corbis/
Tranz; page 25 (right) © Photolibrary; page 26 (left) © Howard
Davies/Corbis/Tranz; page 26 (right) © Wolfgang Kaehler/Corbis/
Tranz; page 29, Photodisc.

Produced through the worldwide resources of the National
Geographic Society, John M. Fahey, Jr., President and Chief
Executive Officer; Gilbert M. Grosvenor, Chairman of the Board.

PREPARED BY NATIONAL GEOGRAPHIC SCHOOL PUBLISHING
Sheron Long, Chief Executive Officer; Samuel Gesumaria,
President; Steve Mico, Executive Vice President and Publisher;
Francis Downey, Editor in Chief; Richard Easby, Editorial Manager;
Margaret Sidlosky, Director of Design and Illustrations; Jim Hiscott,
Design Manager; Cynthia Olson and Ruth Ann Thompson, Art
Directors; Matt Wascavage, Director of Publishing Services; Lisa
Pergolizzi, Production Manager.

MANUFACTURING AND QUALITY CONTROL
Christopher A. Liedel, Chief Financial Officer; Phillip L. Schlosser,
Vice President; Clifton M. Brown III, Director.

EDITOR
Mary Anne Wengel

PROGRAM CONSULTANTS
Dr. Shirley V. Dickson, National Literacy Consultant; James A.
Shymansky, E. Desmond Lee Professor of Science Education,
University of Missouri-St Louis.

National Geographic Theme Sets program developed by Macmillan
Education Australia Pty Limited.

Published by the National Geographic Society
1145 17th Street N.W.
Washington, D.C. 20036-4688

ISBN: 978-1-4263-5140-2

Product# 4P1005147

Printed in Hong Kong.

2011 2010 2009 2008 2007
1 2 3 4 5 6 7 8 9 10 11 12 13 14 15

Contents

Plants
in Their Habitats

Plants grow almost everywhere on Earth. The places where plants grow are called habitats. A plant gets all it needs to grow from its habitat. There are many different habitats on Earth. Four of these are tropical rain forests, deserts, temperate forests, and wetlands.

 ## Key Concepts ••••••••••••••••••••••••••••••••••••

1. Each part of a plant helps it survive.

2. Adaptations help plants survive in their habitats. There are many different habitats on Earth.

3. Plants and animals depend on one another for survival.

Four Kinds of Habitats

Tropical Rain Forests

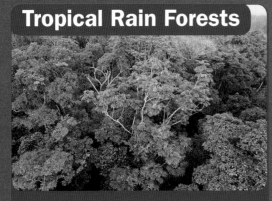

Tropical rain forests are good habitats for plants such as tropical hardwood trees.

Deserts

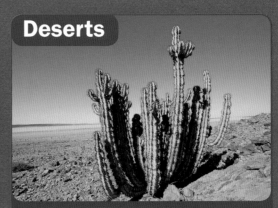

Deserts are good habitats for plants such as cactuses.

4

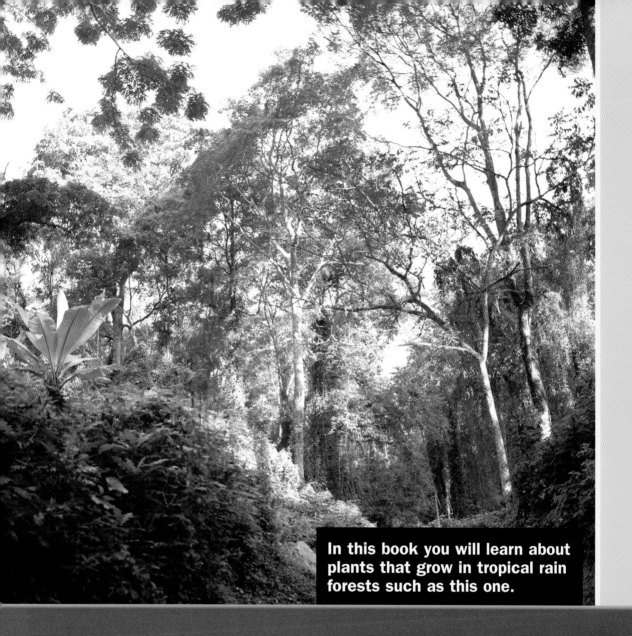

In this book you will learn about plants that grow in tropical rain forests such as this one.

Temperate Forests

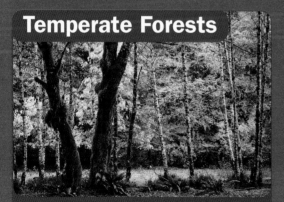

Temperate forests are good habitats for plants such as red alder trees.

Wetlands

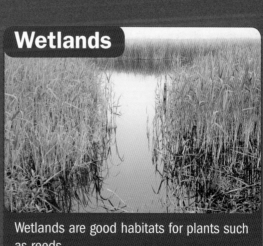

Wetlands are good habitats for plants such as reeds.

Plants of the
Tropical Rain Forest

Take a walk in a tropical rain forest. What do you see? You see a lot of plants. Plants are on the ground, at eye level, and high above your head. It's warm and wet here all the time. Millions of plants live here.

Tropical Rain Forests—Wet and Warm

Tropical rain forests grow in hot, wet places. A tropical rain forest is a good **habitat** for many plants.

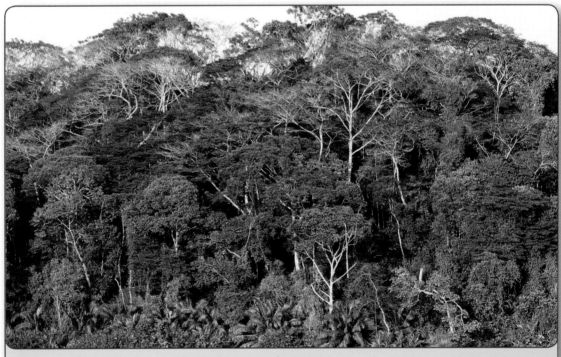

Millions of plants grow in a tropical rain forest.

Most tropical rain forests are found near the **Equator.** These places get direct sunlight all year. Warm winds bring a lot of rain to these places. The largest tropical rain forest is in South America.

A trumpet tree grows well in a hot, wet habitat.

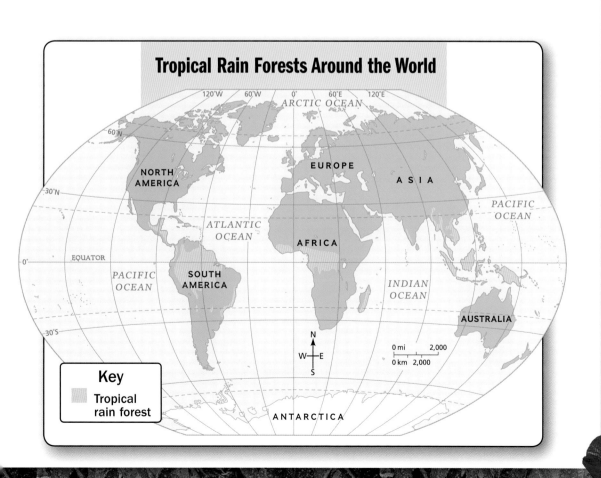

Tropical Rain Forests Around the World

120°W   60°W   0°   60°E   120°E

ARCTIC OCEAN

60°N

EUROPE

NORTH AMERICA

ASIA

30°N

PACIFIC OCEAN

ATLANTIC OCEAN

AFRICA

0°   EQUATOR

PACIFIC OCEAN

SOUTH AMERICA

INDIAN OCEAN

AUSTRALIA

30°S

N
W   E
S

0 mi   2,000
0 km   2,000

ANTARCTICA

Key
Tropical rain forest

Parts of a Plant

Plants have different parts. The main parts of a plant are the roots, stems, leaves, and seeds. Each part helps the plant **survive.**

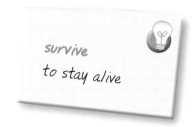

survive
to stay alive

Roots

The roots of most plants are under the ground. Roots help plants survive in two ways. First, roots hold plants in the soil. They keep the plant from falling over. Second, roots take in water and **minerals** from the soil. A plant needs water and minerals to grow.

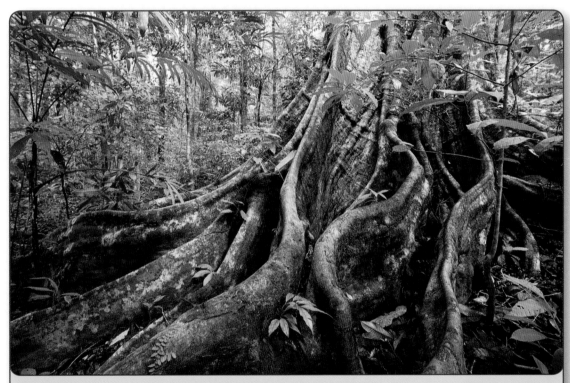

The roots of this sloanea tree spread across the ground. The roots take in water and minerals.

Stems

Stems help plants survive. Stems hold the leaves up to the sunlight. Water and minerals move from the roots to the stems. They then move through the stems to other parts of the plant. Food made by the leaves moves through the stems. The stems move the food to other parts of the plant.

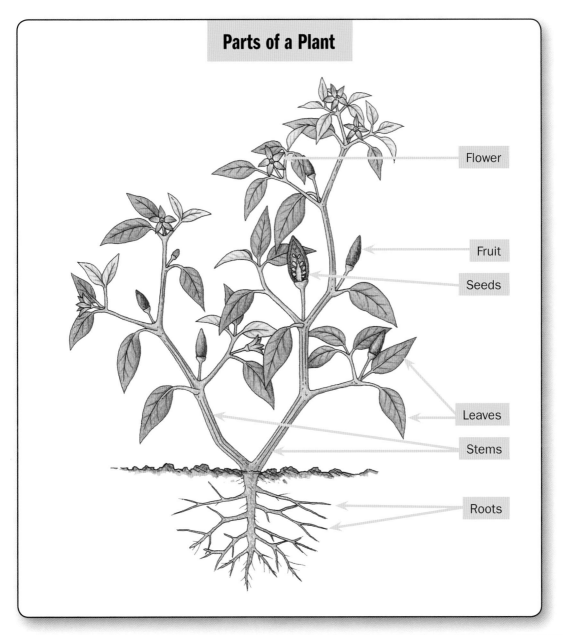

Parts of a Plant

Flower

Fruit

Seeds

Leaves

Stems

Roots

Leaves

Plants' leaves do an important job. Leaves make food for plants. This process is called **photosynthesis.**

Leaves trap energy from sunlight. Leaves also take in a gas from the air. The gas is called carbon dioxide. Plants use the sun's energy to change carbon dioxide and water from the soil into sugar. Plants use this sugar to live and grow.

During photosynthesis plant leaves give off oxygen. People and animals breathe in this oxygen. The plants in a tropical rain forest give off a lot of oxygen.

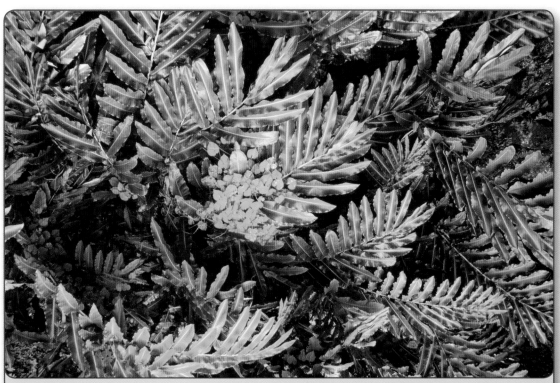

The leaves of these rain forest plants use sunlight, water, and carbon dioxide to make food.

Photosynthesis

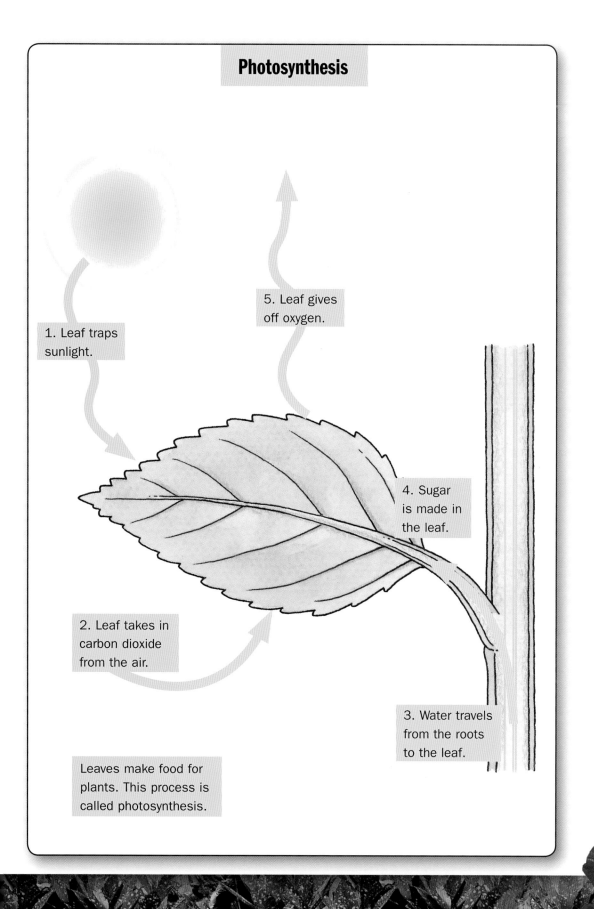

1. Leaf traps sunlight.

5. Leaf gives off oxygen.

4. Sugar is made in the leaf.

2. Leaf takes in carbon dioxide from the air.

3. Water travels from the roots to the leaf.

Leaves make food for plants. This process is called photosynthesis.

Seeds

Seeds are another part of a plant. Many new plants grow from seeds.

Seeds form in the fruit of most plants. A **seed coat,** which is like a skin, protects the seed until it is ready to grow. The seed also stores food and water. This helps the new plant grow until it can make its own food.

Many tropical rain forest plants have fruit. The seeds are inside the fruit.

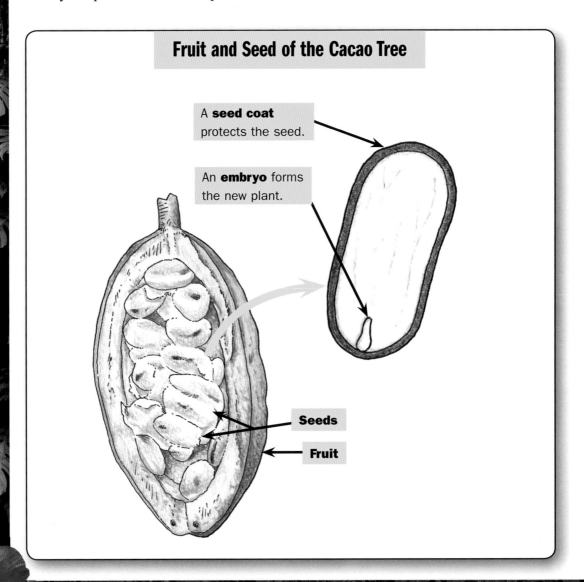

Fruit and Seed of the Cacao Tree

A **seed coat** protects the seed.

An **embryo** forms the new plant.

Seeds

Fruit

Living in a Tropical Rain Forest

An **adaptation** is something that helps a plant survive in its habitat. Tropical rain forest plants have many adaptations. Some help plants live with little sunlight. Others help plants live with poor soil.

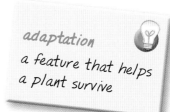

adaptation
a feature that helps
a plant survive

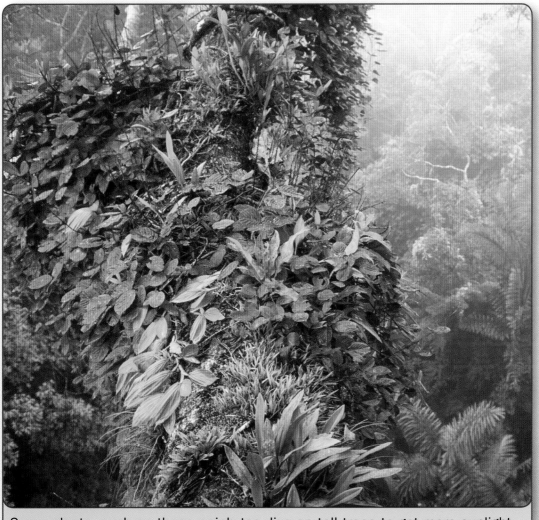

Some plants, such as these epiphytes, live on tall trees to get more sunlight.

Living in Levels

A tropical rain forest has many levels. Plants growing at each level get different amounts of sunlight. The tallest trees get the most sunlight. They stop sunlight from reaching plants on the forest floor.

Some plants that grow on the floor have adaptations that help them get more sunlight. Plants called vines climb up tall trees. This helps them get closer to the sunlight.

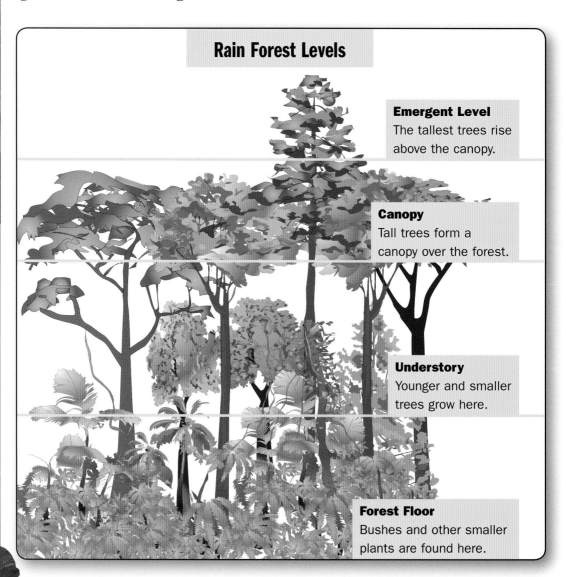

Rain Forest Levels

Emergent Level
The tallest trees rise above the canopy.

Canopy
Tall trees form a canopy over the forest.

Understory
Younger and smaller trees grow here.

Forest Floor
Bushes and other smaller plants are found here.

Living with Poor Soil

The soil in a rain forest is not rich. It does not contain many minerals. Plants have adaptations that help them survive in poor soil. The roots of some trees spread out over the ground. They do not grow down deep. This lets the roots take in minerals from a large area.

Some plants get the minerals they need from insects. Plants trap the insects. A plant may be sticky so an insect that lands on it cannot get away. The insect dies and rots. The plant then uses minerals from the insect's body to help it survive. These plants are called carnivorous plants.

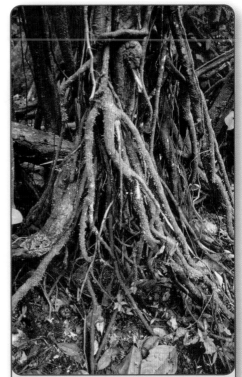

The roots of this rain forest tree gather minerals from a large area.

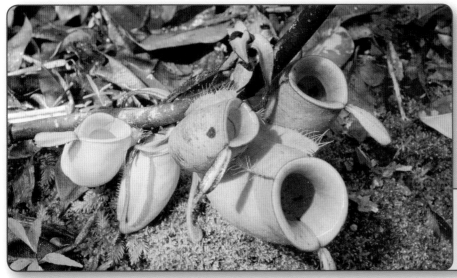

This plant has pitcher-shaped leaves that trap insects.

Living Together

Many plants and animals live in a tropical rain forest. They rely, or **depend,** on one another to survive.

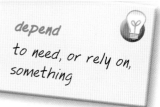

depend
to need, or rely on, something

Plants and Animals in the Rain Forest

Monkeys and pythons live in the rain forest. Monkeys eat fruit for food. Pythons eat monkeys.

Tropical fruit such as jackfruit grow on trees. Monkeys eat the fruit. The monkeys help spread the seeds.

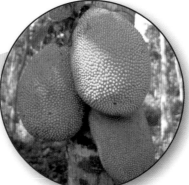

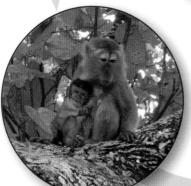

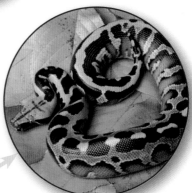

Monkeys live in the trees. They are eaten by pythons.

Plants Provide Food

Animals depend on plants for food. In a rain forest, all kinds of animals eat plants. Animals that eat only plants are called **herbivores.** There are many herbivores in a rain forest. The hawk-headed parrot is a herbivore.

Animals that eat other animals are called **carnivores.** A carnivore depends on plants too. Carnivores eat herbivores. There are many carnivores in a rain forest. The jaguar is a carnivore.

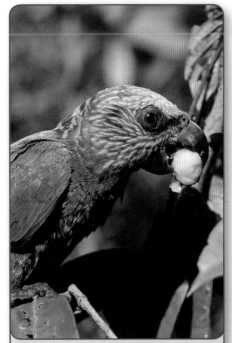

The hawk-headed parrot eats fruit.

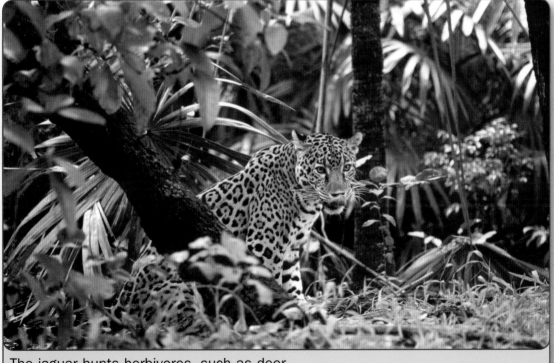

The jaguar hunts herbivores, such as deer.

Animals Spread Seeds

Animals help rain forest plants grow new plants, or **reproduce.** This happens in two ways. An animal eats the fruit and seeds of a plant. The seeds pass through the animal's body. They then come out in the animal's droppings. New plants grow where these seeds fall.

Sometimes, seeds stick to the fur of an animal. The seeds fall off the animal as it moves from place to place. New plants can grow where these seeds land.

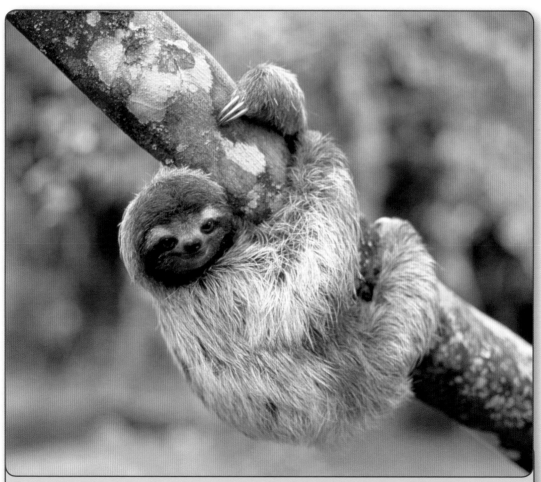

The sloth eats fruit and drops the seeds. This helps spread the seeds of plants.

Think About the **Key Concepts**

Think about what you read. Think about the pictures and diagrams. Use these to answer the questions. Share what you think with others.

1. How do the different parts of a plant help it survive?

2. What happens during photosynthesis?

3. What adaptations help plants survive?

4. How do animals help plants survive?

Labeled Diagram

Diagrams are pictures that show information.
You can learn new ideas without having to read many words. Diagrams use pictures and words to explain ideas.

There are different kinds of diagrams.
This diagram of a black pepper plant is a **labeled diagram.** A labeled diagram is a picture that shows the parts of something. It can give information about each part. Look back at the diagram on page 9. It is a labeled diagram of the parts of a plant.

How to Read a Diagram

1. **Read the title.**
   The title tells you what the diagram is about.

2. **Read the labels.**
   The labels name the parts of the diagram. They may also give information about the parts.

3. **Study the diagram.**
   Use the labels to help you understand the diagram.

4. **Think about what you learned.**
   Decide what new information you learned from the diagram.

A Black Pepper Plant

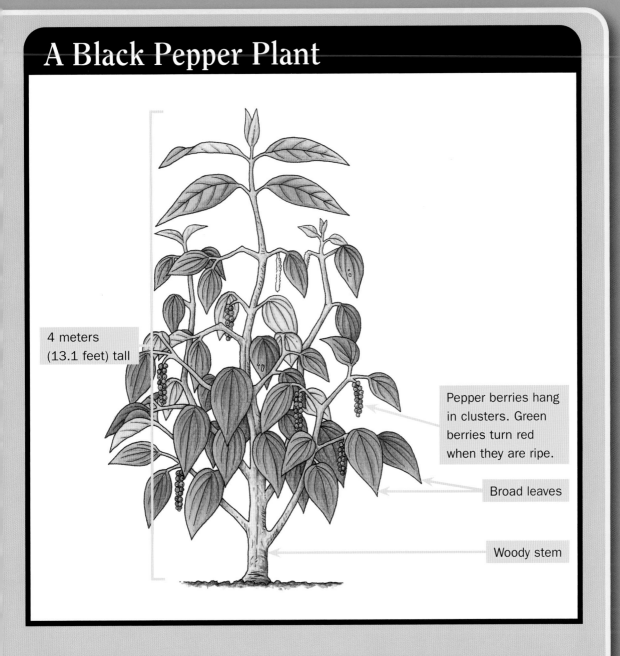

4 meters
(13.1 feet) tall

Pepper berries hang
in clusters. Green
berries turn red
when they are ripe.

Broad leaves

Woody stem

What Have You Learned?

Read the diagram by following the steps on page 20. Write down all
the things you have learned about the black pepper plant. Share the
things you have learned with a classmate. Compare what you learned.
What is the same? What is different?

Reference Sources

The purpose of **reference sources** is to inform. Reference sources can take many forms.

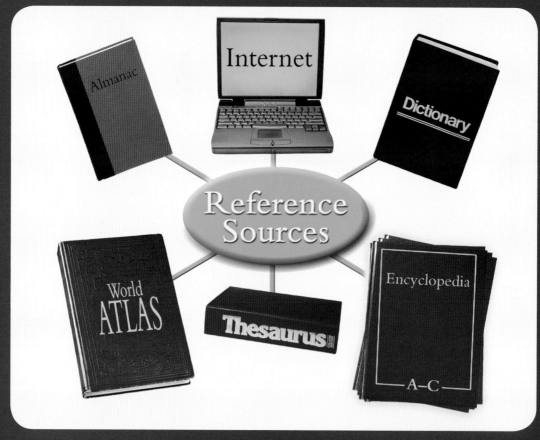

You use different reference sources for different purposes. For example, if you want to know how to spell *cinchona*, use a dictionary. But if you want to know facts about cinchona, use an **encyclopedia.**

You do not read a reference source from beginning to end. You read only the parts that cover topics you want to learn about.

Encyclopedia
of Tropical Rain Forest Plants

This sample shows seven encyclopedia entries. Encyclopedia entries give basic facts about many topics. All the entries in this encyclopedia are about tropical rain forest plants.

Bamboo

- found in most tropical areas
- uses: building, furniture, food
- parts used: stems, shoots

Bamboo is a very tall grass. It has a hollow, woody stem. Its leaves are long and narrow. Bamboo grows very quickly. It can grow to 37 meters (121 feet) tall.

Woody bamboo stems can be used to build houses. People in tropical countries use bamboo to make furniture and weave mats. Some people cook young bamboo shoots as food.

Title names the topic.

List gives facts about the topic.

Text gives important information.

Photographs help you picture what you are reading.

Captions give more information.

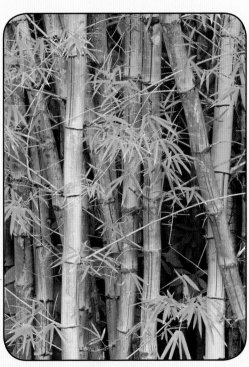

▲ Bamboo grows well in a hot, moist habitat.

Black Pepper

- found in Asia, South America, and Africa
- use: spice
- part used: fruit

Black pepper is a vine. The vine grows green berries. The berries grow on long, hanging stalks. The berries turn red when they are ripe.

Pepper is a popular spice. People use it in cooking. People harvest the unripe green berries and dry them to get black pepper. Ripe red berries are dried to form white pepper.

Brazil Nut

- found in South America
- uses: food, oil, soap
- part used: seeds

The Brazil nut tree is a tall tree. It can grow up to 46 meters (150 feet) tall. The Brazil nut tree produces Brazil nuts. The nuts grow inside round or pear-shaped fruit. There can be 12–24 nuts inside each fruit.

The nuts are good to eat. People also make oil from the nuts. Brazil nut oil is used in soaps and shampoos.

Brazil nut ►

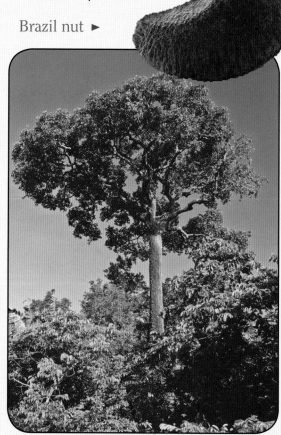

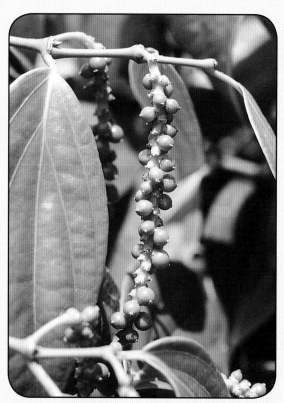

▲ Unripe green berries are picked and dried to get black pepper.

▲ Brazil nut trees stay green all year round.

Cacao

- found in most tropical areas
- uses: chocolate, cocoa
- part used: seeds

The cacao is an evergreen tree. It grows in hot, rainy parts of the world. It grows to 12 meters (39.3 feet) tall. Long pods grow on the trunk and branches of the tree. The pods are filled with light brown beans.

People make cacao beans into cocoa solids and cocoa butter. These are used to make cocoa powder, chocolate bars, and other chocolate products.

Cinchona

- found in South America and Asia
- use: medicine
- part used: bark

Cinchona is an evergreen tree and shrub. It stays green all year. It has sweet-smelling flowers.

Cinchona is used to make medicine. Quinine comes from cinchona bark. People use quinine to treat malaria. It reduces fever. Malaria is a tropical sickness. The cinchona is also called sacred bark.

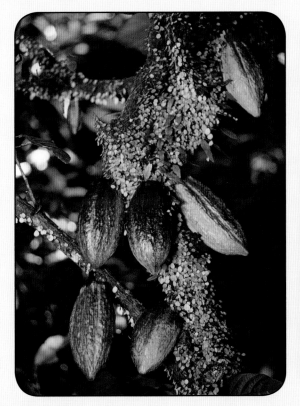

▲ These ripe cacao pods are ready to be picked.

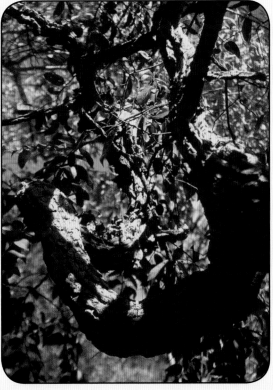

▲ People make medicine from the bark of the cinchona tree.

Rubber

- found in Asia, Africa, and South America
- use: rubber products
- part used: latex

The rubber tree is a large tree. It grows to about 21 meters (70 feet) tall. It has a slim trunk.

People grow rubber trees on large farms called plantations. They cut the trunk to get a white liquid called latex. Latex is made into rubber. Rubber is used to make car tires and other goods.

Vanilla

- found in Mexico, Madagascar, and Asia
- use: flavoring
- part used: pods

The vanilla plant grows on other trees. It uses little roots to attach itself to trees. The plant has orange flowers and grows slender pods. The pods are filled with tiny black seeds. When the pods are dried, they have a lovely smell.

Vanilla is an expensive spice. It is used to flavor ice cream, chocolate, candy, and cake.

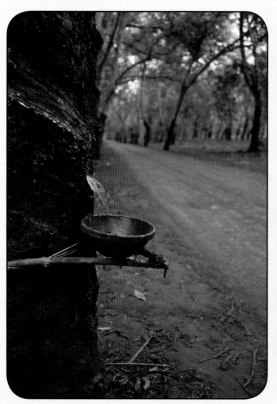

▲ A bowl collects latex from this rubber tree.

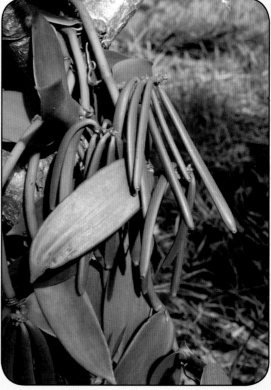

▲ Vanilla pods are long and slender.

Apply the **Key Concepts**

Key Concept 1 Each part of a plant helps it survive.

Activity

Choose a plant from a tropical rain forest and draw it. Label the parts of the plant that help it survive. Write captions that explain how the parts of the plant help it survive.

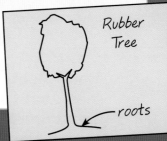

Key Concept 2 Adaptations help plants survive in their habitats. There are many different habitats on Earth.

Activity

Create a two-column chart that explains how plants adapt to the tropical rain forest habitat. Label one column "Habitat Conditions" and the other column "Plant Adaptations."

Habitat Conditions	Plant Adaptations

Key Concept 3 Plants and animals depend on one another for survival.

Activity

Plants and animals help one another survive. List three plant and animal pairs that depend on each other in a tropical rain forest. Explain how each helps the other.

Plant and Animal Pairs

1.

2.

3.

Create Your Own Encyclopedia

Many plants live in tropical rain forests. You have read about some of them. Now it is time to find out about more of them. Get ready to do some research. Then make a book about tropical rain forest plants. You can work with others to make a group book.

1. Study the Model

Look back at pages 23–26. Pick one plant you think is interesting. Now look closely at the entry for that plant. What facts are included? Do these tell about different parts of the plant? How does it reproduce? How does it adapt to the rain forest habitat? These are the kinds of facts you might want to include in your entry.

Encyclopedia Entries

- Each entry is about one person, place, or thing.
- Use a title to say what the entry is about.
- Use pictures with labels to show what things look like.
- Include important facts.

2. Choose Your Topic

You cannot write about what you do not know. Start by looking through books about tropical rain forest plants. Look at the pictures. Read about plants that look interesting. For each plant, ask yourself:

- What is special about this plant?
- What facts are important?
- Does the picture show what the plant looks like?

List the plants that you think are interesting. Then pick the one you would like to learn more about.

3. Research Your Topic

Question

Ask yourself what you want to know. Make a list of questions. Use this list to guide your research. To find facts about your plant, look through books. Look on the Internet.

Take Notes

Keep track of what you find out. Take notes. Use a chart to help you sort your notes. Make copies of pictures you might want to use.

Mahogany

1. What does it look like?

2. Where does it grow?

3. How do people use it?

4.

4. Write a Draft

Look over the facts you found. Now look back at one of the entries on pages 23–26. Use it as a model for writing about your plant. Be sure to use the important facts you collected. Also include any interesting or weird facts about your plant.

5. Revise and Edit

Read your draft. What do you like? What would you like to change? Make these changes. Then read your draft again. This time, fix any mistakes. Look for words that are misspelled. Be sure each sentence starts with a capital letter.

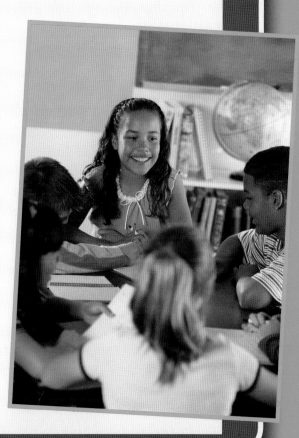

Create Your Own Book

Now you can share your work. Get together with others to make a class book. Follow the steps below.

How to Make a Book

1. Check that each entry has a title.
Check that the title names the plant in the entry.

2. Include a photo or drawing for each entry.
Use a photo or draw a picture of your plant.

3. Add captions to pictures.
Captions and labels tell what pictures are about.

4. Organize the entries alphabetically.
Put each entry in alphabetical order.

5. Number the pages.
Add the page number for each page.

6. Prepare a table of contents.
Look at the table of contents in this book. Now make one for your book.

7. Make a cover.
Talk with your group about what you want on your cover. Choose pictures and decide on a title. Then make your cover.

8. Now bind the pages together.
You can staple the pages together. Or you can punch holes on the left side and tie the pages together with yarn.

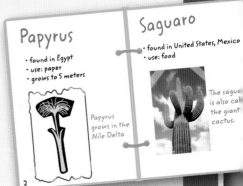

Papyrus
• found in Egypt
• use: paper
• grows to 5 meters

Papyrus grows in the Nile Delta

Saguaro
• found in United States, Mexico
• use: food

The saguaro is also called the giant cactus.

2

Plant Encyclopedia

Glossary

adaptation – a feature that helps a plant survive

carnivores – animals that eat only meat

depend – to need, or rely on, something

Equator – an invisible line around Earth that separates the Northern Hemisphere from the Southern Hemisphere

habitat – a place where a plant or animal usually lives in nature

herbivores – animals that eat only plants

minerals – substances that provide the nutrition plants need to grow

photosynthesis – the process by which plants make food

reproduce – to grow new plants

seed coat – a covering that protects a seed until it is ready to grow

survive – to stay alive

Index